Nutrition for Healthy Hair

Ralph M. Trüeb

Nutrition for Healthy Hair

Guide to Understanding and Proper Practice

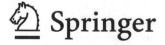 Springer

Ralph M. Trüeb
Center for Dermatology and Hair Diseases Professor Trüeb
Wallisellen
Switzerland

ISBN 978-3-030-59922-5   ISBN 978-3-030-59920-1   (eBook)
https://doi.org/10.1007/978-3-030-59920-1

This Springer imprint is published by the registered company Springer Nature Switzerland AG
The registered company address is: Gewerbestrasse 11, 6330 Cham, Switzerland

Preface

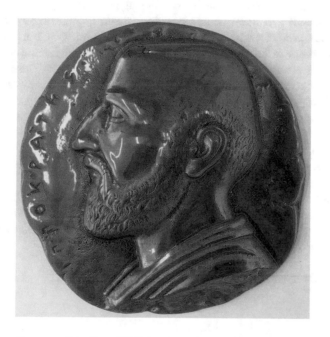

Courtesy of Dr. Harry P. Michaelides, DDS, Chicago, IL, USA

Let food be thy medicine and medicine be thy food.—Hippocrates (460–370 BC)

"Thou shouldst eat to live; not live to eat" is a proverb originally attributed to the classical Greek Athenian philosopher Socrates and later reiterated by the Roman orator Marcus Tullius Cicero. Yet another Ancient Greek, Hippocrates, was among the first to establish the role of diet in health and disease. He proposed lifestyle modifications, including dietary factors, to prevent or treat diseases, and is therefore often quoted with "Let food be thy medicine." And yet, there is hardly another field with so much prejudice, misconception, and debate as diet and health, let alone hair health. In his publication "How Doctors Think," Jerome Groopman from Harvard Medical School focuses on the thinking errors in medicine, and among them ultimately states that "Aside from relatively common dietary deficiencies—lack of vitamin B12 causing pernicious anemia, or insufficient vitamin C giving rise to scurvy—little is known about the effects of nutrition on many bodily functions."

The fact is that quantity and quality of hair are closely related to the nutritional state of an individual. Normal supply, uptake, and transport of proteins, calories, trace elements, and vitamins are of fundamental importance in tissues with a high biosynthetic activity such as the hair follicle. Because hair shaft is composed almost entirely of protein, protein component of diet is critical for production of normal healthy hair. The rate of mitosis is sensitive to the calorific value of diet, provided mainly by carbohydrates. Finally, a sufficient supply of vitamins and trace metals is essential for the biosynthetic and energetic metabolism of the follicle.

Since an important commercial interest lies in the nutritional value of nutritional supplements, a central question that arises is whether increasing the content of a seemingly adequate diet with specific amino acids, vitamins, and/or trace elements may further promote hair growth and quality. Pharmacy aisles and Internet drug-stores are full of nutritional supplements promising full, thick, luscious hair for prices that range from suspiciously cheap to dishearteningly exorbitant. It would appear that unless hair loss is due to a specific nutritional deficiency, there is only so much that nutritional therapies can do to enhance hair growth and quality. And yet, there are a number of factors, such as inborn errors of metabolism, life cycle needs, dietary habits, lifestyle, environmental toxins, age, and comorbidities, that influence hair health to such a degree, that nutritional therapy can boost hair that is suffering from these multifaceted issues.

This book aims at distinguishing facts from fiction, and at providing a sound scientific basis for nutrition-based strategies for healthy hair, at the same time acknowledging the problems and limitations of our current understanding and practice.

Wallisellen, Switzerland   Ralph M. Trüeb

Acknowledgments

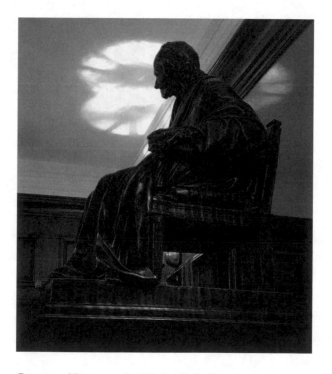

Courtesy of Restaurant Le Voltaire, Paris, France

Appreciation is a wonderful thing: It makes what is excellent in others belong to us as well.—Voltaire (1694–1778)

I would like to acknowledge my brother René François Trüeb, MD, DDS, and his wife, Barbara Hotzenköcherle Trüeb, DDS, who have taught me that food matters: our choice is a responsibility towards ourselves, and a responsibility towards our world.

Finally, I acknowledge my mother Hélène Trüeb Michaelides (01.01.1925–27.05.2020) for having taught me that common sense is more important than common opinion; that truthfulness is more enduring than hypocrisy; that doubt is more enlightening than conviction; that self-consciousness is more enobling that conceit; and that courtesy and candor are more enriching than impertinence and artifice.

Contents

About the Author

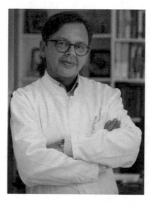

True virtue is nothing else but living in accordance with reason.—Baruch Spinoza (1632–1677)

Ralph M. Trüeb is Professor of Dermatology. He received his MD and Swiss Board Certification for Dermatology and Venerology as well as for Allergology and Clinical Immunology from the University of Zurich, Switzerland. In 1994–95, he spent a year at the University of Texas Southwestern Medical Center at Dallas with Rick Sontheimer and at the Howard Hughes Medical Institute in Dallas with Bruce Beutler to complete his Fellowship in Immunodermatology. After 20 years tenure at the Department of Dermatology, University Hospital of Zurich, where he founded and was head of the Hair Consultation Clinic, he established in 2010 his private Center for Dermatology and Hair Diseases in Zurich, where he offers since 2013 doctors-in-training and dermatologists international traineeships in Medical Trichology/Trichiatry. He is founding President of the Swiss Trichology Study group (founding year: 1999), and past-President of the European Hair Research Society (2008–11). His clinical research interests focus on hair loss, inflammatory phenomena, hair aging and anti-aging, hair and nutrition, hair care and cosmetics, and patient expectation management. He is currently author of 226 peer-reviewed scientific publications and 7 textbooks on hair.

Introduction

1

"To eat is a necessity, but to eat intelligently is an art."

François de La Rochefoucauld (1613–1680)

La Rochefoucauld was a noted French author of maxims. His worldview was clear eyed and urbane. He neither condemned human conduct nor celebrated it with sentimentality. He received the education of the nobleman of his time, with an emphasis on court etiquette, elegance of expression and comportment, and worldly knowledge. Ultimately, he was considered a fine example of the accomplished seventeenth-century French nobleman, and his maxims are timeless and acclaimed up to this day.

The French Art de la Table was in no jeopardy of neglect at the time. The ceremonial public meal or Royal Table was a daily avowal of the king's power and dignity. There was an abundance of dishes, which were brought to the table in services at staggered intervals. The soups and starters were followed by roasts and salads, then puddings, and finally fruits, either fresh or candied. And yet, the menus and dining habits of the king and his court offer insight into the excesses taking their toll not only on the tax payers, but also on the health of the indulgers, while at the same time famine and malnutrition were rampant among the population of approximately 20 million in the seventeenth-century France.

Refinement to the point of excess also characterized the hairstyles at the French court of the time. King Louis XIII (1601–1643) began wearing a wig to cover his thinning hair. Soon, the courtiers followed his example, regardless of their own hair condition. Wearing a long wig became a sign of status and a symbol of wealth and power, with the height, length, and bulk of wigs increasing accordingly, culminating in the long, dark brown wig with loose waves posed by the Sun King Louis XIV (1638–1715) in the most celebrated of his majestic portraits.

© Springer Nature Switzerland AG 2020
R. M. Trüeb, *Nutrition for Healthy Hair*,
https://doi.org/10.1007/978-3-030-59920-1_1

The care for food and the care of the hair obviously share commonalities. Both are deeply rooted in human culture and personal self-cultivation, and require a degree of knowledge, intelligence, and refinement. It has always been acknowledged that the condition of the hair reflects the general condition of health and well-being, and that health and nutrition are closely connected. Therefore, there has always been a popular market for nutritional remedies for beautiful hair. But so far, the science on the effect of nutrition on hair growth and quality has been limited, reduced to the observations in the specific deficiency disorders, rare inborn errors of metabolism, and few supplementation studies.

In the first two chapters of this book, it is reflected upon the history of human nutrition and today's understanding of nutrition basics. In the following two chapters, an overview is given on the hair growth cycle's relation to nutrition and energy, and on the nutritional disorders, both the specific deficiencies and the complex nutritional disorders, and how they may affect the hair. Finally, the last three chapters attempt at separating the chaff from the grain in the practice of nutrition-based interventions for healthy hair through a review of safety and efficacy issues, and conclude with guidance for supplementation by life stage, health risks, and specific hair conditions.

The supply, uptake, and transport of proteins, calories, trace elements, and vitamins are of fundamental importance for survival and function. This applies to both the total organism as a whole and the specific organs, particularly the tissues with a high biosynthetic activity, such as the hair follicle. Ultimately, to eat intelligently, in particular getting the right balance between quantity, quality, and combination of the nutrients in relation to the age, sex, occupation, environmental exposure, and health status, is not only an art, but also a science.

Brief History of Human Nutrition

2

The history of nutrition [1–4] dates back as far as to the dawn of humanity. In the days of the hunters and gatherers, people knew of the necessity of food for survival. It was up to their observational capacity and understanding to figure out which foods were suitable and which could possibly cause illness or even death. The diet of an individual was largely determined by the availability and palatability of foods, and the teachings and techniques that were used to obtain and prepare food came from trial and error, and an incredible capacity of human inventiveness. For humans, a healthy diet includes preparation of food and storage methods that preserve nutrients from oxidation, heat, or leaching, and that reduce risk of foodborne illnesses. Ultimately, the societies throughout the ages have looked at diet and nutrition as a means of healthy living.

American science popularizer Carl Sagan (1934–1996) said, "You have to know the past to understand the present." This chapter aims at reviewing some key historical moments in the development of our understanding of diet and health. Although food and nutrition have been studied for centuries, modern nutritional science is relatively young [5]. Nevertheless, many important insights have been anticipated early on, and as Austrian-born philosopher Ludwig Wittgenstein (1889–1951) said, "Knowledge is in the end based on acknowledgement," while "the problems are solved, not by giving new information, but by arranging what we have known since long" [6].

2.1 Prehistory

In a broader sense, the term prehistory refers to the vast span of time since the beginning of the universe or the appearance of life on Earth, and herewith opens to the realm to genesis. In a more specific sense of historical understanding, it refers to the period since humanlike beings appeared, and encompasses the period between the use of the first stone tools, ca. 3, 3 million years, and the invention of writing

© Springer Nature Switzerland AG 2020
R. M. Trüeb, *Nutrition for Healthy Hair*,
https://doi.org/10.1007/978-3-030-59920-1_2

systems ca. 5300 years ago. Depending on the artifacts representative of the respective ages, it has been divided into the Stone (Paleolithic) Age, the Bronze Age, and the Iron Age.

The Neolithic was a period in the development of human technology beginning about 10,200 BC, with the origin of the Neolithic culture considered to be in Jericho in the Levant about 10,200–8800 BC. Traditionally considered the last part of the Stone Age, the Neolithic followed the last glacial period transitioning into the current warm period, commenced with the beginning of farming, and ended when metal tools became widespread. The Neolithic is a progression of behavioral and cultural characteristics and changes, including the use of wild and domestic crops and of domesticated animals. Early Neolithic farming was limited to a narrow range of plants, which included einkorn wheat, millet and spelt, and the keeping of dogs, sheep, and goats. By about 6900–6400 BC, it included domesticated cattle and pigs, the establishment of permanently or seasonally inhabited settlements, and the use of pottery.

The *Paleolithic diet* is a modern fad diet requiring the consumption of foods presumed to have been the only foods available to and consumed by the humans during the Paleolithic age. The original idea can be traced to a 1975 book by American gastroenterologist Walter L. Voegtlin (1904–1975) [7], and was commented on in a respective New England Journal of Medicine article by Melvin Konner and Stanley Boyd Eaton in 1985 [8], before finally being popularized by Loren Cordain from the Colorado State University, Department of Health and Exercise Science, College of Applied Human Sciences, in his 2002 bestselling book *"The Paleo Diet: Lose Weight and Get Healthy by Eating the Food You Were Designed to Eat"* [9]. Like other fad diets, the Paleo diet is marketed with an appeal to nature and a narrative of conspiracy theories about how nutritional research and development are controlled by an unscrupulously profit-driven food industry. While there is wide variability in the way the paleo diet may be interpreted, the diet typically includes vegetables, fruits, nuts, roots, and meat, and typically excludes foods that humans began eating when they transitioned from hunter-gatherer lifestyles to settled agriculture, including all processed foods of the modern food industry.

So far, there is some preliminary evidence that the Paleolithic diet may assist in controlling weight and waist circumference and in managing chronic diseases. However, more randomized clinical studies with larger populations and duration are necessary to prove health benefits, specifically regarding cardiovascular and metabolic health, before recommending the Paleo diet for treatment of pathologic conditions [10, 11].

As early as the eighteenth century, French philosopher Jean-Jacques Rousseau (1712–1778) developed a spartan theory of food whereby eating "is an imperative for survival, not for enjoyment." Rousseau apparently ate food that required the minimum of preparation [12]. In common with other philosophers of the day, Rousseau looked to a hypothetical state of nature as a normative guide. The state of nature is a concept used in moral and political philosophy, religion, and social contract theories to denote the hypothetical conditions of what the lives of people might have been like before societies came into existence. Philosophers of the state of nature theory deduce that there must have been a time before organized societies existed, and this presumption thus raises questions such as the following: "What was life like before civil society?" Rousseau's answer was this: "The passage from the state of nature to the civil state produces a very remarkable change in man, by substituting justice for instinct in his conduct, and giving his actions morality they had formerly lacked. Then only, when the voice of duty takes the place of physical impulses and right of appetite, does man, who so far had considered only himself, find that he is forced to act on different principles, and to consult his reason before listening to his inclinations. Although in this state he deprives himself of some advantages which he got from nature, he gains in return others so great, his faculties are so stimulated and developed, his ideas so extended, his feelings so ennobled, and his whole soul so uplifted, that, did not the abuses of this new condition often degrade him below that which he left, he would be bound to bless continually the happy moment which took him from it forever, and, instead of a stupid and unimaginative animal, made him an intelligent being and a man" [13]. Rousseau claimed that the stage of human development associated with what he called savages was the best or optimal in human development, between the less-than-optimal extreme of brute animals on the one hand and the extreme of decadent civilization on the other. In his novel *"Julie or The New Heloïse"* (1761) he ultimately writes: "In general I think one could often find some index of people's character in the choice of foods they prefer."

"Philosophers have a long but scattered history of analyzing food … Food is vexing." So predictably, says David M. Kaplan, Associate Professor of Philosophy at the University of North Texas, in his book *"The Philosophy of Food"* (2012): "There is no consensus among philosophers about the nature of food." He notes that even our most essential questions about food, such as what we should eat, whether food is safe, or what is considered good food are "difficult questions because they involve philosophic questions about metaphysics, epistemology, ethics, politics, and aesthetics" [14].

Ultimately, *veganism* is the prototype of dietary behavior that involves ethics, politics, and environmental concern beyond the simple nutritional aspects of food. It is the practice of abstaining from the use of all animal products, particularly in diet, and an associated philosophy that rejects the commodity status of animals as unethical. The vegan diet has become increasingly mainstream in the latter half of the 2010s, and ultimately, the European Parliament defined the meaning of vegan for food labels in 2010, in force as of 2015.

In preliminary clinical research, vegan diets lowered the risk of type 2 diabetes [15], high blood pressure [16], obesity [17], ischemic heart disease, and cancer [18]. On the other hand, eliminating all animal products may increase the risk of deficiencies of vitamins B12 and D, calcium, and omega-3 fatty acids. Many vegans overestimate the health benefits of a vegan diet, which has resulted in victim blaming when vegans fall ill. In fact, staunch critics of veganism questioned the evolutionary legitimacy of the vegan diet, and pointed to long-standing philosophical traditions which held that humans are superior to the animals. And yet, the Bible has taken its stance on this issue in Genesis 1:29,30, stating: "[29]And look! I have given you the seed-bearing plants throughout the earth, and all the fruit trees for your food. [30]And I've given all the grass and plants to the animals and birds for their food." It is only after the great flood that God told Noah: "[2,3]All wild animals and birds and fish will be afraid of you, for I have placed them in your power, and they are yours to use for food, in addition to grain and vegetables" (Genesis 9:2,3).

2.2   Antiquity

The first recorded human nutritional trial is found in the Bible's Book of Daniel 1,8–17:8: "[8]But Daniel made up his mind not to eat the food and wine given to them by the king. He asked the superintendent for permission to eat other things instead. ... [11]Daniel talked it over with the steward who was appointed by the Superintendent to look after Daniel, Hananiah, Misha-el, and Azariah, [12]and suggested a ten-day diet of only vegetables and water; [13]then, at the end of this trial period the steward could see how they looked in comparison with the other fellows who ate the king's rich food, and decide whether or not to let them continue their diet. [14]The steward finally agreed to the test. [15]Well, at the end of the ten days, Daniel and his three friends looked healthier and better nourished than the youths who had been eating the food supplied by the king! [16]So after that the steward fed them only vegetables and water, without the rich foods and wines! [17]God gave these four youths great ability to learn and they soon mastered all the literature and science of the time."

Around 475 BC, pre-Socratic philosopher Anaxagoras of Clazomenae (500–428 BC) in Asia Minor stated that food is absorbed by the human body and, therefore, contains generative compounds or "homeomerics," suggesting the existence of nutrients. A number of early Greek thinkers before and during the time of Socrates are collectively known as the pre-Socratics. Their inquiries spanned the workings of the natural world as well as of human society, to include ethics, and religion, seeking explanations based on natural principles rather than the actions of supernatural gods. They introduced to the West the notion of the world as an ordered arrangement (kosmos) that could be understood through rational inquiry. Coming from the eastern or western fringes of ancient Greece, they were the forerunners of Western philosophy and natural sciences. They sought the material principle of things, and the method of their origin and disappearance. Anaxagoras himself maintained the existence of an ordering principle as well as a material substance, and while regarding the latter as an infinite multitude of imperishable primary elements, he conceived divine reason or mind (nous) as ordering them. To Anaxagoras belongs the credit of first establishing philosophy at Athens.

"Thou shouldst eat to live; not live to eat" is a saying attributed to the Athenian philosopher Socrates (469–399 BC), and later reiterated by the Roman statesman and orator Marcus Tullius Cicero (106–43 BC). Though Socrates himself has not passed down any writings, it is through his disciple Plato's (428/427 or 424/423–348/347 BC) dialogues that he has become renowned for his contribution to the field of ethics, and it is Plato's portrayal of Socrates that lends his name to the concept of Socratic irony. Meanwhile, it was Cicero who introduced the Romans to the chief schools of Greek philosophy, ultimately also distinguishing himself as a philosopher.

Hippocrates of Kos (460–370 BC) was among the first to establish the role of diet in health and disease. He proposed lifestyle modifications, such as diet and exercise, to treat diseases, and is therefore often quoted with "let food be your medicine." However, the quote is an apparent misquotation and its exact origin remains unknown. Nevertheless, Hippocrates is considered one of the most outstanding figures in the history of medicine, and is referred to as the Father of Western Medicine in recognition of his lasting contributions to the science and practice of the diagnosis, treatment, and prevention of disease. Hippocrates revolutionized medicine in ancient Greece, distinguishing it as a discipline from other fields with which it had traditionally been associated, such as philosophy and theurgy (the practice of rituals, sometimes seen as magical in nature, performed with the intention of invoking the action of gods), ultimately establishing medicine as an independent profession [19].

Other than Hippocrates, whose body of work is replete with references to the importance of a healthy regimen involving a balance between food intake and proper exercise, Plato (428–348 BC) was one of the ancient Greek philosophers to address the importance of diet and its contribution to disease [20]. In *The Republic*, Plato writes, "… the first and chief of our needs is the provision of food for existence and life." In *Laws*, he writes, "For there ought to be no other secondary task to hinder the work of supplying the body with its proper exercise and nourishment," and finally in *Timaeus*, "… one ought to control all such diseases … by means of dieting rather than irritate a fractious evil by drugging."

In the second century BC, Cato the Elder (234–149 BC) believed that cabbage could cure all kind of ailments [21]. He was a Roman senator and historian notable for his conservatism and opposition in his eyes to decadent Hellenistic influences [22]. He tried to preserve Rome's ancestral customs. For him, rusticity, austerity, and asceticism were the marks of old Roman inflexible integrity and love of order.

Living at the turn of the millennium, Roman encyclopedist Aulus Celsus (25 BC-50 AD), known for his extant medical work, *De Medicina*, believed in "strong" and "weak" foods (bread for example was strong, as were older animals and vegetables). The *De Medicina* is a primary source on diet, pharmacy, surgery, and related fields, and it is one of the best sources concerning medical knowledge in the Roman world [23, 24].

Roman philosopher Seneca (4 BC–65 AD) was a writer of philosophical works on stoicism. Stoicism became a popular philosophy in this period of imperial arbitrariness, and many upper-class Romans found in it a guiding ethical framework for societal and political involvement. Seneca was strictly opposed to the enormous waste and gluttony of Imperial Rome of his day. He quotes Epicurus (341–270 BC): "If you live according to nature you will never be poor; if according to conventionalism, you will never be rich. Nature demands little, fashion superfluity." Ultimately, he states on the perils of the urban lifestyle: "but now they (women) go bald and are sick in the feet (gout). The nature of women has not changed, but has been overwhelmed by their lifestyle" [25].

Plutarch (45–127) was a Greek historian, biographer, and essayist, who later became a Roman citizen. His literacy accomplishments were enormous. He is most known for his biographical studies of Greek and Latin statesmen and philosophers, but he also authored a number of treatises on matters of ethics. This collection of about 60 in 15 volumes is known as the *"Moralia"* or moral essays. Of particular note is Plutarch's essay *"On the Eating of Animal Flesh,"* Volume 12 of the *Moralia*. With this work he is a forerunner and frequently quoted proponent of ethical vegetarianism. In this essay, Plutarch challenges the idea that man is naturally carnivorous, an excuse so often used today to justify the eating of meat that appears to have been used for its justification in ancient times. Also, in his discussion against meat eating Plutarch maintains that animals deserve ethical consideration because they possess the attributes of intelligence and sentience. Ultimately, Plutarch argued that the eating of meat made the consumer spiritually course. The cruelty by which meat is acquired brutalizes the human character which makes it callous not only to the suffering of nonhuman animals but also to human beings: "Note that the eating of flesh is not only physically against nature, but it also makes us spiritually course and gross by reason of satiety and surfeit." "But apart from these considerations, do you not find here a wonderful means of training in social responsibility? Who could wrong a human being when he found himself so gently and humanely disposed toward other non-human creatures?" [26].

2.3   From Galen to Lind

Despite Cato the Elder's initial protests and preference for cabbage as the panacea, it was in ancient Rome that Greek medicine flourished to an extent to have a profound influence on the future history of Western medicine. Galen of Pergamon (129–200) was arguably the most accomplished of all medical authorities of antiquity. Galen was originally physician to gladiators in Pergamon and Rome, and eventually rose to the rank of physician to the Emperor Marcus Aurelius (121–180) and his three successors. His understanding of medicine was principally influenced by the then-current theory of humourism, a now discredited theory of the makeup and workings of the human body, positing that an excess or deficiency of any of four distinct bodily fluids (blood, yellow bile, black bile, phlegm) in a person directly influences their temperament (sanguine, phlegmatic, choleric, or melancholic) and health. Galen knew and acted on Hippocrates' statement on food medicine. In his treatises, Galen set out his theory that was to be profoundly influential on medicine and described the effects on health of a vast range of foods, from lettuce, lard, and fish to peaches, pickles, and hyacinths. Galen used personal anecdotes to defend his concept of food and food's effect on humors. Each of the three books of *"On the Power of Foodstuffs"* is organized around a specific food group: grains, vegetables and fruits, or meats, giving insight into the variety of foods that were available to Roman citizens, and into the eating habits of the Roman people [27]. Ultimately, Galen thought that for a person to have gout, kidney stones, or arthritis was disgraceful. Most of Galen's teachings were gathered and enhanced in the late eleventh century by the Benedictine monks at the School of Salerno in the *Regimen sanitatis Salernitanum* [28], and for 1500 years it was practically considered heretic to disagree with Galen.

Only in the sixteenth century Belgian anatomist and physician Andreas Vesalius (1514–1564) challenged Galen's authority in medicine. He was followed by piercing thought amalgamated with the era's new philosophy fueled by the mechanics of Galileo Galilei (1564–1642) and Isaac Newton (1643–1727). Flemish chemist, physiologist, and physician Jan Baptist van Helmont (1580–1644) discovered carbon dioxide ("gas sylvestre"), and performed the first quantitative experiments on a willow tree to determine where plants get their mass; Robert Boyle (1627–1691) further advanced chemistry and is regarded as one of the pioneers of the modern experimental method; Venetian physiologist and physician Santorio Santorio (1561–1636) introduced the quantitative approach into medicine and measured body weight; and Dutch physician Herman Boerhaave (1668–1738) modeled the digestive process. Boerhaave was heavily influenced by French mathematician and philosopher René Descartes (1596–1650), who contributed much to the iatromechanical theories [29]. Boerhaave's view on medicine was based on an apparatus-like body philosophy and thus focused attention on materialistic problems rather than on mystical explanations of illness [30]. Along with his pupil, the Swiss anatomist, physiologist, naturalist, and encyclopedist Albrecht von Haller (1708–1777) [31], he is best known for demonstrating the relation of symptoms to lesions. His motto was *simplex sigillum veri* ("the simple is the sign of the true"). Boerhaave's understanding of nutrition was within the limits of contemporary knowledge. As yet, he knew nothing of cells in the modern sense, of enzymes, of hormones, or of metabolic regulations. At the time it was not yet known that matter consists of atoms that combine to form distinct molecules, and that food is composed of such molecules.

James Lind (1716–1794), a physician in the British navy, is generally credited for having performed the first scientific nutrition experiment in 1747, demonstrating that lime juice saved sailors that had been at sea for years from scurvy [32]. Lind's experiment provided one group of sailors salt water, one group vinegar, and one group limes. Those given limes did not develop scurvy by virtue of the vitamin C contained in the fruit. However, the Portuguese explorers at sea, Vasco da Gama (1460s–1524) and Pedro Álvares Cabral (1467–1520), became familiar with curative effects of citrus fruit already on their respective expeditions during the Portuguese golden age of discoveries. Nevertheless, these travel accounts did not prevent further maritime deaths due to scurvy, because of the lack of communication between travelers and those responsible for their health, and because fruits and vegetables could not be kept for long in ships. In 1536, French explorer Jacques Cartier (1491–1557), on his ventures to the St. Lawrence River in North America, used the local natives' knowledge to cure his men of scurvy by boiling the needles of the *arbor vitae* tree (eastern white cedar) to make a decoction that only much later was recognized to contain 50 mg of vitamin C per 100 g. Finally, in 1601 prominent Elizabethan trader and privateer Sir James Lancaster (1554–1618) unintentionally performed an experimental study of lemon juice as a preventive for scurvy. Of his fleet of four ships, after 4 months of sailing, three were devastated by scurvy, while the men on Lancaster's ship the *Red Dragon* remained in better health because every morning they were given three spoonfuls of bottled lemon juice. Nevertheless, it was only from 1796 that lemon juice was issued to all Royal Navy crewmen, giving rise to the slang nickname "limey" for a British person.

2.4   From Lavoisier to the Modern Sciences

Before 1785 many scholars had published their opinions on how food was used in our bodies, but it was only with the "Chemical Revolution" in France at the end of the eighteenth century, with its identification of the main elements and the development of methods of chemical analysis, that old and new ideas began to be tested in a quantitative, scientific way. During the Age of Enlightenment (1715–1789), scientific and medical development increased exponentially. The concept of metabolism, the transfer of food and oxygen into heat and water in the body, creating energy, was discovered in 1770 by French chemist Antoine Laurent de Lavoisier (1743–1794), the "Father of Nutrition and Chemistry" [33]. In collaboration with Armand-Jean-François Seguin (1767–1835) he measured human respiratory output of carbon dioxide, both at rest and when lifting weights, and showed how it increased with activity. Lavoisier also collaborated with the mathematician Pierre-Simon Laplace (1749–1827) in comparing the heat produced by the guinea pig with its production of carbon dioxide, and comparing those results with the heat produced by a lighted candle or charcoal. Heat production was measured calorimetrically, by which the heat evolved was related to the weight of water released from the melting of the ice surrounding the inner chamber where the animal or burning material was housed. The results were consistent enough for them to assume that most of the animal heat was coming from slow combustion of organic compounds within the animal's tissues. In 1793, at the height of the French Revolution, Lavoisier was arrested during the Reign of Terror. On the day of his trial he pleaded for a short stay of execution that would allow him to do one more experiment, but the judge Jean-Baptiste Coffinhal, notorious for his tendency for misplaced witticisms, is alleged to have replied: "The Republic has no need of scientists or chemists; the course of justice cannot be delayed."

In the early 1800s, the elements of carbon, nitrogen, hydrogen, and oxygen, the main components of food, were isolated and soon connected to health. Essential studies into the chemical nature of foods followed: In 1816, French physiologist François Magendie (1783–1855) discovered that dogs fed only carbohydrates (sugar), fat (olive oil), and water died evidently of starvation, but dogs also fed protein survived, identifying protein as an essential dietary component [34]. His most important contributions to science were also his most disputed. Magendie was a notorious vivisector, shocking even many of his contemporaries with the live dissections that he performed at public lectures in physiology. In 1827, British chemist and physician William Prout (1885–1850) was the first person to divide foods into carbohydrates, fat, and protein [35]. French chemist Jean-Baptiste Dumas

(1800–1884) and German chemist Justus von Liebig (1803–1873) disputed over their shared belief that animals get their protein directly from plants. With a reputation as the leading organic chemist of his day and the author of a widely read book entitled *"Animal Chemistry or Organic Chemistry in Its Application to Physiology and Pathology"* [36], Liebig grew rich producing food extracts like beef extract. In the 1860s, French physiologist Claude Bernard (1813–1878) discovered that body fat can be synthesized from carbohydrate and protein, showing that the energy in blood glucose can be stored as fat or as glycogen.

In the early 1880s, Japanese naval physician Kanehiro Takaki (1849–1920) observed that Japanese sailors whose diets consisted almost entirely of white rice developed beriberi, while British sailors and Japanese naval officers did not. Adding vegetables and meat to the diets of Japanese sailors prevented the condition, not because of the increased protein as Takaki assumed, but because it introduced thiamine (vitamin B1) to the diet, later understood as a cure [37]. In the early twentieth century, further research followed into the area of the vitamins. In 1912, Polish biochemist Kazimierz Funk (1884–1967) coined the term "vitamins" as essential factors in the diet. After reading an article by the Dutch physician and professor of physiology Christiaan Eijkman (1858–1930) that indicated that persons who ate brown rice were less vulnerable to beriberi than those who ate only the fully milled product, Funk tried to isolate the substance responsible, and he succeeded. Because that substance was of vital importance, and contained an amine group, he called it "vitamin." Funk was sure that more than one substance like vitamin B1 existed, and in his 1912 article for the Journal of State Medicine, he proposed the existence of at least four vitamins: one preventing beriberi ("antiberiberi"), one preventing scurvy ("antiscorbutic"), one preventing pellagra ("antipellagric"), and one preventing rickets ("antirachitic") [38]. From there, Funk published a book, *The Vitamines*, in 1912. Finally, Christiaan Eijkman received together with English biochemist Sir Frederick Gowland Hopkins (1861–1947) the Nobel Prize for Physiology or Medicine in 1929 for the discovery of vitamins.

2.5   From Hopkins to the Present

Hopkins had for a long time studied how cells obtain energy via a complex metabolic process of oxidation and reduction reactions. In 1912 Hopkins published the work for which he is best known, demonstrating in a series of animal feeding experiments that diets consisting of pure proteins, carbohydrates, fats, minerals, and water fail to support animal growth. This led him to suggest the existence in normal diets of tiny quantities of as-yet unidentified substances that are essential for animal growth and survival. These hypothetical substances he called "accessory food factors," later renamed vitamins. Hopkins is credited with the discovery and characterization of glutathione in 1921 [39]. Glutathione is an antioxidant capable of preventing damage to important cellular components caused by reactive oxygen species such as free radicals, peroxides, lipid peroxides, and heavy metals. Glutathione is not an essential nutrient for humans, since it can be synthesized in the body from the amino acids L-cysteine, L-glutamic acid, and glycine. The sulfhydryl group of the cysteine molecule serves as a proton donor and is responsible for its biological activity. Cysteine is the rate-limiting factor in cellular glutathione biosynthesis, since this amino acid is relatively rare in foods. Systemic bioavailability of orally consumed glutathione is poor because the molecule, a tripeptide, is the substrate of proteases (peptidases) of the alimentary canal, and due to the absence of a specific carrier of glutathione at the level of cell membrane. Because direct supplementation of glutathione is not always successful, supply of the raw nutritional materials used to generate glutathione, such as cysteine and glycine, may be more effective at increasing glutathione levels. Low glutathione is commonly observed in wasting and negative nitrogen balance.

All vitamins were identified between 1913 and 1948 [40], ushering in a half century of discovery focused on single-nutrient-deficiency diseases. The first half of the twentieth century witnessed the identification and synthesis of many of the known essential vitamins and minerals and their use to prevent and treat nutritional deficiency-related diseases including scurvy, beriberi, pellagra, rickets, xerophthalmia, and nutritional anemias. Before 1935, the only source of vitamins was from food. Then, commercially produced tablet of yeast extract vitamin B complex and semisynthetic vitamin C became available, followed, in the 1950, by the mass production and ultimately marketing of vitamin supplements, including multivitamins, launching an entire vitamin supplement industry.

This new science of single-nutrient-deficiency diseases also led to fortification of selected staple foods with micronutrients, such as iodine in salt and niacin (vitamin B_3) and iron in wheat flour and bread. These approaches proved to be effective at reducing the prevalence of a number of specific deficiency disorders, including goiter (iodine), xerophthalmia (vitamin A), rickets (vitamin D), and anemia (iron).

Accelerating economic development and modernization of agricultural, food processing, and food formulation techniques continued to reduce single-nutrient-deficiency diseases globally. In response, nutrition science shifted to the research on the role of nutrition in complex noncommunicable chronic diseases, such as cardiovascular disease, diabetes, obesity, and cancers. Among the most important scientific development of recent decades was the design and completion of multiple, complementary, large nutrition studies, including prospective observational cohorts and randomized clinical trials. Cohort studies provided, for the first time, individual-level, multivariable-adjusted findings on a range of nutrients, foods, and diet patterns and a diversity of health outcomes. Clinical trials allowed further testing of specific questions in targeted, often high-risk populations, in particular effects of isolated vitamin supplements and, more recently, specific diet patterns.

Growing realization of the importance of overall diet patterns has stimulated not only scientific inquiry but also a deluge of empirical, commercial, and popular dietary patterns of varying origin and scientific backing. These range, for example, from flexitarian, vegetarian, and vegan to low carb, paleo, and gluten free. Many of these patterns have specific aims, such as general health, weight loss, and anti-inflammation, and are based on differing interpretations of current evidence.

Additional complexity may arise in nutritional recommendations for general well-being versus treatment of specific conditions. Recognition of complexity is a key lesson of the past. This is common in scientific progress whether in nutrition or in clinical medicine. Initial observations lead to reasonable, simplified theories that achieve certain practical benefits, which are then inevitably advanced by new knowledge and recognition of ever-increasing complexity [5].

Most of what we know about the effect of nutrition on hair stems from observations in those lacking nutrition, specifically deficiencies of protein and calories, biotin, essential fatty acids, iron, and zinc [41]. Trials have indicated that correct nutrition is instrumental for healthy hair growth [42]. Healthy hair requires a complexity of nutrients and a ready supply of oxygen, but comparatively few authoritative studies have trialed ingredients to maintain or promote hair growth and quality. In the 1960s, the role of L-cystine and L-methionine in the production of wool in sheep was investigated, and it was found that enrichment of even what appeared to be a normal diet with sulfur-containing amino acids increased wool production [43, 44]. When considering which dietary supplements could be used for improving hair growth in humans, L-cystine was therefore a candidate. Starting in the 1990s, original clinical studies on the effect of dietary supplements containing L-cystine in combination with nutritional yeast, pantothenic acid, and thiamine were performed in tandem with bioavailability and in vitro studies for the evidence-based marketing of respective nutrient-based medical nutrition therapy for hair growth and quality [45–48]. Finally, animal studies on cigarette smoke-induced hair loss in mice [49], and chemoprotection with L-cystine and vitamin B6 [50], together with the unraveling of molecular mechanisms underlying specific types of hair loss, specifically the role of oxidative stress in androgenetic alopecia [51, 52], and a putative protective role of the glutathione-related detoxification system [50], have issued a deeper understanding into the modes of action of nutritional therapies to restore and maintain healthy hair. *Dum vita est, spes est.*

References

1. Carpenter KJ. A short history of nutritional science: part 1 (1785–1885). J Nutr. 2003;133:638–45.
2. Carpenter KJ. A short history of nutritional science: part 2 (1885–1912). J Nutr. 2003;133:975–84.
3. Carpenter KJ. A short history of nutritional science: part 3 (1912–1944). J Nutr. 2003;133:3023–32.
4. Carpenter KJ. A short history of nutritional science: part 4 (1945–1985). J Nutr. 2003;133:3331–42.
5. Mozaffarian D, Rosenberg I, Uauy R. History of modern nutrition science-implications for current research, dietary guidelines, and food policy. BMJ. 2018;361:k2392.
6. Wittgenstein L (edited by GEM Anscombe and GH Wright. Translated by D Paul and GEM Anscombe). On certainty. Basil Blackwell, Oxford 1969.
7. Voegtlin WL. The stone age diet: based on in-depth studies of human ecology and the diet of man. New York: Vantage Press; 1975.

8. Eaton SB, Konner M. Paleolithic nutrition. A consideration of its nature and current implications. N Engl J Med. 1985;312(5):283–9.
9. The CL, Diet P. Lose weight and get healthy by eating the food you were designed to eat. New York: John Wiley & Sons; 2002.
10. de Menezes EVA, Sampaio HAC, Carioca AAF, Parente NA, Brito FO, Moreira TMM, de Souza ACC, Arruda SPM. Influence of Paleolithic diet on anthropometric markers in chronic diseases: systematic review and meta-analysis. Nutr J. 2019;18:41.
11. Johnson AR. The paleo diet and the American weight loss utopia, 1975–2014. Utop Stud. 2015;26:101–24.
12. Rousseau JJ. The confessions, trans. Angela scholar. Oxford: Oxford University Press; 2000.
13. Rousseau JJ. The social Contract' and other later political writings, trans. Victor Gourevitch. Cambridge: Cambridge University Press; 1997.
14. Kaplan DM, editor. The philosophy of food. Berkeley: University of California Press; 2012.
15. Ajala O, English P, Pinkney J. Systematic review and meta-analysis of different dietary approaches to the management of type 2 diabetes. Am J Clin Nutr. 2013;97(3):505–16.
16. Lopez PD, Cativo EH, Atlas SA, Rosendorff C. The effect of vegan diets on blood pressure in adults: a meta-analysis of randomized controlled trials. Am J Med. 2019;132:875–883.e7.
17. Huang RY, Huang CC, Hu FB, Chavarro JE. Vegetarian diets and weight reduction: a meta-analysis of randomized controlled trials. J Gen Intern Med. 2016;31:109–16.
18. Dinu M, Abbate R, Gensini GF, Casini A, Sofi F. Vegetarian, vegan diets and multiple health outcomes: a systematic review with meta-analysis of observational studies. Crit Rev Food Sci Nutr. 2017;57:3640–9.
19. Yapijakis C. Hippocrates of Kos, the father of clinical medicine, and Asclepiades of Bithynia, the father of molecular medicine. Review. In Vivo. 2009;23:507–14.
20. Skiadas PK, Lascaratos JG. Dietetics in ancient Greek philosophy: Plato's concepts of healthy diet. Eur J Clin Nutr. 2001;55:532–7.
21. Rolando I. Cato's panacea. Minerva Med. 1953;144:548–50.
22. Näf B. Origin of Roman medical criticism and its reception in Rome [article in German]. Gesnerus. 1993;50:11–26.
23. Papavramidou N, Christopoulou-Aletra H. Greco-Roman and byzantine views on obesity. Obes Surg. 2007;17:112–6.
24. Tesařová D. Aulus Cornelius Celsus and a regimen. Cas Lek Cesk. 2018;157:263–7.
25. Wildberger J, Colish ML, editors. Seneca philosophus. Berlin/Boston: Walter de Gruyter GmbH; 2014.
26. Walter KS, Portmess L, editors. Ethical vegetarianism. From Pythagoras to Peter Singer. Albany: State University of New York Press; 1999.
27. Eijk P. A textual note on Galen, on the powers of foodstuffs I 1.3 (P. 202.17 Helmreich). Class Q. 1993;43:506–8.
28. Berardinelli W. Prevention and treatment of obesity; advice of celebrated gluttons and gourmets and the precepts of the regimen Sanitatis Salernitanum. Resen Clin Cient. 1952;21:291–4.
29. Jeune B. Descartes and medicine [article in Danish]. Dan Medicinhist Arbog. 2004:75–117.
30. Scholer AJ, Khan MA, Tandon A, Swan K, Chokshi RJ, Boerhaave H. The Dutch Hippocrates, a Forgotten Father of Medicine. Am Surg. 2018;84:323–5.
31. Conti AA. Albrecht Von Haller: an encyclopaedic cosmopolite in the history of Swiss medicine. [article in Italian]. Clin Ter. 2013;164:e445–8.
32. Baron JH. Who was James Lind, and what exactly did he achieve. J R Soc Med. 2013;106:118.
33. West JB. The collaboration of Antoine and Marie-Anne Lavoisier and the first measurements of human oxygen consumption. Am J Physiol Lung Cell Mol Physiol. 2013;305:L775–85.
34. Wolinsky I. Nutrition in exercise and sport. 3rd ed. Boca Raton, FL: CRC Press; 1997. p. 22.
35. Price C. Probing the mysteries of human digestion. Distillations. 2018;4:27–35.
36. Liebig J, Gregory W. Animal chemistry or organic chemistry in its application to physiology and pathology. Cambridge: John Owen; 1843.
37. Sugiyama Y, Seita A. Kanehiro Takaki and the control of beriberi in the Japanese navy. J R Soc Med. 2013;106:332–4.

38. Funk C. The etiology of the deficiency diseases. Beri-beri, polyneuritis in birds, epidemic dropsy, scurvy, experimental scurvy in animals, infantile scurvy, ship beri-beri, pellagra. Journal of State Medicine. 1912;20:341–68.
39. Simoni RD, Hill RL, Vaughan M. On glutathione. II. A thermostable oxidation-reduction system (Hopkins, F. G., and Dixon, M. (1922) J. Biol. Chem. 54, 527–563). J Biol Chem. 2002;277:e13.
40. Semba RD. The discovery of the vitamins. Int J Vitam Nutr Res. 2012;82:310–5.
41. Gummer CL. Diet and hair loss. Semin Dermatol. 1985;4:35–9.
42. Finner AM. Nutrition and hair: deficiencies and supplements. Dermatol Clin. 2013;31:167–72.
43. Gillespie JM, Reis PJ. Dietary regulated biosynthesis of high-sulfur wool proteins. Biochem J. 1966;98:669–77.
44. Reis PJ, Tunks DA, Sharry LF. Plasma amino acid patterns in sheep receiving abomasal infusions of methionine and cystine. Aust J Biol Sci. 1973;26:635–44.
45. Petri H, Perchalla P, Tronnier H. Die Wirksamkeit einer medikamentösen Therapie bei Haarstrukturschäden und diffusen Effluvien—vergleichende Doppelblindstudie. Schweiz Rundsch Med Prax. 1990;79:1457–62.
46. Budde J, Tronnier H, Rahlfs VW, Frei-Kleiner S. Systemische Therapie von diffusem Effluvium und Haarstrukturschäden. Hautarzt. 1993;44:380–4.
47. Lengg N, Heidecker B, Seifert B, Trüeb RM. Dietary supplement increases anagen hair rate in women with telogen effluvium: results of a double-blind placebo-controlled trial. Therapy. 2007;4:59–6.
48. Hengl T, Herfert J, Soliman A, Schlinzig K, Trüeb RM, Abts HF. Cystine-thiamin-containing hair-growth formulation modulates the response to UV radiation in an in vitro model for growth-limiting conditions of human keratinocytes. J Photochem Photobiol B. 2018;189:318–25.
49. D'Agostini F, Balansky R, Pesce C, et al. Induction of alopecia in mice exposed to cigarette smoking. Toxicol Lett. 2000;114:117–23.
50. D'Agostini F, Fiallo P, Pennisi TM, De Flora S. Chemoprevention of smoke-induced alopecia in mice by oral administration of L-cystine and vitamin B6. J Dermatol Sci. 2007;46:189–98.
51. Bahta AW, Farjo N, Farjo B, Philpott MP. Premature senescence of balding dermal papilla cells in vitro is associated with p16(INK4a) expression. J Invest Dermatol. 2008;128:1088–94.
52. Upton JH, Hannen RF, Bahta AW, Farjo N, Farjo B, Philpott MP. Oxidative stress-associated senescence in dermal papilla cells of men with androgenetic alopecia. J Invest Dermatol. 2015;135:1244–52.

Nutrition Basics

3

Nutrition is the science that interprets the interaction of nutrients and other substances in food in relation to maintenance, growth, reproduction, health, and disease of an organism. Consuming a healthy diet throughout life helps prevent malnutrition and a range of associated diseases and conditions. The exact composition of a healthy diet varies depending on the individual needs, specifically age, gender, degree of physical activity, and general health condition, but also cultural context, regional availability of foods, and dietary customs. Nevertheless, the basic principles of what constitutes a diversified, balanced, and healthy diet remain the same.

With regard to the nutrients a distinction is made between macronutrients which are needed in relatively large amounts and micronutrients which are needed in smaller quantities. The macronutrients consist of the carbohydrates, fiber, fats, protein, and water. Excluding fiber and water, they provide structural material and energy. The micronutrients consist of minerals, vitamins, and others. Dietary minerals represent inorganic chemical elements, while the vitamins are essential nutrients, necessary in the diet for maintenance of a good health status [1].

Unhealthy diet and a lack of physical activity are the leading global risks to health. Rapid urbanization with a change of lifestyles and an increased production of processed food have led to a shift in dietary patterns [2]. People are consuming more foods high in energy, fats, free sugars, or sodium, and many do not eat enough fruit, vegetables, and dietary fiber, particularly whole grains [3].

As a principle, energy intake (calories) should be in balance with energy expenditure. Evidence indicates that total fat should not exceed 30% of total energy intake to avoid unhealthy weight gain. Intake of saturated fats should be less than 10% of total energy intake and trans fats to less than 1% of total energy intake, with a shift in fat consumption away from saturated fats and trans fats to unsaturated fats, and towards the elimination of industrial trans fats. Finally, limiting intake of free sugars to less than 10% of total energy intake is part of a healthy diet. And a further reduction to less than 5% of total energy intake is suggested for additional health benefits [1].

© Springer Nature Switzerland AG 2020
R. M. Trüeb, *Nutrition for Healthy Hair*,
https://doi.org/10.1007/978-3-030-59920-1_3

Malnutrition refers to insufficient, excessive, or imbalanced consumption of nutrients by an organism. In developed countries, the diseases of malnutrition are most often associated with nutritional imbalances or excessive consumption, while in the developing countries, malnutrition is caused by poor access to a range of nutritious foods or nutrition illiteracy.

The U.S. Food and Nutrition Board sets Estimated Average Requirements (EARs) and Recommended Dietary Allowances (RDAs) for vitamins and minerals. EARs and RDAs are part of Dietary Reference Intakes. As well, the U.S. Food and Nutrition Board sets tolerable upper intake levels (known as ULs) for vitamins and minerals when evidence is sufficient. ULs are set at a safe fraction below amounts shown to cause health problems. ULs are again part of Dietary Reference Intakes. The European Food Safety Authority also reviews the same safety questions and sets its own ULs.

Health disorders caused by improper nutrient consumption, including effects on hair, are listed in Table 3.1

The U.S. Food and Nutrition Board Recommended Dietary Allowances (RDAs) for vitamins and minerals [4] are listed in Table 3.2. The EARs are the estimated average expected to satisfy the needs of 50% of the people, and it is the AI (adequate intake) where no RDA has been established.

In addition to vitamins, there are yet other biologically active molecules that have been recognized in plants and are therefore called phytochemicals. What triggered the investigation into these compounds was the observation of health benefits in people who were eating whole foods compared to those who were eating micronutrient-deficient refined foods and relying on dietary supplements for the source of vitamins and minerals. Phytochemicals exert multifaceted health benefits, with a variety of functions, including antioxidant activity, hormonal actions, and antibacterial effects. Finally, the beneficial effects of phytochemicals are believed to result from synergistic actions of multiple constituents, many of which have yet to be identified, as opposed to the actions of the isolated compounds.

Foods derived from animals and those that have been processed and refined are practically devoid of phytochemicals. Color is a prominent indicator of a significant quantity of specific phytochemicals present in a food, such as red (lycopene), yellow-green (zeaxanthin), red-purple (anthocyanin), orange (β-carotene), orange-yellow (flavonoids), green (glucosinolate), and with-green (allyl sulfides).

While there are no established Dietary Refence Intakes (DRIs) for the phytochemicals, consuming a colorful variety of fruits, vegetables, whole grains, and nuts will provide with a good supply of phytochemicals.

Plant-derived phytochemicals that have been studied for symptom relief of hair loss include caffeine, green tea (*Camellia sinensis* L.), procyanidin B-2 isolated

Table 3.1 Health disorders caused by improper nutrient consumption

Nutrients	Deficiency	Tolerable Upper Intake Level (UL) and Toxicity
Macronutrients:		
Calories (4 kcal/g from carbohydrates and from proteins, 9 kcal/g form fats, and 7 kcal/g from alcohol)	Starvation, marasmus (emaciated appearance, loss of body fat), hair loss	Calories requirements vary throughout life and are altered in disease states. Excess lead to: obesity, diabetes mellitus, cardiovascular disease
Simple carbo-hydrates (mono-and disaccharides)	The monosaccharides (glucose, fructose, galactose) are the building blocks for all carbohydrates, and energy demands will determine whether they are used for immediate energy or stored as glycogen. The brain has no stored supply of glucose, and therefore is dependent on a minute-to-minute supply of glucose from the blood for proper functioning.	Obeslty, dlabetes mellitus,cardiovascular disease
Complex carbo-hydrates (polysaccharides)	The important polysaccharides in human nutrition include: starch, glycogen,and dietary fiber.	Obesity, diabetes mellitus, cardiovascular disease (especially high glycemic index foods) A high-fiber diet containing phytic acid (legumes, wheat bran, and seeds) may bind iron, calcium, magnesium, and zinc making them unavailable for absorption
Proteins	Kwashiorkor (fatty liver, generalized edema), hair loss, pigment dilution	Excess dietary protein does not build up muscle; only exercise with enough protein to support growth can do that. Excess dietary protein results in inflammation and apoptosis in the glomerular cells of the kidney
Saturated fatty acid	Fatty acids are a concentrated fuel source for the human energy system. A large amount can be stored in relatively little space within the adipose tissue. Low testosterone levels, vitamin deficiencies.	Obesity, cardiovascular disease
Unsaterated fatty acid	Fat-soluble vitamin deficiency	Obesity, cardiovascular disease
Trans-fatty acids	Trans fats are unnecessary in human nutrition and pose a great number of negative health consequences	Obesity, cardiovascular disease

(continued)

Table 3.1 (continued)

Micronutrients:		
Vitamin A (retinol, retinal, and retinoic acid)	Night blindness, xerophthalmia, keratomalacia, dry skin, hyperkeratosis, impaired immunity, susceptibility to epithelial infection	UL: 3'000 mcg/day Hair loss, bone pain, liver damage (liver scirrhosis, portal hypertension), birth defects (teratogen during pregnancy)
Vitamin B1 (thiamin)	Beriberi (deficiency disease), gastrointestinal: loss of appetite, indigestion, central nervous: fatigue Wernicke-(Korsakoff)'s encephalopathy, nerve damage, paralysis, cardiovascular: heart failure, edema of legs	Toxicity unknown, therefore UL not set
Vitamin B2 (riboflavin)	Ariboflavinosis (deficiency disease), angular stomatitis, glossitis, ocular irritation, scaly flexural dermatitis	Toxicity unknown, therefore UL not set
Vitamin B3 (niacin, nicotinamide, nicotinic acid, vitamin PP)	Pellagra (deficiency disease), 4 D's: dermatitis, diarrhea, dementia, death	UL: 35 mg/day Skin flushing, liver damage (at doses > 2 g/day)
Pantothenic acid (vitamin B5)	Unknown due to widespread distribution in all foods	Toxicity unknown, therefore UL not set
Vitamin B6 (pyridoxine)	Microcytic hypochromic anemia, hyperirritability, neuritis, possibly convulsions	UL: 100 mg/day Uncoordinated movement, nerve damage
Biotin (vitamin B7, vitamin B8, vitamin H)	Erythematous periorofacial macular rash, seborrheic-like dermatitis, neurological symptoms; depression, lethargy, hallucination, numbness and tingling of the extremities, hair loss (alopecia)	Toxicity unknown, therefore UL not set May interfere with avidin-based laboratory testing systems
Folate (folic acid, folacin, vitamin B9)	Megaloblastic anemia, neural tube defects	UL: 1'000 mg/day May mask symptoms of vitamin B12 deficiency
Choline	Fatty liver disease. Possibly cancer, neural tube defects, and dementia	No UL established Depressed blood pressure, fishy body odor, sweating, excessive salivation
Vitamin B12 (cobolamin)	Pernicious anemia, glossitis, neuropathy, premature hair graying	Toxicity unknown, therefore UL not set

Table 3.1 (continued)

Vitamin C (ascorbic acid)	Scurvy (deficiency disease), tissue bleeding, e.g. bleeding gums, easy bruising, pinpoint perifollicular skin hemorrhage, joint bleeding, weakened bones, poor wound healing, loss of teeth	UL: 2'000 mg/day Osmotic diarrhea
Vitamin D (cholecalciferol, ergocalciferol)	Rickets and growth retardation in children, osteomalacia in aduts, possibly increased incidence of several autoimmune diseases	UL: 4'000 IU/day (in children under age of 9 years: 1'000 IU/day) Dehydration, vomiting, constipation, hypercalcemia, calcification of soft tissue, kidney damage
Vitamin E (α-tocopherol)	Hemolytic anemia (particularly in premature infants), nerve damage, retinopathy	UL: 1'000 mg/day Inhibition of vitamin K activity in blood clotting (excessive bleeding)
Vitamin K	Bleeding tendency, poor bone growth	No UL established Decreased effect of oral anticoagulants (warfarin, coumarin)
Omega-3 fatty acids (alpha-linolenic acid, eicosapentaenoic acid EPA, and docosahexaenoic acid DHA)	Hair loss, infertility, low blood platelet levels, impaired vision, comprised brain function, growth retardation in children	No UL established Hemorrhages, Hemorrhagic stroke, reduced glycemic control among diabetics
Omega-6 fatty acids (linoleic acid, and others)	Dry skin	No UL established Cardiovascular disease, cancer
Cholesterol	Asteatotic eczema (on statins)	No UL established Cardiovascular disease
Macrominerals:		
Calcium	Osteoporosis, tetany, carpopedal spasm, laryngospasm, cardiac arrhythmias	Fatigue, depression, confusion, nausea, vomiting, constipation, pancreatitis, increased urination, kidney stones
Magnesium	Hypertension	Weakness, nausea, vomiting, impaired breathing, and hypotension
Potassium	Hypokalemia, cardiac arrhythmias	Hyperkalemia, palpitations
Sodium	Hyponatremia	Hypernatremia, hypertension

(continued)

Table 3.1 (continued)

Trace minerals:		
Iron	Most common nutritional deficiency in the world. Iron-deficiency anemia, cheilosis, glossitis, esophageal webs (Plummer-Vinson/Paterson-Brown-Kelly syndrome), koilonychia Hair loss	Liver cirrhosis (in hemochromatosis) cardiovascular disease, cancer
Iodine	Goiter, hypothyroidism	Iodine toxicity (goiter, hypothyroidism)
Copper	Anemia-like symptoms, neutropenia, bone abnormalities, hypopigmentation, impaired growth, increased incidence of infections, osteoporosis, hyperthyroidism, and abnormalities in glucose and cholesterol metabolism.	Liver cirrhosis (Wilson's disease), worsening of Alzheimer's disease
Selenium	Kashin-Beck disease (China)	Selenosis, garlic odor on the breath, gastrointestinal disorders, sloughing of nails, fatigue, irritability, and neurological damage. Hair loss
Zinc	Acrodermatitis enteropathica, depressed growth, diarrhea, impotence and delayed sexual maturation, eye and skin lesions, impaired appetite, altered cognition, impaired host defense properties, defects in carbohydrate utilization, and reproductive teratogenesis. Hair loss	Copper deficiency, anosmia

from apple juice (*Malus pumila*), purified polyphenols from *Ecklonia cava* (Ec) sourced from marine brown alga, clover extract, raspberry ketone, capsaicin from red chili, rosemary oil, onion juice, saw palmetto, and Korean red ginseng extract. The demand for non-medicinal treatments of hair loss lends itself to a more holistic approach, including oral treatments. A small number of in vivo oral supplement-based treatments of hair loss have been reported so far in the literature and, similarly to the clinical studies of topical treatments, the robustness of the methods and data is variable [review in 6].

Table 3.2 The U.S. Food and Nutrition Board Recommended Dietary Allowances [5]

Nutrient	EAR	Highest RDA/ AI	Unit	Top common sources, 100 grams, U.S. Department of Agriculture (USDA)
Vitamin A	625	900	μg	cod liver oil,liver,dehydrated red sweet peppers, veal, dehydrated carrots
Thiamin (B₁)	1.0	1.2	mg	fortified breakfast cereals, energy bars, vegetarian, and baby food products
Riboflavin (B₂)	1.1	1.3	mg	fortified food products, lamb liver, spirulina
Niacin (B₃)	12	16	mg	fortified food products, baker's yeast, rice bran, instant coffee, fortified beverages
Pantothenic acid (B₅)	NE	5	mg	fortified food and beverage products, dried shiitake mushrooms, beef liver, rice bran
Vitamin B₆	1.1	1.3	mg	fortified food and beverage products, rice bran, fortified margarines, ground sage
Biotin (B₇)	NE	30	μg	organ meats, eggs, fish, meat, seeds, nuts
Folate (B₉)	320	400	μg	baker's yeast, fortified food and beverage products, poultry liver
Cobalamin (B₁₂)	2.0	2.4	μg	shellfish, beef, animal liver, fortified food and beverage products
Vitamin C	75	90	mg	fortified beverages, dried sweet peppers, raw acerola, dried chives and coriander,rose hips, fortified food products
Vitamin D	10	15	μg	cod liver oil, mushrooms (if exposed to ultraviolet light), halibut, mackerel, canned sockeye salmon
α-tocopherol (Vitamin E)	12	15	mg	wheat germ oil, fortified food and beverage products, hazelnut oil, fortified peanut butter, chili powder
Vitamin K	NE	120	μg	dried spices, fresh parsley, cooked and raw kale, chard, other leaf vegetables

(continued)

Table 3.2 (continued)

Choline	NE	550	mg	egg yolk, organ meats from beef and pork, soybean oil, fish roe
Calcium	800	1000	mg	fortified cereals, beverages, tofu, energy bars, and baby foods, dried basil and other spices, dried whey, cheese, milk powder
Chloride	NE	2300	mg	table salt
Chromium	NE	35	µg	broccoli, turkey ham dried apricots, tuna, pineapple, grape juice
Copper	700	900	µg	animal liver, seaweed products, dried shiitake mushrooms, oysters, sesame seeds, cocoa powder, cashews, sunflower seeds
Fluoride	NE	4	mg	public drinking water, where fluoridation is performed or natural fluorides are present, tea, raisins
Iodine	95	150	µg	iodized salt, kelp, cod
Iron	6	18	mg	dried thyme and other spices, fortified foods, including baby foods, animal organ meats
Magnesium	350	420	mg	crude rice bran, cottonseed flour,hemp seeds, dried spices, cocoa powder, fortified beverages
Manganese	NE	2.3	mg	fortified beverages and infant formulas, ground cloves and other dried spices, chickpeas, fortified breakfast cereals
Molybdenum	34	45	µg	legumes, grain products, nuts and seeds
Phosphorus	580	700	mg	baking powder, instant pudding, cottonseed meal, hemp seeds, fortified beverages, dried whey
Potassium	NE	4700	mg	baking powder, dried parsley and other spices, instant tea and instant coffee, dried tomatoes, dried sweet peppers, soy sauce

Table 3.2   (continued)

Selenium	45	55	μg	Brazil nuts and mixed nuts, animal kidneys, dried eggs, oysters, dried cod
Sodium	NE	1500	mg	table salt, baking soda, soup bouillon cube, seasoning mixes, onion soup mix, fish sauce
Zinc	9.4	11	mg	oysters, fortified breakfast cereals, baby foods, beverages, peanut butter, and energy bars, wheat germ

EAR Estimated Average Requirement, *RDA* Recommended Dietary Allowance, *AI* adequate intake

3.1   The Food Pyramid

Hundred years ago, Wilbur O. Atwater (1844–1907) charted a new course for nutrition education by using the scientific process to develop dietary guidance to improve public health and well-being. Each of the areas of research, nutrient requirements, food composition, food consumption, and consumer economics proved essential components in the development of dietary guidance. The emerging science of nutrition was translated into recommendations for a healthful diet by Caroline Hunt (1865–1927) in 1916 in the first USDA food guide. Research involved development of a new food guide and a graphic to illustrate it. Although the time since the release of the new Food Guide Pyramid has been short, its wide acceptance by the professional community, industry, and the media promises to make it an effective nutrition education tool [7].

A food pyramid is a triangular diagram representing the optimal number of servings to be eaten each day from each of the basic food groups.

A food group is a collection of foods that share similar nutritional properties or biological classifications. Nutrition guides typically divide foods into food groups and recommend daily servings of each group for a healthy diet. The most common food groups include dairy, fruits, grains, beans and legumes, meat, confections, vegetables, and water.

A serving size or portion size is the amount of a food or drink that is generally served. As of 2017, it was not clear if controlling the serving size, called "portion control," was an effective way to change the amount of food or drink that people consume. However, evidence from a systematic review of 72 randomized controlled trials indicates that people consistently eat more food when offered larger portion, package, or tableware sizes rather than smaller size alternatives [8].

Sweden's National Board of Health and Welfare originally developed the idea of basic foods that were both affordable and nutritious, and supplemental foods that added nutrition missing from the basic foods. Anna-Britt Agnsäter, chief of the test kitchen for Kooperativa Förbundet (a cooperative Swedish retail chain), held a lecture the next year on how to illustrate these food groups. Attendee Fjalar Clemes suggested a triangle displaying basic foods at the base. Agnsäter developed the idea into the first food pyramid, which was introduced to the public in 1974. The pyramid was divided into basic foods at the base, including milk, cheese, margarine, bread, cereals and potato, a large section of supplemental vegetables and fruit, and an apex of supplemental meat, fish, and egg.

The World Health Organization (WHO), in conjunction with the Food and Agriculture Organization, published guidelines that can effectively be represented in a food pyramid relating to objectives to prevent obesity, chronic diseases, and dental caries based on meta-analysis.

The USDA food pyramid was created in 1992 and divided into six horizontal sections containing depictions of foods from each section's food group. It was updated in 2005 with colorful vertical wedges replacing the horizontal sections.

Controversies prompted the creation of alternative pyramids for specific audiences, particularly the Mediterranean pyramid in 1993, and some Vegetarian Diet Pyramids. Following the results of nutrition studies published in peer-reviewed scientific journals more closely, the Harvard School of Public Health proposed a healthy eating pyramid, which includes calcium and multivitamin supplements as well as moderate amounts of alcohol, as an alternative to the Food Guide Pyramid.

In their book *"Fantastic Voyage: Live Long Enough to Live Forever"* (2004), Ray Kurzweil and Terry Grossman M.D. point out that the guidelines provided in the Harvard Pyramid fail to distinguish between healthy and unhealthy oils. In addition, whole-grain foods are given more priority than vegetables, which should not be the case, as vegetables have a lower glycemic load. Other observations are that fish should be given a higher priority due to its high omega-3 content, and that high-fat dairy products should be excluded. As an alternative, the authors postulate a new food pyramid, emphasizing low glycemic-load vegetables, healthy fats such as avocados, nuts and seeds, lean animal protein, fish, and extra virgin olive oil.

According to WHO recommendations a healthy diet contains:

- **Fruits, vegetables, legumes (e.g., lentils, beans), nuts and whole grains (e.g., unprocessed maize, millet, oats, wheat, brown rice)**: Eating at least 400 g, or five portions, of fruits and vegetables per day reduces the risk of noncommunicable disease, and helps ensure an adequate daily intake of dietary fiber. Potatoes, sweet potatoes, cassava, and other starchy roots are not classified as fruits or vegetables.
- **Less than 10% of total energy intake from free sugars which is equivalent to 50 g (or around 12 level teaspoons) for a person of healthy body weight consuming approximately 2000 calories per day, but ideally**

less than 5% of total energy intake for additional health benefits: Most free sugars are added to foods or drinks by the manufacturer, cook, or consumer, and can also be found in sugars naturally present in honey, syrups, fruit juices, and fruit juice concentrates. Consuming free sugars increases the risk of dental caries, while excess calories from foods and drinks high in free sugars contribute to unhealthy weight gain, overweight, and obesity. Sugar intake can be reduced by limiting the consumption of foods and drinks containing high amounts of sugars (e.g., sugar-sweetened beverages, sugary snacks, and candies), and eating fresh fruits and raw vegetables as snacks instead of sugary snacks.

- **Less than 30% of total energy intake from fats**: Unsaturated fats (found in fish, avocado, nuts, sunflower, canola, and olive oils) are preferable to saturated fats (found in fatty meat, butter, palm and coconut oil, cream, cheese, ghee, and lard) and trans fats of all kinds, including both industrially produced trans fats (found in processed food, fast food, snack food, fried food, frozen pizza, pies, cookies, biscuits, wafers, margarines, and spreads) and ruminant trans fats (found in meat and dairy foods from ruminant animals, such as cows, sheep, goats, camels, and others). It is suggested to reduce the intake of saturated fats to less than 10% of total energy intake and trans fats to less than 1% of total energy intake. In particular, industrially produced trans fats are not part of a healthy diet and should be avoided. Fat intake can be reduced by changing cooking habits to remove the fatty part of meat; using vegetable oil (not animal oil); boiling, steaming, or baking rather than frying; limiting the consumption of foods containing high amounts of saturated fats (e.g., cheese, ice cream, fatty meat); and avoiding processed, baked, or fried foods containing industrially produced trans fats.
- **Less than 5 g of salt (equivalent to approximately 1 teaspoon) per day (6) and use iodized salt**: People are often unaware of the amount of salt they consume. Most salt comes from processed foods, particularly ready meals; processed meats like bacon, ham, and salami; cheese and salty snacks; or food consumed frequently in large amounts, such as bread. Salt is also added to food during cooking (bouillon, stock cubes, soy sauce, and fish sauce) or at the table (table salt). Salt consumption can be reduced by not adding salt, soy sauce, or fish sauce during the preparation of food; not having salt on the table; limiting the consumption of salty snacks; and choosing products with lower sodium content. Some food manufacturers are reformulating recipes to reduce the salt content of their products, and it may be helpful to check food labels to see how much sodium is there in a product. Finally, potassium, which can mitigate the negative effects of elevated sodium consumption on blood pressure, can be increased again with consumption of fresh fruits and vegetables.

3.1.1 Superfoods

The social media often publish lists of so-called superfoods. By definition, a super-food is supposed to have health benefits as a result of some part of its nutritional analysis or its overall nutrient density [9]. Some of the nutrients that certain super-foods contain include antioxidants, thought to ward off cancer; healthy fats, thought to prevent heart disease; fiber, thought to prevent diabetes and digestive problems; or phytochemicals, the chemicals in plants responsible for deep colors and smells, which can have numerous health benefits. Not surprisingly, the "superfoods" have a mysterious tendency towards the exotic, obscure, or highly perishable in compari-son to equally nourishing and pleasant foodstuffs of lesser celebrity, which means they are usually only available at a greater expense and/or from a limited number of specialized merchants. Currently, superfood-based powders, juices, and elixirs are aggressively promoted by self-proclaimed health gurus with a self-educational background and economical conflicts of interests while targeting the populace at the heart of its unspoken apprehensions and remorse with regard to lifestyle, nutrition, and health, and seeking for easy solutions. The consumption of superfoods is far more prevalent among higher socioeconomic groups. Ultimately, the associations between socioeconomic position and the consumption of "superfoods" seem to be partially driven by a process of social distinction [10].

Some of the foods that have garnered the "superfood" label are Açaí berries (*Euterpe oleracea*), apple cider vinegar, blueberries (*Vaccinium* spp.), brewer's yeast, chia seeds (*Salvia hispanica*), cranberries *(Vaccinium* spp.), curry (turmeric, *Curcuma longa*, in particular), goji berries or Chinese wolfberries (*Lycium bar-barum*) , green tea (*Camellia sinensis*), jiaogulan (*Gynostemma pentaphyllum*), and pomegranate juice (*Punica granatum*).

Among the extreme claims used to market goji berries is the unsupported story by a Chinese man named Li Qing Yuen (1677–1933), who was said to have con-sumed the berries daily, and lived to the age of 256 years [11]. He spent most of his life in the mountains; worked as a herbalist, selling lingzhi, goji berry, wild ginseng, he shou wu, and gotu kola along with other Chinese herbs; and lived off a diet of these herbs and rice wine. In 1927, the National Revolutionary Army General Yang Sen (1884–1977) invited him to his residence in Wan Xian, Sichuan. Yang Sen was also known as a Taoist master and ultimately published a book about Li Qing Yuen titled *"A Factual Account of the 250 Year-Old Good-Luck Man,"* in which he described Li's appearance: "He has good eyesight and a brisk stride; Li stands seven feet tall, has very long fingernails, and a ruddy complexion."

Fact is that the term "superfood" is not used by qualified nutrition scientists or dietitians, many of whom even dispute that particular foods have the health benefits claimed by their advocates. The use of the term is largely a marketing tool. In fact, there are no set criteria for determining what is and what is not a superfood, accord-ing to the American Heart Association.

In 2007, the marketing of products as superfoods was prohibited in the European Union unless accompanied by a specific authorized health claim supported by cred-ible scientific research. The Dutch food safety organization Voedingscentrum specifically noted that the health claims marketers used to sell goji berry, hemp seed, chia seed, and wheatgrass were not scientifically proved. Ultimately, the organization warned that people who consumed such foods in large quantities may develop an impaired, one-sided diet. Moreover, while the food itself might be healthful, the processing might not be. For example, green tea has several antioxidants. But green tea processed and marketed in the United States is generally cut with inferior teas and brewed with copious amounts of sugar. Similarly, many whole grains are processed in a way to be more palatable and less healthful. For example, instant whole-grain oats are as unhealthy as overly processed white bread in that they quickly spike sugar levels in the bloodstream once consumed, promoting insulin resistance, obesity, and diabetes.

Nutrition literacy [12] and common sense teach us that the ideal diet is one that is largely plant based with a wide variety of fruits, vegetables, and whole grains, and a critical choice of healthful animal products, with minimal industrial processing.

3.1.2 Functional Foods

A functional food is a food given an additional function related to health promotion or disease prevention by adding new ingredients or more of existing ingredients. Functional foods are designed to have physiological benefits and/or reduce the risk of chronic disease beyond basic nutritional functions, and may be similar in appearance to conventional food and consumed as part of a regular diet.

Such foods are also referred to as "nutraceuticals" or "designer foods." General recommendations for functional food intake do not exist since the scientific evidence on which to base such recommendations is lacking. Studies are being performed on the value of botanical antioxidants, carotenoids, green tea polyphenols, flavonoid-rich nutrients, omega-3 fatty acids, and soy for skin protection [13].

3.1.3 Prebiotics, Probiotics, Synbiotics

The human organism lives in coherence with millions of bacteria, both in the intestine and on the surface of the body. The intestinal bacteria both provide a protective barrier against pathogens and actively participate in the regulation of immune responses, while the microbiota of the skin are characterized by a complex network between the microbes and the skin surface, with specific profiles of the resident flora depending on the skin site.

Probiotics are defined as live microorganisms that are promoted with the claim that they may provide health benefits when consumed, generally by improving or restoring the intestinal flora. The original theory is generally attributed to 1908 Nobel Prize in Medicine or Physiology laureate Élie Metchnikoff (1845–1916), who postulated that yoghurt-consuming Bulgarian peasants lived longer. He developed a theory that aging is caused by toxic bacteria in the gut, a belief that went back at least to ancient Egyptians, and that lactic acid could prolong life [14].

Metchnikoff is also credited by some authors with originally coining the term gerontology for the emerging study of aging and longevity [15]. The interest in probiotics has originally been largely confined to intestinal pathologies; however, there is increasing evidence suggesting that oral probiotics may also have systemic effects, including the skin. Among the skin health benefits attributed to probiotics is their capacity to improve atopic dermatitis [16], and to accelerate skin recovery from UV exposure, thus contributing to photoprotection [17].

Borde and Åstrand raised the potential of the impact of the modern society's processed Western diet on gut integrity in leading to increased intestinal permeability as a driver of increased allergies and autoimmune diseases, including alopecia areata. The authors hypothesize that there may be a common root cause of diseases with T cell-driven autoimmunity originating from chronic inflammation, and that the gut is the most commonly exposed area, with a particular focus on the gut microbiome. In summary, the authors see a link between alopecia areata and a dysfunctional gastrointestinal system which raises the hypothesis that underlying intestinal inflammation may drive the priming and dysregulation of immune cells that eventually lead to hair follicle destruction in the genetically susceptible individuals. While it remains important to resolve local inflammation and to restore the immune privilege of hair follicles, they believe that the root cause needs to be eradicated by long-term interventions to suppress the force driving the disease. Having a balanced microbiome is thus essential for a tight epithelial barrier and a functional and regulatory immune system. Specifically, a high intake of fibers affects the makeup of the intestinal microbiota, primarily increasing short-chain fatty acid concentrations that have beneficial immunomodulatory effects, such as increasing T regulatory cell numbers and function [18].

Given the multitude of bacteria in the gastrointestinal tract, it seems unlikely that ingestion of only one probiotic will have a major therapeutic effect. Therefore, current research has turned to the prebiotics, defined as the indigestible substances that activate the growth of host probiotic bacteria. Ultimately, current trends aim at combining prebiotics with probiotics, an association called synbiotics, for a maximum effect.

Inspired by the progresses made in prebiotic and probiotic food supplements, the understanding of potential beneficial effects from prebiotic cosmetics has been further developed. Considerable efforts are made to substantiate cosmetic product claims with significant results, even though the beneficial effects of cosmetics are more difficult to substantiate than those of therapeutics, where the study endpoints are better defined. Basically, the aim of prebiotic cosmetics is to rebalance the skin microflora. Ouwehand et al. [19] originally proposed dairy strains of propionibacteria for cosmetic use, and demonstrated antimicrobial activity against the skin pathogens *M. furfur*, *C. albicans*, and *S. aureus*. In a study on volunteers suffering from scalp seborrheic dermatitis a 4-week daily application of a 5% lotion of *Vitreoscilla filiformis*, an apathogenic bacteria isolated from a thermal spring which traditionally has been used in the treatment of skin diseases, showed significant reduction in the clinical scores as well as in the self-evaluated pruritus [20]. Therefore, *V. filiformis* was proposed as an active ingredient for an anti-dandruff shampoo.

Traditionally, the medical focus has been either on hair loss, or on the condition of the hair scalp in terms of specific dermatological conditions. In fact, the proximate structural arrangement of the scalp and hair leads to an interdependent relationship between the two. The protective benefits of the hair to the scalp, such as ultraviolet radiation screening, moisture retention, and mechanical shielding, are obvious, while the role of the scalp as an incubatory environment for the pre-emerging hair fiber has been underestimated [21]. In fact, the scalp is characterized by a high density of terminal hair follicles with numerous sebaceous glands that contribute to a specific microenvironment. Ecologically, sebaceous areas have greater species richness than dry ones, with implications both for skin physiology and pathologic conditions. There is ample evidence from data involving collections and characterization of hair samples from various unhealthy scalp conditions to help establish a link between scalp health and hair growth and quality. Most of the published data are epidemiological in nature comparing hair obtained from individuals with dandruff or seborrheic dermatitis [22–28], atopic dermatitis [29], and psoriasis [30–36] with that from a control group of healthy scalp individuals. The most common manifestation to hair emerged from an unhealthy scalp is an altered cuticle with evidence of surface pitting, roughness, cuticle rigidity, or breakage, and in some cases shine reduction. In addition to the physical changes, there are biochemical alterations observed in hair emerged from an unhealthy scalp, with both protein and lipid components affected, most commonly by oxidative damage. Finally, a number of observations have found that premature hair loss may be caused by the poor scalp health associated with either dandruff and seborrheic dermatitis or psoriasis, indicating that the effect on the pre-emerging hair fiber may alter the anchoring force of the fiber with the follicle, as evidenced by an increased proportion of both catagen and telogen [37], and of dysplastic anagen hairs (anagen hairs devoid of hair root sheaths) [38] in the trichogram (hair pluck). Today, it is understood that scalp care products for dandruff and seborrheic dermatitis, atopic dermatitis, and psoriasis exert their benefits by controlling scalp *Malassezia* levels. Given the observations on the role of oxidative stress in premature hair loss and the part that *Malassezia* spp. play in generating oxidative stress [39–42], it is likely that products with *Malassezia* active control, either antimicrobials such as ketoconazole [43, 44] or zinc pyrithione [45] or prebiotics, would demonstrate some hair loss prevention benefits.

3.1.4   Medical Nutrition Therapy

Medical foods, called "food for special medical purposes" in Europe, are foods that are specially formulated and intended for the dietary management of a disease that has distinctive nutritional needs that cannot be met by normal diet alone. Normally, individuals obtain the necessary nutrients their bodies require through normal daily diets that process the foods accordingly within the body. Nevertheless, there are circumstances such as disease, distress, and stress that may prevent the body from obtaining sufficient nutrients through diets alone. In such conditions, a dietary supplementation specifically formulated for their individual condition may be required to fill the void created by the specific condition.

In order to be considered a medical food the product must be a food for oral ingestion or tube feeding; must be labeled for the dietary management of a specific medical disorder, disease, or condition for which there are distinctive nutritional requirements; and must be intended to be used under medical supervision [46].

Basically, medical nutrition therapy is the therapeutic approach to treating medical conditions and their associated symptoms via the use of a specifically tailored diet devised and monitored by a medical doctor physician or registered dietitian nutritionist. Medical nutrition can benefit people with various medical conditions such as cancer, chronic obstructive pulmonary disease, diabetes mellitus, eating disorders, food allergies, gastrointestinal disorders, immune system disorders such as HIV/AIDS, inherited disorders of metabolism, involuntary weight loss, kidney disease, aging-related sarcopenia, surgery recovery, pregnancy, and osteoporosis. Many of these chronic medical conditions may also affect hair growth and quality, either through the medical condition itself or through associated specific nutritional imbalances.

Finally, according to the European Directive 2004/27/EC, an amendment to the Directive 2001/83/EEC, a medicinal product is defined as any substance or combination of substances presented as having properties for treating or preventing disease in human beings, or any substance or combination of substances which may be used in or administered to human beings either with a view of restoring, correcting, or modifying physiological functions by exerting a pharmacological, immunological, or metabolic action or for making a medical diagnosis [47].

3.2   World Nutrition Facts

Despite significant progress over the recent decades, poor nutrition remains a universal problem, with one in three people on the planet affected by some form of malnutrition. Undernutrition, specifically inadequate energy or nutrients, continues to affect more than 150 million children worldwide, while rates of overweight and obesity are rising in all countries and expected to affect 1 in 2 people by 2030. Ultimately, poor diet is now the number one risk factor driving the world's burden of disease.

In instances of protein and calorie malnutrition, deficiency of essential amino acids, of trace elements, and of vitamins, hair growth and pigmentation may be impaired [48, 49]. In general, malnutrition is due to one or more of the following factors: inadequate food intake, food choices that lead to dietary deficiencies, and illness that causes increased nutrient requirements, increased nutrient loss, poor nutrient absorption, or a combination of these factors.

It appears that on a typical Western diet, the hair follicle should have no problem in producing an appropriate hair shaft. Nevertheless, vitamin and nutritional deficiencies are not uncommonly observed in adolescent females and young women with eating disorders (anorexia and bulimia nervosa), and are especially common in the elderly population. There is evidence that with age, the needs for types and quantities of nutrients may change, and it has been found that as many as 50% of older adults have a vitamin and mineral intake less than the recommended dietary allowance, and as many as 30% of the elderly population have subnormal levels of vitamins and minerals [50].

References

1. Nix S. Williams' basic nutrition and diet therapy. 15th ed. St. Louis, Missouri: Elsevier; 2017.
2. Whitney E, Rolfes SR. Understanding nutrition. 13th ed. Belmont, CA: Wadsworth, Cengage Learning; 2013.
3. Ian CN, James WPT. A life course approach to diet, nutrition and the prevention of chronic diseases. Public Health Nutr. 2004;7(1A):101–21.
4. https://ods.od.nih.gov/Health_Information/Dietary_Reference_Intakes.aspx
5. Dietary Reference Intakes: The Essential Guide to Nutrient Requirements http://www.nap.edu/catalog/11537.html
6. Daniels G, Akram S, Westgate GE, Tamburic S. Can plant-derived phytochemicals provide symptom relief for hair loss? A critical review. Int J Cosmet Sci. 2019;41:332–45.
7. Welsh S. Atwater to the present: evolution of nutrition education. J Nutr. 1994;124(9 Suppl):1799S–807S.
8. Shemilt I, Marteau TM, Jebb SA, Lewis HB, Wei Y, Higgins JPT, Ogilvie D, Cochrane Public Health Group Portion. Package or tableware size for changing selection and consumption of food, alcohol and tobacco. Cochrane Database Syst Rev. 2015;2015(9):CD011045.
9. Fitzgerald M. It's a bird! It's a plane! It's superfood!. Diet cults: The surprising fallacy at the core of nutrition fads and a guide to healthy eating for the rest of US. New York: Pegasus Books; 2014.
10. Oude Groeniger J, van Lenthe FJ, Beenackers MA, Kamphuis CB. Does social distinction contribute to socioeconomic inequalities in diet: the case of 'superfoods' consumption. Int J Behav Nutr Phys Act. 2017;14:40.
11. Young RD, Desjardins B, McLaughlin K, Poulain M, Perls TT. Typologies of extreme longevity myths. Curr Gerontol Geriatr Res. 2010;2010:1–12.
12. Cullen T, Hatch J, Wharf Higgins WMJ, Sheppard R. Food literacy: definition and framework for action. Can J Diet Pract Res. 2015;76:140–5.
13. Simmering R, Breves R. Prebiotic cosmetics. Functional food for skin works: intervention studies in humans and animal models. In: Krutmann J, Humbert P (eds.). Nutrition for healthy skin. Strategies for clinical and cosmetic practice. Berlin Heidelberg: Springer; 2011. p. 137ff.
14. Brown AC, Valiere A. Probiotics and medical nutrition therapy. Nutr Clin Care. 2004;7:56–68.
15. Martin DJ, Gillen LL. Revisiting gerontology's scrapbook: from Metchnikoff to the spectrum model of aging. Gerontologist. 2013;54:51–8.
16. Lee J, Seto D, Bielory L. Meta-analysis of clinical trials of probiotics for prevention of pediatric atopic dermatitis. J Allergy Clin Immunol. 2008;121:116–21.
17. Peguet-Navarro J, Dezutter-Dambuyant C, Buetler T, Leclaire J, Smola H, Blum S, Bastien P, Breton L, Gueniche A. Supplementation with oral probiotic bacteria protects human cutaneous immune homeostasis after UV exposure-double blind, randomized, placebo controlled clinical trial. Eur J Dermatol. 2008;18:504–11.
18. Borde A, Åstrand A. Alopecia areata and the gut-the link opens up for novel therapeutic interventions. Expert Opin Ther Targets. 2018;22:503–11.
19. Ouwehand AC, Båtsman A, Salminen S. Probiotics for the skin: a new area of potential application? Lett Appl Microbiol. 2003;36:327–31.

20. Guéniche A, Cathelineau AC, Bastien P, Esdaile J, Martin R, Queille Roussel C, Breton L. Vitreoscilla filiformis biomass improves seborrheic dermatitis. J Eur Acad Dermatol Venereol. 2008;22:1014–5.
21. Trüeb RM, Henry JP, Davis MG, Schwartz JR. Scalp condition impacts hair growth and retention via oxidative stress. Int J Trichol. 2018;10:262–70.
22. Sinclair RD, Schwartz JR, Rocchetta HL, Dawson TL Jr, Fisher BK, Meinert K, Wilder EA. Dandruff and seborrheic dermatitis adversely affect hair quality. Eur J Dermatol. 2009;19:410–1.
23. Kim KS, Shin MK, Park HK. Effects of scalp dermatitis on chemical property of hair keratin. Spectrochim Acta A Mol Biomol Spectrosc. 2013;109:226–31.
24. Schwartz JR, Henry JP, Kerr KM, Mizoguchi H, Li L. The role of oxidative damage in poor scalp health: ramifications to causality and associated hair growth. Int J Cosmet Sci. 2015;37(Suppl 2):9–15.
25. Piérard-Franchimont C, Xhauflaire-Uhoda E, Loussouarn G, Saint Léger D, Piérard GE. Dandruff-associated smouldering alopecia: a chronobiological assessment over 5 years. Clin Exp Dermatol. 2006;31:23–6.
26. Piérard-Franchimont C, Xhauflaire-Uhoda E, Piérard GE. Revisiting dandruff. Int J Cosmet Sci. 2006;2:311–8.
27. Pitney L, Weedon D, Pitney M. Is seborrhoeic dermatitis associated with a diffuse, low-grade folliculitis and progressive cicatricial alopecia? Australas J Dermatol. 2016;57:e105–7.
28. Kim KS, Shin MK, Ahn JJ, Haw CR, Park HK. Investigation of hair shaft in seborrheic dermatitis using atomic force microscopy. Skin Res Technol. 2011;17:288–94.
29. Kim KS, Shin MK, Kim JH, Kim MH, Haw CR, Park HK. Effects of atopic dermatitis on the morphology and water content of scalp hair. Microsc Res Tech. 2012;75:620–5.
30. Kim KS, Shin MK, Ahn JJ, Haw CR, Park HK. A comparative study of hair shafts in scalp psoriasis and seborrheic dermatitis using atomic force microscopy. Skin Res Technol. 2013;19:e60–4.
31. Shuster S. Psoriatic alopecia. Arch Dermatol. 1990;126:397.
32. Runne U, Kroneisen-Wiersma P. Psoriatic alopecia: acute and chronic hair loss in 47 patients with scalp psoriasis. Dermatology. 1992;185:82–7.
33. Wyatt E, Bottoms E, Comaish S. Abnormal hair shafts in psoriasis on scanning electron microscopy. Br J Dermatol. 1972;87:368–73.
34. Headington JT, Gupta AK, Goldfarb MT, Nickoloff BJ, Hamilton TA, Ellis CN, Voorhees JJ. A morphometric and histologic study of the scalp in psoriasis. Paradoxical sebaceous gland atrophy and decreased hair shaft diameters without alopecia. Arch Dermatol. 1989;125:639–42.
35. Plozzer C, Coletti C, Kokelj F, Trevisan G. Scanning electron microscopy study of hair shaft disorders in psoriasis. Acta Derm Venereol Suppl (Stockh) Suppl. 2000;211:9–11.
36. Kumar B, Soni A, Saraswat A, Kaur I, Dogra S. Hair in psoriasis: a prospective, blinded scanning electron microscopic study. Clin Exp Dermatol. 2008;33:491–4.
37. Schoorl WJ, van Baar HJ, van de Kerkhof PC. The hair root pattern in psoriasis of the scalp. Acta Derm Venereol. 1992;72:141–2.
38. Stanimirović A, Skerlev M, Stipić T, Beck T, Basta-Juzbasić A, Ivanković D. Has psoriasis its own characteristic trichogram? J Dermatol Sci. 1998;17:156–9.
39. Niwa Y, Sumi H, Kawahira K, Terashima T, Nakamura T, Akamatsu H. Protein oxidative damage in the stratum corneum: Evidence for a link between environmental oxidants and the changing prevalence and nature of atopic dermatitis in Japan. Br J Dermatol. 2003;149:248–54.
40. Kurutas EB, Ozturk P. The evaluation of local oxidative/nitrosative stress in patients with pityriasis versicolor: a preliminary study. Mycoses. 2016;59:720–5.
41. Nazzaro-Porro M, Passi S, Picardo M, Mercantini R, Breathnach AS. Lipoxygenase activity of Pityrosporum in vitro and in vivo. J Invest Dermatol. 1986;87:108–12.
42. Später S, Hipler UC, Haustein UF, Nenoff P. Generation of reactive oxygen species in vitro by Malassezia yeasts [Article in German]. Hautarzt. 2009;60:122–7.

43. Piérard GE, Piérard-Franchimont C, Nikkels-Tassoudji N, et al. Improvement in the inflam-matory aspect of androgenetic alopecia A pilot study with an antimicrobial lotion. J Dermatol Treat. 1996;7:153–7.
44. Piérard-Franchimont C, De Doncker P, Cauwenbergh G, Piérard GE. Ketoconazole shampoo: effect of long-term use in androgenic alopecia. Dermatology. 1998;196:474–7.
45. Berger RS, Fu JL, Smiles KA, Turner CB, Schnell BM, Werchowski KM, Lammers KM. The effects of minoxidil, 1% pyrithione zinc and a combination of both on hair density: a random-ized controlled trial. Br J Dermatol. 2003;149:354–62.
46. Freijer K, Volger S, Pitter JG, Molsen-David E, Cooblall C, Evers S, Hiligsmann M, Danel A, Lenoir-Wijnkoop I. ISPOR Nutrition Economics Medical Nutrition Terms & Definitions Working Group's Leadership TeamMedical Nutrition Terminology and regulations in the United States and Europe-a scoping review: report of the ISPOR Nutrition Economics Special Interest Group. Value Health. 2019;22:1–12.
47. Karajiannis H, Fish C. Legal aspects: how do food supplements differ from drugs, medical devices, and cosmetic procedures? In: Krutman J, Humbert P, editors. Nutrition for healthy skin. Strategies for clinical and cosmetic practice. Berlin Heidelberg: Springer; 2011. p. 171.
48. Gummer CL. Diet and hair loss. Semin Dermatol. 1985;4:35–9.
49. Finner AM. Nutrition and hair: deficiencies and supplements. Dermatol Clin. 2013;31:167–72.
50. Johnson KA, Bernard MA, Funderberg K. Vitamin nutrition in older adults. Clin Geriatr Med. 2002;18:773–99.

The Hair Cycle and Its Relation to Nutrition

4

Much in the same way as Lord Shiva Nataraja (Fig. 4.1) performs the dance in which everything is created, maintained, and dissolved, for production and maintenance of hair in a good condition, the hair follicle is subject to a constant turnover in the course of perpetual cycles through phases of proliferation in anagen,

Fig. 4.1 Shiva Nataraja performing the cosmic dance (courtesy of Dr. Sundaram Murugusundram, Chennai, India)

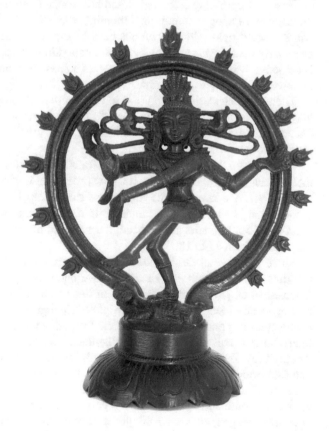

involution in catagen, and resting in telogen, with regeneration in the successive hair cycle (Fig. 4.2).

The stoic face of Shiva represents his neutrality, thus being in balance. The snake swirling around his waist is kundalini, the divine force thought to reside within everything. The dwarf on which Nataraja dances is the demon Apasmara (Muyalaka, as known in Tamil), which symbolizes the victory of awareness over ignorance [1].

Ultimately, understanding the basics of the hair cycle and its requirements enables insights into the principles of hair growth and shedding in health and in disease.

It is a major characteristic of anagen (duration: 2–6 years) that not only the hair shaft is growing, but also most epithelial hair follicle compartments undergo proliferation, with the hair matrix keratinocytes showing the highest rate of proliferation. It represents the phase of the cycle with the highest mitotic and biochemical activity, and therefore the most vulnerable to insults. At the same time, the duration of the anagen phase determines the percentage of hair growing at any given time point and the length of the produced hair shaft. During catagen (duration: 2 weeks), hair follicles enter a process of involution that is characterized by a burst of programmed cell death (apoptosis) in the majority of follicular keratinocytes. The resulting shortening of the regressing epithelial strand is associated with an upward movement of the follicle. In telogen (duration: 3 months), the hair shaft matures into a club hair, which is held tightly in the bulbous base of the follicular epithelium, before it is eventually shed. It was unresolved whether shedding of the telogen hair (teloptosis) is an active, regulated process or represents a passive event that occurs at the onset of subsequent anagen, as the new hair grows in [2, 3] (Fig. 4.2a).

There are considerable variations in the length of these phases depending on the body site location, with the duration of anagen determining the type of hair produced, particularly its length (vellus, intermediate, terminal). In general, the anagen phase is longer in women than in men.

On the scalp, hairs remain in anagen for a 2- to 6-year period of time, whereas that of telogen is approximately 100 days, resulting in a ratio of anagen to telogen hairs of 9:1. On average, the amount of new scalp hair formation matches the amount that is shed, thereby maintaining a consistent covering. With a range of 75,000 to 150,000 hairs on the head, the reported average daily telogen hair shedding varies from 35 to 180 hairs.

Since the original description of the hair growth cycle, additional phenomena relevant to hair growth and shedding have been recognized (Fig. 4.2b): In 1996, Guarrera et al. [4] observed that anagen hairs may fail to replace telogen hairs in androgenetic alopecia. By using the phototrichogram, a novel phenomenon was discovered: emptiness of the hair follicle following teloptosis. Rebora and Guarrera later chose to call this phenomenon kenogen, deriving from the Greek word for "empty" [5]. During kenogen, the hair follicle rests physiologically, but duration and frequency were shown to be greater in androgenetic alopecia, possibly accounting for baldness [6]. In addition to the classical cycle, the hair follicle may follow an alternative route during which the telogen phase, not accompanied by a coincident new early anagen, ends with teloptosis leaving the follicle empty. In 2002, Stenn

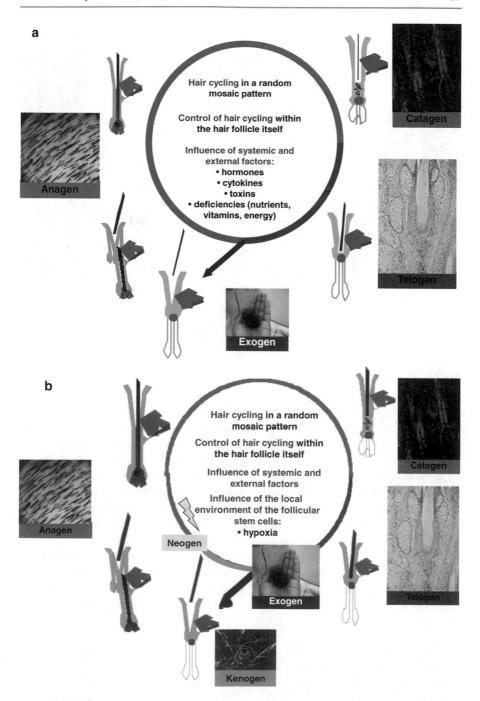

Fig. 4.2 (**a–c**) Hair cycle. (**a**) As originally described. (**b**) Extended concept, including kenogen, exogen, and neogen. (**c**) Derangements of the hair cycle: mitotic arrest, synchronization phenomena, shortening of anagen duration

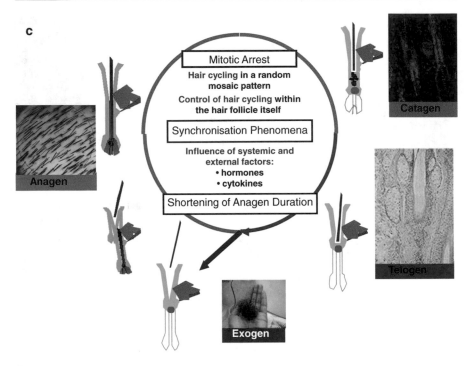

Fig. 4.2 (continued)

et al. [7] recognized the shedding phase of the hair growth cycle to be a uniquely controlled final step in the hair cycle involving a specific proteolytic step, and renamed it exogen. Finally, in 2013 Bernard et al. [8] identified hypoxia markers in the human hair follicle stem cells, and proposed hypoxia signaling mediated by the hypoxia-inducible transcription factor HIF1 to be important for reentry of the follicle into a new hair cycle in the course of a novel neomorphogenic hair cycle phase that they named neogen. Ultimately, it was further hypothesized that molecules that mimic hypoxic signaling may figure as a new approach to sustain hair growth and cycling, such as stemoxydine, a molecule developed by L'Oréal.

Cyclic hair growth activity occurs in a random mosaic pattern with each follicle possessing its own individual control mechanism over the evolution and triggering of the successive phases, including the local milieu at the level of stem cells. In addition, a number of systemic and environmental factors may have influence, such as:

- Hormones
- Cytokines and growth factors
- Toxins
- Deficiencies of nutrients, vitamins, and energy (calories)

4.1   Pathologic Dynamics of Hair Loss as They Relate to the Hair Cycle

Many factors can lead to a pathologically increased hair loss. Whatever the cause, the follicle tends to behave in a similar way. To grasp the meaning of this generalization requires understanding the varied derangements of the hair cycle underlying hair loss, i.e., mitotic arrest (dystrophic anagen effluvium), synchronization phenomena (telogen effluvium), shorting of anagen duration (Fig. 4.2c), and their causes.

4.1.1   Dystrophic Anagen Effluvium

Dystrophic anagen effluvium is hair loss that results from the shedding of large numbers of hairs from the anagen phase of growth. It is a major characteristic of anagen that the epithelial hair follicle compartment undergoes proliferation, with the hair matrix keratinocytes showing the highest proliferative activity in building up the hair shaft. The common pathogenesis which unites the different etiologies of dystrophic anagen effluvium is a direct insult to the rapidly dividing bulb matrix cells. The abrupt cessation of mitotic activity leads to the weakening of the partially keratinized proximal portion of the hair shaft, its narrowing and subsequent breakage within the hair canal, and shedding (Fig. 4.3a). The morphological consequence is the dystrophic anagen hair with a tapered proximal end and lack of root sheath (Fig. 4.3b). Hair loss is usually dramatic, involving 90% of affected hairs that are shed within days to few weeks of the inciting event. The hair loss may be diffuse in chemotherapy-induced alopecia (Fig. 4.3c) and toxic alopecia or focal in radiation-induced alopecia (Fig. 4.3d) [9].

Causes for dystrophic anagen effluvium are listed in Table 4.1.

Nutritional causes of dystrophic anagen effluvium are rare, and related to the exposure to either heavy metals or toxic plants.

Heavy metals are capable of disrupting the formation of the hair shaft through covalent binding with the sulfhydryl groups in keratin: thallium, mercury, arsenic, copper, cadmium, and bismuth. A study conducted by Piérard [10] in Belgium in 1979 reported diffuse alopecia related to ingestion of toxic metals in 36 of 78 patients with diffuse alopecia. Copper was involved in 17 alopecias, arsenic in 12, mercury in 5, and cadmium in 2. The leading cause, copper intoxication, was found to be related to ingestion of tap water containing a high concentration of copper salts, presumably from low pH, presence of chelating agents, or connection of electrical ground wires to copper water pipes, which caused sufficient flow of electrical current to ionize the metal.

Arsenic is a chemical element with the symbol As. It occurs in many minerals, usually in combination with sulfur and metals, but also as a pure elemental crystal. Orpiment (Fig. 4.4a) is a deep-colored, orange-yellow arsenic sulfide mineral with formula As_2S_3. Orpiment was traded in the Roman Empire and was used as a medicine in China [11], even though it is very toxic. Because of its striking color, it was of interest to alchemists, both in China and the West, searching for a way to make gold. For centuries, orpiment was ground down and used as a pigment in painting, and was one of the few clear, bright-yellow pigments available to artists until the nineteenth century. However, its extreme toxicity meant that its use as a pigment ended when cadmium yellows, chromium yellows, and organic dye-based colors were introduced during the nineteenth century. Mixed with slaked lime, orpiment is still commonly used in rural India as a depilatory.

The primary use of arsenic is in alloys of lead, for example in car batteries and ammunition. Arsenic is a common dopant in semiconductor electronic devices, and the optoelectronic compound gallium arsenide is the second most commonly used semiconductor after doped silicon. Furthermore, arsenic and its trioxide are used in the production of pesticides, treated wood products, herbicides, and insecticides, though these applications are declining due to the toxicity of arsenic.

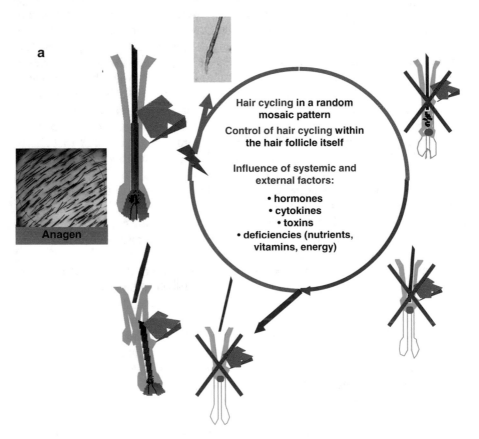

Fig. 4.3 (**a–e**) Dystrophic anagen effluvium. (**a**) Abrupt cessation of mitotic activity of the hair cycle. (**b**) Dystrophic anagen hair with a tapered proximal end and lack of root sheath (light microscopy). (**c**) Chemotherapy-induced alopecia. (**d**) Transient radiation-induced alopecia areata-like alopecia following neuroradiologically guided embolization procedure. (**e**) Permanent radiation-induced alopecia following a single dose above 1200 cGy, or a fractionated dose above 4500 cGy

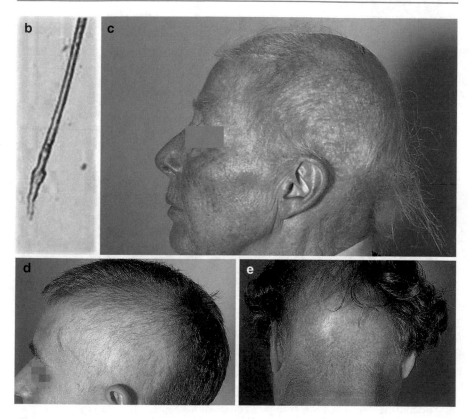

Fig. 4.3 (continued)

Table 4.1 Causes for dystrophic anagen effluvium

• Antineoplastic drugs (chemotherapy induced alopecia)
• X-ray (radiation induced alopecia)
• Immunologic injury (alopecia areata)
• Environmental or occupational exposure to toxins (toxic alopecia)

Arsenic comprises about 1.5 ppm (0.00015%) of the Earth's crust as the 53rd most abundant element. Typical background concentrations of arsenic do not exceed 3 ng/m³ in the atmosphere, 100 mg/kg in soil, and 10 µg/L in freshwater. Nevertheless, arsenic contamination of groundwater is a problem that affects millions of people across the world, specifically in Bangladesh and neighboring countries. The arsenic in the groundwater is of natural origin, and is released from the sediment into the groundwater. Other countries in Southeast Asia, such as Vietnam, Cambodia, and Thailand, have geological environments that produce groundwater with a high arsenic content. The Chao Phraya River in Bangkok, Thailand (Fig. 4.4b), contains high

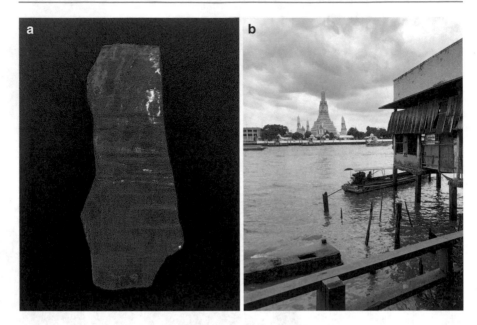

Fig. 4.4 (**a**, **b**) Arsenic. (**a**) Orpiment. (**b**) Chao Phraya river, Bangkok, Thailand (courtesy of Dr. Chuchai Tanglertsampan)

levels of naturally occurring dissolved arsenic without being a public health problem because much of the public uses bottled water. In Pakistan, more than 60 million people are exposed to arsenic-polluted drinking water indicated by a respective report: of more than 1200 samples more than 66% exceeded the WHO minimum contamination level [12]. Finally, arsenic is itself a constituent of tobacco smoke [13].

In the Victorian era, "white arsenic" (arsenic trioxide) was mixed with vinegar and chalk and eaten or was rubbed into the faces and arms of women to improve their complexion making their skin paler. During the eighteenth through early twentieth centuries, arsenic compounds were used as medicines, including arsphenamine (neosalvarsan) by Paul Ehrlich (1854–1915) and arsenic trioxide (Fowler's solution) by Thomas Fowler (1736–1801) for treatment of syphilis and psoriasis, respectively. In subtoxic doses, soluble arsenic compounds act as stimulants, and were once popular in small doses as a medicine in the mid-eighteenth to nineteenth centuries.

Arsenic has been linked to epigenetic changes, i.e., gene expression that occurs without changes in DNA sequence. These include DNA methylation, histone modification, and RNA interference. Toxic levels of arsenic cause significant DNA hypermethylation of tumor-suppressor genes p16 and p53, thus increasing the risk of carcinogenesis. Long-term exposure to arsenic has thus been linked to cancers of the bladder, kidney, liver, prostate, skin, lungs, and nasal cavity [14].

Acute arsenic intoxication today is usually the result of an accidental ingestion or exposure, industrial accidents, or suicidal or homicidal intentions. Symptoms are nausea, vomiting, abdominal pain, and a garlic odor on the breath, along with hypotension, cyanosis, shortness of breath, delirium, seizures, coma, acute tubular necrosis of the kidney, and hemolysis. One to three weeks after ingestion of the arsenic, polyneuritis may become evident, approximately at 6 weeks Mees' transverse white nail lines [15] may appear, while a diffuse hair loss occurs usually within 1–2 months after exposure.

Mercury (Hg) is yet another elemental metal that may cause intoxication with dermatologic symptoms and hair loss. It is the only metallic element that is liquid at standard conditions for temperature and pressure. A complete explanation of mercury's extreme volatility delves deep into the realm of quantum physics. Mercury dissolves many metals such as gold and silver to form amalgams. Mercury occurs in deposits throughout the world mostly as cinnabar (mercuric sulfide). The red pigment vermilion is obtained by grinding natural cinnabar or synthetic mercuric sulfide.

In Ancient China, mercury use was thought to prolong life, and maintain generally good health. The first emperor of China, Qín Shǐ Huáng Dì (259–210 BC), allegedly buried in a tomb that contained rivers of flowing mercury on a model of the land he ruled, representative of the rivers of China, died by drinking a mercury and powdered jade mixture formulated by Qin alchemists who intended to give him eternal life, but caused liver failure, mercury poisoning, and brain death. The ancient Greeks used cinnabar (mercury sulfide) in ointments; the ancient Egyptians and the Romans used it in cosmetics. The alchemists thought of mercury as the first matter from which all metals were formed, and believed that different metals could be produced by varying the quality and quantity of sulfur contained within the mercury. The purest of these was gold, and mercury was called for in attempts at the transmutation of base (or impure) metals into gold, which was the goal of the alchemists [16].

Mercury and its compounds have historically been used in medicine, until the toxic effects of mercury and its compounds were more widely understood. Mercury(I) chloride (calomel) has been used in traditional medicine as a diuretic, topical disinfectant, and laxative. Mercury(II) chloride (mercuric chloride or corrosive sublimate) was used to treat syphilis along with other mercury compounds, although it was so toxic that sometimes the symptoms of its toxicity were confused with those of the syphilis it was believed to treat. Blue mass, a pill or syrup in which mercury was the main ingredient, was prescribed throughout the nineteenth century for numerous conditions including constipation, depression, childbearing, and toothaches [17]. In the early twentieth century, mercury was administered to children yearly as a laxative and dewormer, and it was used in teething powders for infants. The mercury-containing organohalide merbromin (Mercurochrome) as a disinfectant is still widely used but has been banned in some countries such as the United States [18].

Mercury has further been used in thermometers, barometers, manometers, sphygmomanometers, float valves, mercury switches, mercury relays, fluorescent lamps, and other devices, though concerns about the element's toxicity have led to mercury-based technologies being largely phased out in clinical environments in favor of alternatives.

Mercury remains in use in amalgam for dental restoration. The use of dental amalgams was first documented in a Chinese Tang Dynasty medical text written by Su Gong (苏恭) in 659, and appeared in Germany in 1528 [19]. In the 1800s, amalgam became the dental restorative material of choice for its low cost, ease of application, strength, and durability [20]. However, concerns have been raised about the potential for mercury poisoning with dental amalgam, specifically neurotoxic and/or neuropsychological effects, but major health and professional organizations regard amalgam as safe [21–23]. In fact, mercury levels in blood and urine correlated with the number of amalgam surfaces in one study, indicating the release of mercury from dental amalgam restorations [24]. However, the mercury levels were far below those where negative health effects would be expected, and they were similar in patients with complaints self-related to dental amalgam restorations and healthy control individuals, so that the mercury was not found to be a likely cause of the impaired health reported by patients. In another study, assays of mercury in urine samples of patients complaining of dental amalgam-related symptoms indicated that the exposure was far below the levels at which symptoms could be indicated by psychometric tests [25, 26]. Psychologic investigation indicated that the symptoms were rather of psychosomatic origin [27–29]. All patients had experienced important psychic traumata in close correlation with the first appearance of symptoms [30].

An industrial disaster of catastrophic dimensions was the dumping of mercury compounds into Minamata Bay, Japan, resulting in an estimated over 3000 people suffering of severe mercury poisoning symptoms, deformities, or death from what became notoriously known as Minamata disease. Japanese writer and activist Michiko Ishimure (1927–2018) won in 1973 Asia's highest award for literature and journalism, the Ramon Magsaysay Award, for publicizing the politically explosive issue in her writings (*Paradise in the Sea of Sorrow*, 1969).

Fish and shellfish have a natural tendency to concentrate mercury in their bodies, often in the form of methylmercury, a highly toxic organic compound of mercury. Species of fish that are high on the food chain, such as shark, swordfish, king mackerel, bluefin tuna, albacore tuna, and tilefish, contain higher concentrations of mercury than others. As mercury and methylmercury are fat soluble, they primarily accumulate in the viscera, though they are also found in the muscle tissue [31]. When this fish is consumed by a predator, the mercury level is accumulated. Since fish are less efficient at depurating than accumulating methylmercury, fish-tissue concentrations increase over time. Therefore, species that are high on the food chain accumulate body burdens of mercury that can be ten times higher than the species they consume. This process is called biomagnification. Mercury poisoning happened this way in Minamata disease [32].

Some skin-whitening products contain the toxic mercury(II) chloride as the active ingredient. When applied, the chemical readily absorbs through the skin into the bloodstream, and symptoms of mercury poisoning may come from the use of mercury-containing cosmetic products [33]. The use of skin-whitening products is especially popular among Asian women. In Hong Kong in 2002, two products were discovered to contain between 9000 and 60,000 times the recommended dose [34].

Cases of mercury poisoning have also been reported in Germany from the use of mercury-containing (about 5–6% Hg) hair bleaches. Loss of weight, stomatitis, hearing and sensory loss, and emotional disturbances have accompanied the cardinal signs of nail discoloration and loss of hair. The mercury content of nails was extremely high (1720 mg/L). The urinary level of mercury after dimercaprol injection was 1.97 mg/L, about 400 times above the upper limit of normal (0.005 mg/L) [35].

The signs of acute mercury poisoning can first appear only weeks to months after exposure, and are primarily neurological: sensory impairment, constriction of visual fields, hearing impairment, ataxia, and speech disturbance (Hunter-Russell syndrome).

Two cases of reversible alopecia associated with elevated blood mercury levels and early menopause have recently been reported. Recommendation to alter diet, including fish intake, was followed by reversal of alopecia, along with decrease in blood mercury levels. The authors suggest that development of alopecia in the setting of mild mercury intoxication should be considered in women complaining of hair loss (Fig. 4.5). Its relationship to early menopause is unclear but deserves

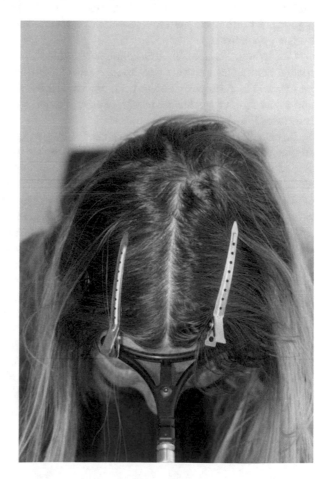

Fig. 4.5 Female in menopause complaining of hair loss with elevated mercury levels in urine (68.7 μg/g)

further research [36]. The development of alopecia in relation to subclinical mercury intoxication had so far not been reported in the medical literature despite its discussion in the popular press.

A peculiar presentation of chronic exposure of infants to inorganic mercury compounds from teething powders has been described as *acrodynia*, *pink disease*, or *Feer's disease*, and consists of a condition of pain and dusky pink discoloration in the hands and feet. Affected children may also show red cheeks and nose, red lips, loss of hair, teeth, and nails, transient rashes, hypotonia, and photophobia [37].

Cadmium (Cd) is a naturally occurring toxic heavy metal with common exposure in industrial workplaces and plant soils, and from smoking. Unlike most other metals, cadmium is resistant to corrosion and has therefore been used as a protective plate on other metals, notably on steel. Cadmium compounds are also used as red, orange, and yellow pigments, to color glass, and to stabilize plastic. However, industrial cadmium use is decreasing because it is toxic, and nickel-cadmium batteries have been replaced by lithium-ion batteries.

Cadmium exposure is a risk factor associated with a large number of illnesses including renal disease, hypertension, and cardiovascular diseases. Studies show a significant correlation between cadmium exposure and occurrence of disease in human populations.

One hypothesis holds that cadmium is an endocrine disruptor and some experimental studies have shown that it can interact with different hormonal signaling pathways. For example, cadmium can bind to the estrogen receptor alpha [38, 39] and affect signal transduction along the estrogen and MAPK signaling pathways at low doses [39–41].

Inside cells, cadmium ions act as a catalytic hydrogen peroxide generator. This sudden surge of cytosolic hydrogen peroxide causes increased lipid peroxidation and additionally depletes ascorbate and glutathione stores. Hydrogen peroxide can also convert thiol groups in proteins into nonfunctional sulfonic acids and is also capable of directly attacking nuclear DNA. This oxidative stress causes the afflicted cell to manufacture large amounts of inflammatory cytokines [42].

Ingestion of any significant amount of cadmium causes immediate poisoning and damage to the liver and the kidneys. Acute, usually industrial, exposure to cadmium fumes may cause flu-like symptoms including chills, fever, and muscle ache. Inhaling cadmium-laden dust quickly leads to respiratory tract and renal symptoms which can be fatal, often from renal failure. Demineralization of bones leads to osteomalacia and osteoporosis resulting in pain in the joints and the back, and increase of risk of fractures [43].

Heavy metal poisoning with cadmium and bismuth in a glass worker was characterized by severe alopecia and extensive nonhealing cutaneous lesions [44].

The tobacco plant readily takes up and accumulates heavy metals, such as cadmium, from the surrounding soil into its leaves. These are readily absorbed into the user's body following smoke inhalation [45]. Tobacco smoking is the most important single source of cadmium exposure in the general population. Absorption of cadmium through the lungs is more effective than through the gastrointestinal tract [46]. On average, cadmium concentration in the blood of smokers is four or five times greater than in nonsmokers. Smoke-induced risk of osteoporosis may be partly mediated by cadmium from tobacco smoke [47].

In the nonsmoking population, food is the greatest source of exposure. High quantities of cadmium can be found in crustaceans, mollusk, offal, and algae products. However, with grains, vegetables, starchy roots, and tubers being consumed in much greater quantity in the United States, they are the source of the greater dietary exposure, since plants bioaccumulate metal toxins like cadmium. When composted to form organic fertilizers, they may yield a product which can contain high concentrations of metal toxin (e.g., over 0.5 mg/kg fertilizer).

For a single exposure by ingestion, gastric decontamination by emesis or gastric lavage may be beneficial soon after exposure. Chelation therapies to remove cadmium are not effective, so the most important action is to prevent exposure.

Zinc, copper, calcium, iron, and selenium with vitamin C are used to treat cadmium intoxication.

Thallium (from Greek θαλλός, thallos, meaning "a green shoot or twig") was discovered 1861 by flame spectroscopy, from which the name derives due to thallium's bright green spectral emission lines. The odorless and tasteless thallium sulfate was once widely used as rat poison and ant killer. Due to safety concerns, this use was banned in 1972 in the United States with other countries following this example in subsequent years.

Thallium salts were formerly used in the treatment of scalp ringworm due to its ability to epilate hair [48], and to reduce the night sweating in patients with tuberculosis. Again, this use has been limited due to the narrow therapeutic index, along with the development of improved treatments for these conditions.

Other applications of thallium have been in optics, electronics, and cardiac perfusion imagery prior to the introduction of technetium-99m for this purpose. According to the United States Environmental Protection Agency (EPA), man-made sources of thallium pollution include gaseous emission of cement factories, coal-burning power plants, and metal sewers. The main source of elevated thallium concentrations in water is the leaching of thallium from ore-processing operations.

Thallium and its compounds are extremely toxic. It is a cumulative poison which is absorbed through the skin, pulmonary tree, or gastrointestinal tract. Thallium binds to sulfhydryl groups in mitochondrial membranes at intracellular sites. Studies have implicated alterations in keratin formation as the mechanism for thallium-induced alopecia, since keratin contains a significant portion of the sulfur in hair, and the alteration in the formation of this protein may lead to hair loss through hair breakage (it is this effect that led to the use of thallium as a depilatory before its toxicity was properly appreciated). Accordingly, experimental alopecia from thallium in rats could be reduced with the addition of 1–2% cystine [49].

Among the distinctive effects of thallium poisoning are hair loss and damage to peripheral nerves [50]. Alopecia is the most common symptom and usually begins 10 days after ingestion as a diffuse shedding of dystrophic anagen hairs [51]. Even repeated low-dose exposure to thallium may lead to alopecia and proximal nail plate erosion (Fig. 4.6) [52].

Fig. 4.6 Erosion of the proximal nail plate from thallium intoxication

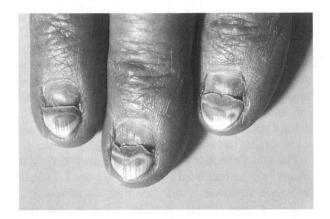

Thallium was once an effective homicidal weapon and has been called the "poisoner's poison," since it is colorless, odorless, and tasteless, and its slow-acting, painful, and wide-ranging symptoms are often suggestive of a host of other medical conditions.

There are two main methods of removing thallium from humans: First, Prussian blue, which is a solid ion exchange material, absorbs thallium. Up to 20 g per day of Prussian blue is fed by mouth to the person, and it passes through their digestive system and comes out in the stool. Second, hemodialysis and hemoperfusion are also used as indicated to remove thallium from the blood serum. At later stage of the treatment additional potassium is used to mobilize thallium from the tissue.

The diagnosis of heavy metal toxicity requires clinical suspicion, observation of presenting symptoms including acute alopecia [53], obtaining a thorough history of potential exposure (occupational, environmental, accidental), and results of laboratory tests. In a study performed by Piérard, toxic metals in abnormal amount in blood and urine were observed when >10% of hair bulbs were dystrophic in trichogram examinations [10]. Therefore, an unexplained dystrophic anagen effluvium with dystrophic anagen rates >10% in the trichogram should prompt further investigations. These include measuring urine, blood, or hair levels of the suspected heavy metals. Chemical hair analysis may prove useful for retrospective purposes when blood and urine are no longer expected to contain a particular contaminant, and are primarily used for forensic purposes [54].

The results of such forensic studies on hair have also been of particular historical interest when performed on hair clippings of famous personalities, such as Beethoven (1770–1827) [55] and Napoleon (1769–1821) [56], where high levels of lead and arsenic, respectively, were detected.

Cases of diffuse alopecia occurring after the ingestion of plants or plant parts have also been reported.

A group of plants have been classified as *seleniferous plants* by virtue of their content in selenocystathionine, a selenium-containing analogue of the sulfur amino acid cystathionine. They include *Lecythis ollaria* (coco de mono), *Astragalus pectinatus* (narrowleaf milkvetch), and *Stanleya pinnata* (desert prince's plume). The plants are toxic by virtue of their high content in selenium resulting in selenium intoxication with inhibition of the anagen phase of the hair cycle. While human intoxication with seleniferous plants is rare, there have been reports from South America, and the United States, where selenium poisoning has been associated with hair loss in Native Americans [57–59]. The cytotoxic effect can be reversed by administration of L-cystine.

Hair loss has also been reported following ingestion of parts of the *Leucaena glauca* plant, a low scrubby tree of tropical and subtropical North America having white flowers tinged with yellow resembling mimosa and long flattened pods. The sudden loss of hair of native women following the consumption of seeds has been attributed to the toxic amino acid leucenol or mimosine [60], believed to interfere either with keratinization by competitively displacing alanine or with mitosis similar to the effect of cytotoxic chemicals [61].

Colchicum autumnale (autumn crocus) is a toxic autumn-blooming flowering plant that resembles the crocus, but is a member of the Colchicaceae plant family, unlike the true crocuses which belong to the Iridaceae family. Despite its vernacular name of meadow saffron, Colchicum autumnale is not the source of saffron, which is obtained from the saffron crocus (*Crocus sativus*), while that plant too is sometimes called autumn crocus as well making the confusion complete. Colchicum plants may be fatally poisonous, and have been mistaken by foragers for wild garlic (*Allium ursinum*), which they vaguely resemble. In spite of its toxicity, the species is commonly cultivated as an ornamental in temperate areas. The bulb-like corms of *Colchicum autumnale* contain colchicine, a useful drug with a narrow therapeutic index.

The autumn crocus has been used as early as 1500 BC to treat joint swelling [62]. Today, colchicine is approved in many countries for the treatment of gout and familial Mediterranean fever.

The symptoms of colchicine poisoning resemble those of arsenic, while no antidote is known. With overdoses, colchicine becomes toxic as an extension of its cellular mechanism of action via binding to tubulin [63]. Cells so affected undergo impaired protein assembly with reduced endocytosis, exocytosis, and cellular motility, culminating in multi-organ failure.

Diffuse alopecia has been reported in patients treated for psoriasis with colchicine in doses of 2–3 mg daily [64]. Typically, there is an increased number of telogen hair, while morphological changes in anagen hairs can also be seen, depending on the severity of the intoxication. Anagen effluvium within 7–14 days of taking colchicine has been reported following colchicine poisoning in a suicide attempt [65]. The mechanism involved in colchicine-induced hair loss is assumed to result from an antimitotic effect.

Gloriosa superba (flame lily) is yet another species of flowering plant from the family of the Colchicaceae. As with other members of the Colchicaceae, this plant contains high levels of colchicine. It also contains the alkaloid gloriocine. The plant is toxic enough to cause human fatalities if ingested, and has been used to commit both murder [66] and suicide. Every part of the plant is poisonous, especially the tuberous rhizomes. Poisonings can occur when the tubers are mistaken for sweet potatoes or yams and then eaten. Within a few hours of ingestion, a victim may experience nausea, vomiting, numbness, tingling around the mouth, burning in the throat, abdominal pain, and bloody diarrhea, which leads to dehydration. As the toxic syndrome progresses, rhabdomyolysis, ileus, respiratory depression, hypotension, coagulopathy, hematuria, altered mental status, seizures, coma, and ascending polyneuropathy may occur. Longer term effects include peeling of the skin and anagen effluvium [67]. One case report described a woman who accidentally ate the tubers and experienced generalized hair loss over her entire body, including complete alopecia [68].

More recently, hair loss from anagen effluvium associated with *cucurbit* poisoning has been reported by Assouly [69]. Cucurbita (Latin for gourd) is a genus of herbaceous vines in the gourd family, originally native to the Andes and Mesoamerica, with species grown worldwide for their edible fruit, variously known as squash, pumpkin, or gourd. Cucurbita fruits are large and fleshy, with fruit size varying considerably from 4 cm in wild specimens to well over 300 kg in domesticated specimens. The current world record was set in 2014 by Beni Meier of Switzerland with a 1054.0 kg pumpkin. Halloween is widely celebrated in the United States with jack-o-lanterns made of large orange pumpkins carved with ghoulish faces and illuminated from inside with candles.

A natural toxin contained in cucurbits with the function as a defense against herbivores and taste deterrent is the cucurbitacins. They are chemically classified as triterpenes. They and their derivatives have been found in many plant families, in some mushrooms, and even in some marine mollusks. They make wild cucurbits and most ornamental gourds bitter to taste. Ingesting too much cucurbitacin can cause stomach cramps, diarrhea, and even collapse. While the process of domestication has largely removed the bitterness from cultivated varieties, there are occasional reports of cucurbitacin causing illness in humans. In laboratory research, cucurbitacins have cytotoxic properties. A particularly bitter taste of the potentially toxic specimen must alert the consumer as well as the physician who treats the patient.

4.1.2 Telogen Effluvium

Telogen effluvium is by far the commonest cause of hair loss, and results from increased shedding of hairs from the telogen phase of the hair cycle. An increase in the percentage of follicles in telogen >20% leads to increased shedding of hairs in telogen. This can be due to either synchronization phenomena of hair cycling (Fig. 4.7a), with hair thinning usually seen at the temples (Fig. 4.7b) and shedding of hairs in the hundreds in telogen effluvium (Fig. 4.7c), or a decrease of anagen-phase duration in androgenetic alopecia. While a number of attempts have been made with respect to the underlying pathologic dynamics of telogen effluvium and its classification, the original classification by Headington from 1993 [70] remains unabated and the most comprehensive. On the basis of changes in different phases of the follicular cycle, Headington proposed the classification of telogen effluvium

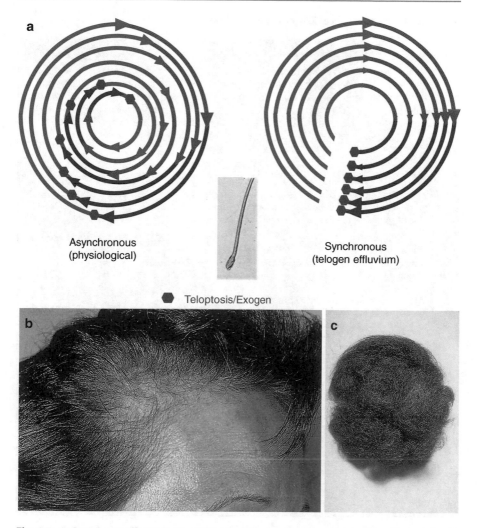

Fig. 4.7 (**a, b**) Telogen effluvium. (**a–c**) Telogen effluvium from synchronization of hair cycle: (**a**) Synchronization of hair cycle, (**b**) temporal thinning, (**c**) shedding of hair in the hundreds

into five functional types depending on changes in different phases of the hair cycle (Table 4.2).

While telogen effluvium represents a monomorphic reaction pattern of the hair follicle to a variety of causes, the underlying pathologic dynamics is more diverse. Headington's classification represents the most rational of all proposals and has proven its validity. It covers all clinical types of telogen effluvium, such as postfebrile, posttraumatic, and postinterventional telogen effluvium (immediate anagen release); postpartum telogen effluvium (delayed anagen release); shedding phase upon initiation of topical minoxidil treatment (immediate telogen release); and seasonal hair shedding (delayed telogen release) [71]. Moreover, Headington's

Table 4.2 Functional types of telogen effluvium. From [70]

Immediate anagen release

Follicles that would normally complete a longer cycle by remaining in anagen prematurely enter telogen. It is a very common form of telogen effluvium, typically occurring after periods of physiologic stress including episodes of high fever. In fever, the pyrogens, basically circulating cytokines, drive the hair follicle keratinocytes into apoptosis initiating catagen with following telogen. Because the shedding is dependent on transition from anagen through catagen and telogen with subsequent release of telogen hairs, hair loss occurs 3 to 4 months after the inciting event.

Delayed anagen release

Hair follicles remain in prolonged anagen rather than cycling into telogen. When finally released from anagen, the clinical sign of increased shedding of telogen hair will be found. This type of telogen effluvium underlies post partum hair loss.

Immediate telogen release

Hair follicles normally programmed for release of the club hair after an interval of usually 100 days after the end of anagen, are prematurely stimulated to cycle into anagen. There is premature teloptosis. This type of telogen effluvium underlies the shedding of hair upon initiation of therapy with topical minoxidil (shedding phase).

Delayed telogen release

Hair follicles remain in prolonged telogen rather than being shed and recycling into anagen. When finally teloptosis sets in, again the clinical sign of increased shedding of club hairs is observed. This process underlies moulting in mammals and probably also seasonal shedding of hairs in humans or mild telogen effluvia following travel from low-daylight to high-daylight conditions.

Short anagen

Finally, a short anagen phase duration (without synchronization) results in a slight but persistent telogen effluvium in association with decreased hair length: This may occur in hereditary hypotrichosis, ectodermal dysplasia (tricho-dental syndrome), and as an isolated disorder in otherwise healthy children, as originally described by Barraud-Klenosvek and Trüeb. Far more frequent is acquired progressive shortening of anagen due to androgenetic alopecia.

ingenious classification predicted the existence of a short anagen syndrome, which was only later confirmed by the original report of the condition as congenital hypotrichosis due to short anagen by Barraud-Klenovsek and Trüeb in 2000 [72] (Fig. 4.8a,b).

4.1.3   Performing the Trichogram as a Diagnostic Test

The trichogram or hair pluck test is a semi-invasive technique for hair analysis on the basis of the hair growth cycle. Studies on the dynamics of the follicular cycle have largely depended on the microscopic evaluation of plucked hairs with quantitative measuring of the number of individual hair roots. The method was introduced

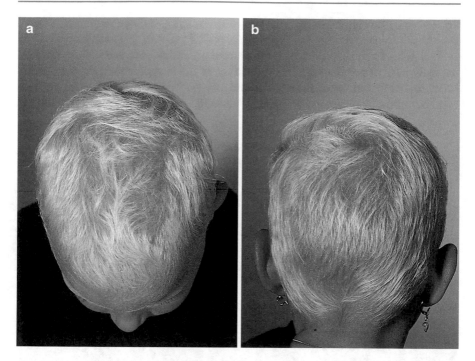

Fig. 4.8 (**a**, **b**) Short anagen hair

in 1957 by van Scott et al. as an indicator of hair growth in studies with cytotoxic agents [73] and radiation [74]. In 1964, the term trichogram was initially used by Pecoraro [75] to describe the normal hair growth parameters, such as the growth rate, shaft diameter, and telogen rate in children and adults. Subsequently, the trichogram technique was developed and standardized to serve as a diagnostic tool for evaluation of hair loss in daily clinical practice [76]. For this purpose, it is simple to perform, repeatable, and reasonably reliable under standardized conditions. Since in 95% of cases hair loss is due to a disorder of hair cycling, trichogram measurements serve as a standard method for quantifying the hair in its different growth cycle phases as it relates to the pathologic dynamics underlying the loss of hair. The percentage of hair roots in anagen, catagen, or telogen reflects either synchronization phenomena of the hair cycle or alterations in the duration of the respective growth cycle phases, while the presence of pathologic dystrophic hair roots signalizes a massive insult to the hair follicle in anagen.

The trichogram technique involves the forceful plucking of 50–100 hairs with a forceps from specific sites of the scalp. Ultimately, the objective of trichogram measurements is to evaluate and count the status of individual hair roots and to establish the ratio of anagen to telogen roots. The reliability of trichogram measurements relies on the adherence to strict standards in obtaining the hair samples.

The materials necessary for performing a trichogram include a tail comb, hair clips, artery forceps covered with rubber tube, a pair of scissors, microslides

76 × 26 mm, cover glasses 50 × 24 mm, Eukitt, xylol, a dissecting needle, and a binocular microscope with variable objectives (2.5 and 4.0) (Fig. 4.9a).

Epilation of hair samples for the trichogram is performed at least 5 days after the last hair wash to avoid an artificial reduction of the telogen count. To avoid additional loss of telogen hairs, the hairs should also not be cut, curled, waved, or backcombed during that period. Epilation is carried out from two specified sites: in

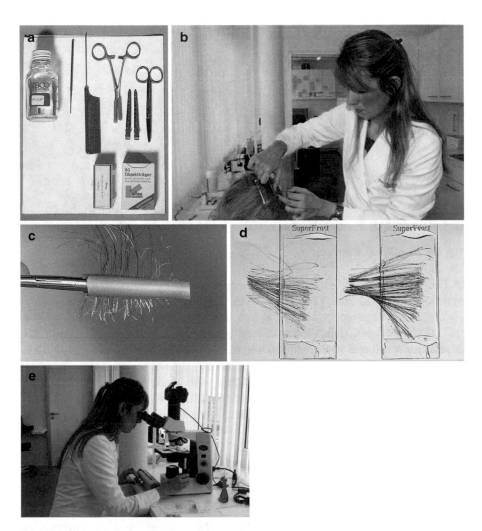

Fig. 4.9 (a–e) Performing the trichogram. (a) Materials. (b–e) Procedure: (b) The hair is parted and fixed with clips. Along the parting line, a bundle of hairs is lifted parallel along the course of the hair and grasped close to the scalp with the forceps which jaws are covered with the rubber tubes. (c) A sharp quick pull and exact plucking in the direction of the emergence angle of the hairs from the scalp are important to obtain a reliable hair sample. (d) Embedding of epilated hairs occurs immediately to prevent dehydration of the hair roots. Correctly embedded hair roots are suitable for unlimited storage. (e) Light microscopic evaluation of the hair root patterns

diffuse effluvium or androgenetic alopecia frontal (2 cm behind the forehead and 2 cm lateral) and occipital (2 cm lateral from the occipital protuberance), and in circumscribed alopecias, such as alopecia areata or trichotillomania, one sample is taken from the border zone and the control from the normal-appearing contralateral region. Within the chosen area for epilation, the hair is parted and fixed with clips (Fig. 4.9b). Along the parting line, a bundle of approximately 50–100 hairs is lifted parallel along the course of the hair and grasped close to the scalp with the forceps whose jaws are covered with the rubber tubes. The forceps jaws are pressed together to the maximum and the tuft of hair is then epilated (Fig. 4.9c). A sharp quick pull and exact plucking in the direction of the emergence angle of the hairs from the scalp are important to obtain a reliable hair root pattern. Slow or hesitant traction, or wrong pulling direction, may induce distortions or alterations of the plucked hairs complicating interpretation.

Embedding of epilated hairs occurs immediately to prevent dehydration of hair roots. A few drops of Eukitt (after condensation, dilute with xylol) is given on two marked microslides. The tuft of hairs is taken with thumb and pointing finger; the roots are dipped in the embedding material (Eukitt), cut off 2 cm above the roots, and arranged in a fast manner with the dissecting needle in a parallel position before being covered. Correctly embedded hair roots are suitable for unlimited storage (Fig. 4.9d).

The light microscopic evaluation can be done when the embedding material no longer runs, usually after 10 min (Fig. 4.9e).

The act of plucking scalp hair may cause slight discomfort to the patient and may leave a small linear bald patch, which is why the frontal epilation site is better chosen contralateral to the natural hair part of the patient. The patient should be reassured that plucked hairs grow back after 3–6 weeks.

Furthermore, the trichogram needs critical interpretation. It provides information about the hair growth capacity, it detects disturbances of hair growth, and it detects toxic effects to the hair structure, induced by chemicals or drugs. In addition, the appearance and the size of the hair bulb are also important as atrophy and shrinkage reflect reduced growth activity. Finally, simultaneous microscopic examination of the hair shaft morphology may help identify abnormalities of the hair shaft.

In every stage of the hair cycle the hair root is characterized by a typical morphologic structure that is easy to recognize.

4.1.3.1 Anagen with Root Sheaths

Anagen hairs are not normally seen in daily hair collections or epilated with a simple hair pull, with the exception of loose anagen hair that presents with anagen hairs devoid of hair root sheaths. Since anagen hairs are normal-growing hairs they must be forcibly plucked from the scalp. The normal anagen hair root has a large base with an equally large diameter throughout. The bulb tip is usually pigmented and the adjacent hair shaft has a white coating composed of both the inner and outer root sheaths (Fig. 4.10a).

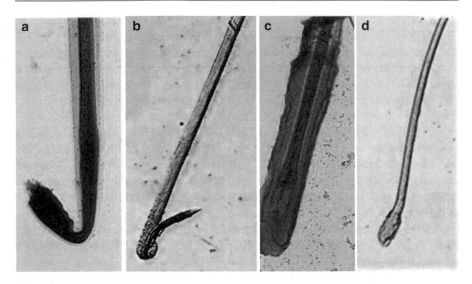

Fig. 4.10 (a–d) Physiological hair root forms. (a) Anagen with root sheath. (b) Anagen devoid of root sheath (they are also called dysplastic hairs). (c) Catagen. (d) Telogen. Their percental distribution is relevant to diagnosis

4.1.3.2 Anagen Devoid of Root Sheaths (Dysplastic Anagen Hair)
These represent an epilation artifact in thin but obviously growing anagen hairs, with a diminished matrix diameter and devoid of hair root sheaths. The lower end of the hair shaft is usually wavy or bent like the handle of a bishop's crozier (Fig. 4.10b).

4.1.3.3 Catagen
The hair root in catagen generally has an equal diameter throughout or can become narrower towards the base. The hair roots look like club hair in the telogen phase, but still shows root sheaths, which increasingly become shorter (Fig. 4.10c).

4.1.3.4 Telogen
Telogen hairs are those hairs shed with daily combing. Telogen bulbs are normally epilated with a simple hair pull. When increased numbers of telogen hairs are shed, this suggests the diagnosis of telogen effluvium. The telogen hair root is characteristically club shaped, unpigmented, and with smooth contours, and has no attached root sheath structure (Fig. 4.10d).

4.1.3.5 Dystrophic Anagen
Under normal circumstances, dystrophic roots appear very seldom. Basically, they represent thin, nongrowing anagen hairs. Any pathologic condition that causes rapid cessation of mitosis in the hair matrix results in tapering of the diameter of the hair shaft that breaks off at the narrowest level with a pencillike broken-end tip (Fig. 4.3b).

4.1.3.6 Broken-Off Hairs

They represent normally growing anagen hairs that have broken off on plucking. They can be easily recognized, since the broken ends appear smooth with a remaining diameter equal to that of the hair shaft.

4.1.3.7 Miniature Hairs

In addition to hairs of normal diameter, patients with androgenetic alopecia have a second population of hairs in the androgen-dependent area resulting from progressive narrowing and shortening of the hair shaft. These hairs represent terminal-to-vellus hair transformation. They are approximately 1 cm long and often have finely tapered tips. By definition vellus hairs have a shaft diameter of <40 μm.

Normally a maximum of 15% of scalp hair bulbs are in telogen and 85% are in anagen, and a maximum of 20% of scalp hair bulbs are anagen hairs devoid of hair root sheaths (dysplastic anagen hairs). Trichograms with >10% broken-off hairs cannot be evaluated correctly. Unless they are due to fragile hair, plucking should be repeated. The normal distribution pattern of hair roots in the trichogram of the scalp is summarized in Table 4.3.

The trichogram is diagnostic for telogen effluvium if more than 20% of bulbs are in telogen. An increase of the frontal telogen rate together with a normal occipital telogen rate is diagnostic for androgenetic alopecia, while an increase of the occipital telogen rate is diagnostic for diffuse telogen effluvium. Normal telogen rates neither support nor exclude the diagnosis of androgenetic alopecia. The trichogram is rather performed for the diagnosis of diffuse telogen effluvium or dystrophic anagen effluvium, since frontal telogen rates may be normal in female androgenetic alopecia. Dermoscopic examination of the central hair part has proven to be more sensitive for the diagnosis of early female androgenetic alopecia than the trichogram based on the detection of diversity of hair shaft diameters [78]. Despite the enthusiasm that has recently arisen for dermoscopy of the hair and scalp (trichoscopy) as a diagnostic tool, so far, only in the diagnosis of early female androgenetic alopecia dermoscopy has proven to be superior to the respective other diagnostic

Table 4.3 Normal distribution pattern of hair roots in the trichogram of the scalp. From [77]

Hair Roots	Percent
Anagen with root sheaths	60-80 %
Anagen without root sheaths (dysplastic anagen)	5 -20 %
Catagen	1-3 %
Telogen	12-15 %
Dystrophic anagen	< 2 %
Broken-off hairs	5-6 %

procedures. As a diagnostic procedure, trichoscopy remains to be understood as representing an integral part of a comprehensive dermatological examination to include the personal history, clinical examination, trichogram, biopsy, microbiology, and blood tests [79].

>10% dystrophic hairs are indicative of dystrophic anagen effluvium. If the cause is not obvious from the patient's history (chemotherapy, radiation), toxicologic studies (heavy metals and plant toxins) may be indicated. In a completed anagen effluvium in which only a few hairs remain on the scalp, all the epilated hairs are telogen bulbs (Fig. 4.11), such as may be seen in alopecia areata evolving to alopecia totalis.

In children, and in persons with thin hair, the rate of dysplastic anagen can occasionally reach >50%. Frontal increase in % anagen hairs devoid of hair root sheaths >20% is also seen in androgenetic alopecia and may represent a subtle clue to the diagnosis when telogen rates are still normal.

A rate of >80% (usually 90–100%) anagen hairs devoid of hair root sheaths (Fig. 4.12a) is diagnostic of loose anagen hair, a condition predominantly observed in children that is characterized by easily pluckable anagen hairs [80]. Additionally, there may be variation in hair texture, and the hair is often dry and lusterless (Fig. 4.12b). Ultrastructural studies show longitudinal grooves and a ruffled cuticle resembling floppy sock appearance of the hair shaft (Fig. 4.12c). The presence of these alterations supports the hypothesis of some abnormality of the root sheath adversely affecting anchoring of the anagen hair in the follicle.

Sometimes, inadequate epilation technique can also lead to an increase in the number of dysplastic hairs.

In trichotillomania, 100% of the hair bulbs are in anagen, since the patient plucks the loose telogen hair.

Broken-off hair may amount up to a maximum of 10% of the total number. Their prevalence is higher either when the hair is fragile or when the plucking technique was not adequate. A light microscopic hair shaft examination is indicated to exclude an underlying hair fragility disorder.

Presence of >13% miniature hairs is indicative of androgenetic alopecia.

Fig. 4.11 In a completed anagen effluvium in which only a few hairs remain on the scalp, all the epilated hairs are telogen bulbs

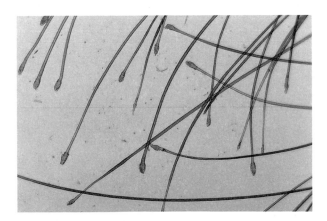

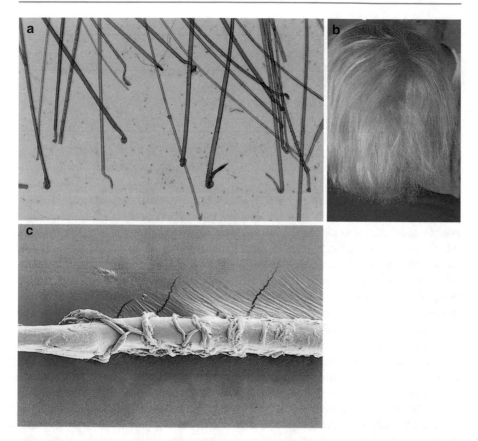

Fig. 4.12 (**a–c**) Loose anagen hair. (**a**) Trichogram. (**b**) Clinical presentation. (**c**) Ruffled cuticle resembling floppy sock appearance of the hair shaft (scanning electron microscopy)

4.1.4   Value of Multielement Hair Analysis

A number of commercial laboratories are committed to providing multielement hair analyses in which a single test is used to determine values for many minerals simultaneously. This type of analysis is particularly used by alternative medicine fields with the claim that hair analyses can help diagnose a wide variety of health problems, and can be used as a basis for prescribing natural chelation therapy, mineral, trace elements, and/or vitamin supplements. However, these uses remain debated for the following reasons [81–83]:

- Most commercial hair analysis laboratories have not validated their analytical techniques by checking them against standard reference materials.
- Hair mineral content can be affected by exposure to various substances such as shampoos, bleaches, and hair dyes. No analytic technique enables reliable determination of the source of specific levels of elements in hair as bodily or environmental.

- The level of certain minerals can be affected by the color, diameter, and rate of growth of an individual's hair; the season of the year; the geographic location; and the age and gender of the individual.
- Normal ranges of hair minerals have not been defined.
- For most elements, no correlation has been established between hair level and other known indicators of nutrition status. It is possible for hair concentration of an element to be high even though deficiency exists in the body, and vice versa.

Seidel et al. [84] assessed commercial laboratories performing hair mineral analysis in the United States. A split hair sample taken from near the scalp of a single healthy volunteer was submitted for analysis to six commercial US laboratories, which analyze 90% of samples submitted for mineral analysis in the United States. Main outcome measures were agreement of test results for each analyte, laboratory reference ranges, laboratory characteristics, and interpretation of health implications. The investigators found laboratory differences in highest and lowest reported mineral concentrations for the split sample to exceed tenfold for 12 minerals, and statistically significant ($P < 0.05$) extreme values were reported for 14 of the 31 minerals that were analyzed by 3 or more laboratories. Variations also were found in laboratory sample preparation methods and calibration standards. Laboratory designations of normal reference ranges varied greatly, resulting in conflicting classifications (high, normal, or low) of nearly all analyzed minerals. Laboratories also provided conflicting dietary and nutritional supplement recommendations based on their results. The authors concluded that hair mineral analysis from these laboratories was unreliable, and recommend that healthcare practitioners refrain from using such analyses to assess individual nutritional status or suspected environmental exposures.

In a same attempt, Drasch and Roider [85] sent hair samples from two volunteers to seven laboratories in Germany, which commercially offer hair mineral analysis. 6 weeks later, another identical part from the hair sample of the volunteer 1 was sent to all seven labs. Altogether, of 50 elements analyzed, 23 was by all seven labs. For comparability, only the results for the elements analyzed by all seven labs were assessed. The intra-laboratory reproducibility was evaluated by the two identical hair samples from volunteer 1. On the average, the reproducibility seemed to be sufficient (median ±9.48% to ±20.59%), but for individual elements there were unacceptable out-rulers up to 100%. Only one lab classified all elements of the first and the second analyses of the identical hair sample in the same category (below, within, or above normal range). The others grouped 4–7 elements as different. The interlaboratory comparability was assessed by the results of the hair samples of both volunteers. For the sample of volunteer 1 at least the results of 6 out of 23 elements were within an acceptable range of ±30% from the consensus value (= mean of all seven labs). For volunteer 2 this was only the case for two elements. Differences of more than 100% were found for most other elements. Moreover, in the majority of the tested elements there was no comparability of the classification to the respective reference ranges of the different laboratories. For example, for volunteer 1 only 3 elements out of 23 were identically classified by all seven labs. As neither the analytical results nor the classification to the individual reference ranges by the laboratories corresponded in tolerable borders, conclusions, drawn from these results, were deemed not to be valid. Hair mineral analysis from these laboratories proved unreliable. Therefore, the authors recommend to refrain from using such analyses to assess individual nutritional status or suspected environmental exposure.

4.2   Nutritional Requirements for Hair Growth and Pigmentation

The quantity and quality of hair are closely related to the nutritional state of an individual. Normal supply, uptake, and transport of proteins, calories, trace elements, and vitamins are of fundamental importance in tissues with a high biosynthetic activity such as the hair follicle. Because hair shaft is composed almost entirely of protein, protein component of diet is critical for production of normal healthy hair. The rate of mitosis is sensitive to the calorific value of diet, provided mainly by carbohydrates stored as glycogen in the outer hair root sheath of the follicle. Finally, a sufficient supply of vitamins and trace metals is essential for the biosynthetic and energetic metabolism of the follicle [86, 87].

4.2.1   Protein and Calories

Debate exists regarding protein intake requirements. The amount of protein required in an individual's diet is determined by overall energy intake, body's need for nitrogen and essential amino acids, body weight and composition, rate of growth of the individual, physical activity level, individual's energy and carbohydrate intake, and presence of illness or injury. Physical activity and exertion as well as larger muscular mass increase the need for protein. Requirements are also higher during childhood for growth and development, during pregnancy and lactation, or when the body needs to recover from malnutrition, trauma, or after an operation.

In case of lack of energy through nutrition, the body utilizes protein from the muscle mass to meet energy needs, eventually leading to muscle wasting. If the individual's intake of protein is inadequate, then muscle will also waste as more vital cellular processes, such as respiration enzymes and blood cells, recycle muscle protein for their proper requirements.

Recommended dietary allowance in grams of protein needed per day are listed in Table 4.4.

The generally accepted daily protein dietary allowance, measured as intake per kilogram of body weight, is 0.8 g/kg [88]. However, this recommendation is based on structural requirements, but disregards the use of protein for energy metabolism. This requirement is for a normal sedentary person, while several studies have come

Table 4.4 Recommended dietary allowance (RDA) in grams of protein per day

• Children ages 1-3	13 grams of protein per day
• Children ages 4-8	19 grams of protein per day
• Children ages 9-13	34 grams of protein per day
• Girls ages 14 -18	46 grams of protein per day
• Boys ages 14 -18	52 grams of protein per day
• Women ages 19-70+	46 grams of protein per day
• If pregnant or breastfeeding	71 grams of protein per day
• Men ages 19-70+	56 gram of protein per day

to the conclusion that active people and athletes may require more elevated protein intake due to increase in muscle mass and sweat loss, as well as need for body repair, and energy source. Suggested amounts vary between 1.6 and 1.8 g/kg, while a proposed maximum daily protein intake would be at least 10%, but not more than 35% of energy requirements, i.e., approximately 2–2.5 g/kg.

Food energy is the chemical energy that is derived from food through the process of cellular respiration. Organisms derive food energy from carbohydrates, fats, and proteins, as well as from organic acids, polyols, and ethanol present in the diet.

Using the International System of Units, scientists measure energy in joules (J) and kilojoule (kJ) or calories and kilocalorie (kcal or Cal) that is equal to 4184 J.

Fats and ethanol have the greatest amount of food energy per gram, 37 kJ/g and 29 kJ/g (8.8 kcal/g and 6.9 kcal/g), respectively. Proteins and most carbohydrates both have about 17 kJ/g (4 kcal/g).

Recommendations in the United States are 2600 and 2000 kcal (10,900 and 8400 kJ) for men and women, respectively, between 31 and 35 years at a physical activity level equivalent to walking 2–5 km (per day at 5–6 km/h (in addition to the light physical activity associated with typical day-to-day life) [89].

Older people and those with sedentary lifestyles require less energy; children and physically active people require more.

For young children, estimated caloric needs range from 1000 to 2000 kcal per day. The recommended caloric intake for older children and adolescents, on the other hand, varies greatly from 1400 to 3200 kcal per day. Boys in general require higher caloric intake than girls [89].

The skin epithelium and its organelles use glycogen as well as glucose as the source of energy. The human hair follicle engages in glutaminolysis and aerobic glycolysis to generate its energy [90]. 90% of the glucose is metabolized to lactate, and only 10% is oxidized. Also glutamine is largely metabolized to lactate rather than oxidized. No glucose-fatty acid cycle operates in the hair follicle, while a glucose-glutamine cycle does exist [91].

In sheep, it has been estimated that 630 kJ of metabolizable energy is required to produce 1 g of clean dry wool (containing 24 kJ gross energy) and 0.27 g of wool grease containing 11 kJ gross energy [92].

4.2.2 Micronutrients (Vitamins, Minerals)

Because the body needs vitamins and minerals only in small amounts, they are called micronutrients. In fact, the total volume of micronutrients that a healthy individual normally requires each day would barely fill a teaspoon. And yet, all micronutrients are essential to life.

Although each vitamin has its specific metabolic profile, general functions of vitamins relevant to the hair include the following:

- Component of coenzymes
- Antioxidant
- Hormone that affects gene expression
- Component of cell membrane

By definition, a *vitamin* is defined by the following two characteristics: (1) It is a vital organic substance that is not a carbohydrate, fat, or protein, and it is necessary to perform a specific metabolic function or to prevent a specific deficiency disease, and (2) it cannot be synthesized by the body in sufficient quantities to maintain health, so that it must be supplied by the diet.

As a rule, several of the B vitamins represent part of coenzymes that in turn are integral parts of enzymes that metabolize glucose, fatty acids, and amino acids to extract energy. Some vitamins, specifically C and D, are involved in tissue building, while the vitamins A, C, and E also act as antioxidants to protect cell structures and to prevent damages caused by free radicals.

When a vitamin deficiency becomes severe, the specific function of that vitamin becomes apparent since it no longer performs its function. This also applies to hair growth and quality, where vitamins play fundamental roles in energy metabolism, tissue remodeling, and cell protection.

The way our bodies digest, absorb, and transport the vitamins depends on their solubility. Traditionally, the vitamins are classified into the fat- and water-soluble vitamins. The fat-soluble vitamins are A, D, E, and K, while the water-soluble vitamins are C and B vitamins.

In general, the absorption of the fat-soluble vitamins depends on the presence of dietary fat, and fat-soluble vitamins are stored in the liver and adipose tissue for long periods of time with implications for their potential cumulative toxicity.

Meanwhile, the intestinal tract easily absorbs the water-soluble vitamins, and with the exception of the vitamins B12 (cobalamin) and B6 (pyridoxine), the body does not store water-soluble vitamins, and therefore depends on the frequent intake of foods that are rich in water-soluble vitamins.

Vitamin A represents a group of unsaturated nutritional organic compounds that include retinol, retinal, retinoic acid, and several provitamin A carotenoids (most notably β-carotene). Vitamin A has multiple functions: it is important for skeletal and soft-tissue growth, strength of epithelial tissue, immunity, and good vison [93]. Vitamin A deficiency is the leading cause of preventable blindness in children worldwide due to xerophthalmia. Vitamin A is also an important antioxidant.

In dermatology, vitamin A, or more specifically retinoic acid, helps maintain skin health by switching on genes and differentiating keratinocytes into mature epidermal cells [94]. For the treatment of severe acne, the most prescribed retinoid drug is 13-*cis* retinoic acid (isotretinoin). It reduces the size and secretion of the sebaceous glands. Isotretinoin reduces bacterial numbers in both the ducts and skin surface as a result of the reduction in sebum, a nutrient source for bacteria. In addition, isotretinoin reduces inflammation via inhibition of chemotactic responses of monocytes and neutrophils [95]. Isotretinoin has also been shown to initiate remodeling of the sebaceous glands by triggering changes in gene expression that selectively induce apoptosis [96]. Since isotretinoin is an important teratogen and bears a number of potential side effects (increase in blood lipids, elevation of liver transaminases), its use requires professional supervision.

Dietary vitamin A occurs either as retinol derived from animal products or as provitamin A or β-carotene, which is a pigment in yellow, orange, and deep green fruits and vegetables, that the body converts into active vitamin A (retinol). Fish liver oil, liver, egg yolk, butter, and cream are sources of natural vitamin A, while collard greens, kale, spinach, carrots, sweet potatoes, pumpkins, melon, and apricots represent some good sources of β-carotene.

Vitamin D (calciferol) is a prohormone rather than a vitamin, and was originally classified as a vitamin by its discoverers when they cured rickets with fish oil [97]. In fact, the activated form of vitamin D, calcitriol, acts with two other hormones, parathyroid hormone and calcitonin, to control calcium and phosphorus absorption and metabolism. Cholecalciferol is the chemical name for vitamin D_3 in its inactive form, often shortened to calciferol. Upon exposure to ultraviolet light, the human organism is able to convert the precursor 7-dehydrocholesterol found in the epidermal layer of the skin into cholecalciferol or calciferol. Calciferol must be activated in two successive hydroxylation reactions in the liver and the kidneys to 1,25-dihydroxycholecalciferol or 1,25-dihydroxyvitamin D_3, also known as calcitriol. Calcitriol stimulates the intestinal absorption, renal reabsorption, and osteoclastic resorption of calcium and phosphorus to maintain blood calcium und phosphorus homeostasis.

Rickets is the disease of childhood that features softening of the bones from inadequate intake of vitamin D and insufficient exposure to sunlight. In addition to causing skeletal malformations, inadequate vitamin D intake prevents children in building up their critical bone mass, thereby contributing to the later development of osteoporosis and osteomalacia in adulthood.

A number of other chronic conditions have been attributed to vitamin D deficiency, including muscle weakness, type 2 diabetes, neurologic disorders, and several autoimmune diseases, and there has been a hype for respective supplementations with vitamin D. However, one meta-analysis covering over 350,000 people concluded that vitamin D supplementation in unselected community-dwelling individuals did not reduce skeletal (total fracture) or nonskeletal outcomes (myocardial infarction, ischemic heart disease, stroke, cerebrovascular disease, cancer) by more than 15% [98]. In fact, a 2019 meta-analysis found that there may be an increased risk of stroke when taking both calcium and vitamin D [99]. Nevertheless, vitamin D deficiency is widespread in the European population [100]. Therefore, research is currently assessing vitamin D intake levels in association with disease rates and policies of dietary recommendations, food fortification, vitamin D supplementation, and sun exposure.

Fatty fish (salmon, sockeye), fish oil, cod liver, and vitamin D fortified milk and dairy products are the food sources of vitamin D. Excessive dietary intake of vitamin D (hypervitaminosis D) can be toxic, resulting in fragile bones, kidney stones, calcification of soft tissues, and elevated blood calcium concentrations with calcium deposits in the kidney nephrons interfering with kidney function.

Vitamin E (tocopherol) was originally identified as a substance that was necessary for animal reproduction; therefore its name is derived from Greek τόκος (tókos) meaning "childbirth" and φέρειν (phérein) meaning "to bring," and an -ol ending to indicate its alcohol functional group [101]. Tocopherol became known as the antisterility vitamin, but it was soon recognized that it had this effect only in rats.

The most vital function of vitamin E is its tissue antioxidant action. As it is fat soluble, vitamin E is incorporated into cell membranes, which are therefore protected from oxidative damage. Alpha-tocopherol, either naturally extracted from plant oils or, most commonly, derived as the synthetic tocopheryl acetate, is sold as a popular dietary supplement, either by itself or incorporated into a multivitamin product, and in oils or lotions for use on skin. Although there is widespread use of topical tocopheryl acetate for improved wound healing and reduced scar tissue, reviews have concluded that there is insufficient evidence to support these claims [102, 103]. A report on vitamin E sales volume in the United States documented a 50% decrease between 2000 and 2006 [104] with a potential reason being a meta-analysis that concluded that high-dosage (≥400 IU/d for at least 1 year) vitamin E was associated with an increase in all-cause mortality [105].

Dermatologic uses for vitamin E have been treatment of granuloma annulare [106], cutaneous lupus erythematosus [107], epidermolysis bullosa [108], yellow nail syndrome [109], and protection from hemolysis and headache associated with dapsone treatment [110, 111]. High-dose vitamin E failed to prevent alopecia induced by doxorubicin [112].

Dietary sources of vitamin E are vegetable oils, specifically wheat germ, soybean, and safflower (also rich sources of polyunsaturated fatty acids), nuts, seeds, and fortified cereals.

Vitamin K is involved in two well-recognized functions in the organism: blood clotting and bone development. The most well-recognized function of vitamin K is its involvement in the blood clotting process. The vitamin is essential for the maintenance of normal blood concentrations of four blood clotting factors: prothrombin (factor II), factors VII, IX, and X. In addition, several proteins involved in bone metabolism require vitamin K-dependent modifications to function: osteocalcin or bone Gla protein (BGP), matrix Gla protein (MGP), periostin, and Gla-rich protein (GRP) [113]. In these, vitamin K is involved in the modification of the glutamic acid residues to form calcium-binding γ-carboxyglutamic acid residues and bone crystals. Also, vitamin K is essential for the biological activity of the growth arrest-specific protein 6 (Gas6). Gas6 was originally found as a gene upregulated by growth-arrested fibroblasts, and is thought to be involved in the stimulation of cell proliferation.

Average diets are usually not lacking in vitamin K, and primary vitamin K deficiency is therefore rare in healthy adults, unless the small intestine is heavily damaged, e.g., with Crohn's disease, resulting in malabsorption of the molecule. Secondary vitamin K deficiency can occur in people with bulimia, those on stringent diets, and those taking anticoagulants.

Vitamin K includes two natural vitamers: vitamin K1 (phytomenadione) and vitamin K2 (menaquinone). A particular at-risk group for deficiency are those subject to decreased production of K2 by normal intestinal microbiota, as seen with broad-spectrum antibiotic use. Finally, the elderly have a reduction in vitamin K2. The vitamin has a protective effect on bone mineral density with a reduced risk of hip, vertebral, and non-vertebral fractures. These effects appear to be accentuated when combined with vitamin D, and in the setting of osteoporosis

Vitamin K1 is found chiefly in leafy green vegetables such as spinach, swiss chard, lettuce, and Brassica vegetables (cabbage, kale, cauliflower, broccoli, brussels sprouts) and often the absorption is greater when accompanied by fats such as butter or oils. Avocados, kiwifruit, and grapes also contain vitamin K.

Vitamin K2 can be found in eggs, dairy, and meat, as well as fermented foods such as cheese and yogurt [114].

Vitamin K deficiency has been defined as a vitamin K-responsive hypoprothrombinemia with increased prothrombin time and risk of bleeding. Symptoms of K1 deficiency include anemia, bruising, nosebleeds, bleeding of the gums, and heavy menstrual bleeding in women, and symptoms of K2 deficiency are osteoporosis and coronary heart disease.

The blood anticoagulant warfarin works by blocking the recycling of vitamin K, so that the body and tissues have lower levels of active vitamin K, and thus a deficiency of vitamin K [115]. A well-recognized unwanted effect of anticoagulant therapy with warfarin is hair loss.

The prothrombin time (PT), along with its derived measures of prothrombin ratio (PR) and international normalized ratio (INR), is the assay used to determine the clotting tendency of blood, in the measure of warfarin dosage, liver damage, and vitamin K status.

Vitamin K is one of the treatments for bleeding events caused either by overdose of the anticoagulant drug warfarin (Coumadin®) or by poisoning with the rodenticide coumarin. Warfarin overdose has been observed in Munchausen syndrome [116], dementia, and suicidal intention [117].

Vitamin C (ascorbic acid) is essentially involved in the repair of tissue in terms of its antioxidant activity, and is a cofactor of a number of enzymes. Therefore, the metabolically active tissues contain greater concentrations of ascorbic acid. Vitamin C is necessary to build up and preserve strong tissues by virtue of its involvement in collagen synthesis. Moreover, collagen remodeling is involved in the hair cycle, and collagen, specifically collagen type 17A1/BP180, has been shown to be important in the differentiation of hair follicle-associated pluripotent stem cells [118].

Similar to vitamin E in function, vitamin C works to protect the tissues from damage caused by free radicals; moreover vitamin C restores vitamin E's antioxidant function. In general, vitamin C acts as an antioxidant by donating electrons to various enzymatic and nonenzymatic reactions. Doing so converts vitamin C to an oxidized state that in turn can be restored to a reduced state by glutathione and NADPH-dependent enzymatic mechanisms.

The enzymes that require ascorbic acid perform a variety of functions, such as (1) the conversion of the neurotransmitter dopamine to norepinephrine; (2) the synthesis of the mitochondrial fatty acid transporter carnitine involved in extracting energy from fatty acids; (3) the oxidation of phenylalanine in tyrosine, a precursor of neurotransmitters and hormones, such as the catecholamines and the thyroid hormones, and to the pigment melanin; (4) the metabolism of tryptophan and folate; and (5) the maturation of some bioactive neural and endocrine peptides. In addition, ascorbic acid facilitates the absorption of nonheme iron by preserving it in bioactive reduced ferrous form (Fe^{2+}) making it available for hemoglobin production to help prevent iron deficiency.

Normal skin contains high concentrations of vitamin C, which supports important and well-known functions, stimulating collagen synthesis and assisting in antioxidant protection against UV-induced photodamage [119]. L-ascorbic acid 2-phosphate, a derivative of l-ascorbic acid, has been shown to promote elongation of hair shafts in cultured human hair follicles and induce hair growth in mice [120]. The mechanism of action is believed to be via the secretion of insulin-like growth factor 1 from dermal papilla cells through phosphatidylinositol 3-kinase [121].

Epidemiological evidence indicates 5% prevalence for vitamin C deficiency and 13% prevalence for suboptimal status even in industrialized countries [122].

Ultimately, the cardinal symptoms of vitamin D deficiency (scurvy) relate to vitamin C's important contribution to collagen synthesis in the respective connective tissues of ligaments, tendons, bone, cartilage, tooth dentin, and capillary walls [123]. The blood vessels are particularly dependent on vitamin C's role in collagen synthesis to help maintain resistance of stretching of their walls while blood runs through them. The vitamin C-dependent enzymes propyl hydroxylase and lysyl hydroxylase are necessary for the hydroxylation of proline and lysine before they are added during collagen synthesis. Since iron is a cofactor for both enzymes, vitamin C is required to maintain the iron atoms in their active ferrous (Fe^{2+}) form.

The best food sources of vitamin C are citrus fruits, bell peppers, and kiwis; others include berries, broccoli, tomato juice, and other green and yellow vegetables.

The vitamin C is readily oxidized upon exposure to air and heat, and therefore special care must be given to the handling of its food sources.

Since 1954 Nobel Prize laureate for Chemistry Linus Pauling originally popularized the concept of high-dose vitamin C as prevention and treatment of the common cold in 1970, and a few years later proposed vitamin C to prevent cardiovascular disease, and at 10 g/day initially (10 days) administered intravenously and thereafter orally to cure late-stage cancer [124], the megadosing theory has now to a large degree been discredited, following controversial doctor, businessman, and vitamin salesman Matthias Rath in Germany and British book writer and entrepreneur Patrick Holford who both have been accused of unsubstantiated treatment claims for treating cancer and HIV infection with megadose vitamin C. Nevertheless, the lack of conclusive evidence has not stopped individual physicians with a primary commercial interest from prescribing intravenous ascorbic acid to thousands of people with cancer and other conditions.

Since cigarette smoke, either for the smoker or anyone inhaling second-hand smoke [125], is an environmental source of free radicals that may disrupt the normal structure of DNA, proteins, carbohydrates, and fatty acids, and eventually result in an increased risk of cancer and cardiovascular disease, in addition to the general recommendation of abstaining from smoking and exposure, an extra consumption of 35 mg of vitamin C per day has been recommended to help avert the additional free radical damage caused.

Although excessive intakes of the water-soluble vitamin C are efficiently secreted in the urine, levels of more than 2000 mg/day may result in osmotic diarrhea. Theoretically, high vitamin C intake may cause excessive absorption of iron. A summary of reviews of iron supplementation in healthy subjects did not report this problem but left as untested the possibility that individuals with hereditary hemochromatosis might be adversely affected. Finally, despite the long-standing issue that vitamin C may increase the risk of kidney stones [126], reviews came to the conclusion that the data from epidemiological studies do not support an association between excess ascorbic acid intake and kidney stone formation in apparently healthy individuals [127]. Nevertheless, one large, multi-year trial did report a nearly twofold increase in kidney stones in men who regularly consumed a vitamin C supplement [128], so that the question arises whether at least individuals with renal disease may be at a particular risk of kidney stone formation associated with excessive vitamin C intake.

The *B vitamin complex* (also called *B vitamins*) encompasses a group of eight vitamins that have an important job in the metabolism of cells. They represent separate vitamins that often can be found together and are found in meat, milk, whole grains, and fresh vegetables. They are required for growth, and proper functioning of nerves and muscles.

Well-known medical syndromes caused by deficiency of B vitamins are beriberi (vitamin B1), Wernicke-Korsakoff syndrome (vitamin B1), ariboflavinosis (vitamin B2), pellagra (niacin), pernicious anemia (vitamin B12), and neural tube defects (folate).

Of the B vitamins, riboflavin, biotin, folate, and vitamin B12 deficiencies have been associated with impairment of hair growth or color [129].

Vitamin B1 (thiamin) is a component of the coenzyme thiamine pyrophosphate, which is involved in metabolic reactions that ultimately provide the body with energy in the form of adenosine triphosphate (ATP). Therefore, vitamin B1 is particularly necessary for the healthy function of systems in need of energy due to constant action, such as the nervous system, cardiovascular system, and gastrointestinal tract. A deficiency will have downstream effects on energy availability.

Due to this effect on energy metabolism, vitamin B1 is a popular supplement in nutritionals for hair, although hair loss has not been reported as a symptom of a respective single-deficiency disorder of vitamin B1. Nevertheless, in an in vitro assay Hengl et al. [130] demonstrated that thiamine had a positive impact on metabolic activity and proliferation of normal human epidermal keratinocytes in culture in a dose-dependent manner.

Increased vitamin B1 intake is necessary in conditions that increase total kilocalorie needs above the average daily energy requirement, specifically during pregnancy and lactation. Pregnant women with hyperemesis gravidarum are at a particular risk for vitamin B1 deficiency due to losses from vomiting [131]. It has also been proposed that vitamin B1 deficiency may play a role in the poor development of the infant brain with an increased risk of sudden infant death syndrome (SIDS) [132]. Diseases that accelerate glucose metabolism, such as fever, also increase the organism's requirement of vitamin B1.

In Western countries, vitamin B1 deficiency is seen mainly in alcohol-misuse disorder. Alcohol inhibits the absorption of vitamin B1. Also at risk are older adults, persons with HIV/AIDS or diabetes, and persons who have had bariatric surgery. Vitamin B1 deficiency has also been associated with the long-term use of high doses of diuretics, particularly furosemide in the treatment of heart failure [133].

Vitamin B1 is found in a wide variety of processed and whole foods, with edible seeds, legumes, rice, pork, and processed foods, such as breakfast cereals, having among the highest contents. And yet, vitamin B1 deficiency is a distinct possibility when food intake is markedly curtailed, e.g., with chronic alcoholism (Wernicke-Korsakoff encephalopathy) or highly inadequate diets. Originally, beriberi (Singhalese for "I can't, I can't") was identified as chronic vitamin B1 deficiency in Asian countries that relied heavily on the consumption of polished white rice as a food staple. In addition, vitamin B1 in foods can be degraded in a number of ways: some raw fish contain a thiamine-degrading enzyme (thiaminase), and sulfites which are added as a preservative to foods will attack thiamine at the methylene bridge in the structure, cleaving the pyrimidine ring from the thiazole ring.

Vitamin B2 (riboflavin) is required by the body for cellular respiration. It is active in its coenzyme form flavin adenine dinucleotide (FADI) and flavin mononucleotide (FMN) required for macronutrient metabolism to produce ATP via the Krebs cycle and the electron transport chain. Other metabolic reactions involving vitamin B2 are the conversion of the amino acid tryptophan to niacin (vitamin B3), and of retinal to retinoic acid, and synthesizing of the active form of folate.

Nutritional sources of vitamin B2 are milk, cheese, eggs, leaf vegetables, liver, kidneys, lean meats, legumes, mushrooms, and almonds. The milling of cereals results in a substantial loss of vitamin B2, so that white flour is enriched in some countries by addition of vitamin B2. The enrichment of bread and ready-to-eat breakfast cereals contributes significantly to the dietary supply of vitamin B2. Polished rice is not usually enriched, because the vitamin's yellow color would make the rice visually unacceptable to the major rice-consuming populations. However, most of the flavin content of whole brown rice is retained if the rice is parboiled prior to milling.

Vitamin B2 requirements are related to total energy requirements depending on the age, level of physical exercise, body size, metabolic rate, and rate of growth. Vitamin B2 is continuously excreted in the urine of healthy individuals, making deficiency relatively common when dietary intake is insufficient.

While deficiency is uncommon in countries that have wheat flour, bread, pasta, corn meal, or rice enrichment regulations, mild deficiencies can exceed 50% of the population in Third World countries and in refugee situations. Subclinical deficiency has also been observed in women on oral contraception, in the elderly, in people with eating disorders, in chronic alcoholism, in HIV, in inflammatory bowel disease, in diabetes, and in chronic heart disease. The Celiac Disease Foundation points out that a gluten-free diet may be low in vitamin B2 as enriched wheat flour and wheat foods comprise a substantial dietary contribution to total vitamin B2 intake. Flours from teff, millet, chestnut, buckwheat, and amaranth are better sources of B group vitamins than flours from corn and rice [134].

Areas of the body with rapid cell regeneration are most affected by vitamin B2 deficiency, and yet there is a paucity of literature on the effect of vitamin B2 deficiency on hair growth and shedding [135], probably due to the low frequency of the condition in developed countries. Typical symptoms of vitamin B2 include cracked lips and mouth corners; a swollen, red tongue; burning and tearing of eyes; and a peculiar scaly, greasy dermatitis of the skin folds.

Vitamin B2 deficiency is usually found together with other nutrient deficiencies, particularly of water-soluble vitamins, and may then have an indicator function for associated deficiencies that may also be relevant to the condition of the hair.

Niacin (vitamin B3) is part of two coenzymes: in line with the theme among the B vitamin functions with regard to macronutrient metabolism, the role of the one of the niacin-containing coenzymes, nicotinamide adenine dinucleotide (NAD), is similar to that of the respective coenzymes containing vitamins B1 and B2, while the other niacin-containing coenzyme, nicotinamide adenine dinucleotide phosphate (NADP), is involved in DNA repair and steroid hormone synthesis.

Meat is a good source of niacin. In addition, niacin is obtained in the diet from a variety of whole and processed foods, with highest contents in fortified packaged foods, whole-grain breads, and ready-to-eat cereals. Peanuts are another good source of niacin.

Niacin-deficiency disorder (pellagra) was once common in the United States and parts of Europe during the early twentieth century in regions where corn which is low in niacin was the staple food. Lack of niacin may also be observed in pandemic deficiency diseases, which are caused by a lack of the five crucial vitamins niacin, vitamin C, vitamin B1, vitamin D, and vitamin A, and are usually found in areas of widespread poverty and malnutrition. Today, in the developed countries the disorder is mainly seen in chronic alcoholism.

Supplemental niacin and its amide form nicotinamide, respectively, are primarily used to treat niacin deficiency (pellagra), high blood cholesterol, and various dermatological indications, including non-melanoma cancer prophylaxis, blistering disorders, acne vulgaris, and cosmetic indications [136]; however in the latter the possible side effects and consequences of excessive nicotinamide exposure such as the development of diabetes, Parkinson's disease, and hepatotoxicity are to be taken into consideration [137]. The UL for niacin is 35 mg/day based on a distinctive skin flushing caused by high supplemental intake. Flushing usually lasts for about 15–30 min, though it can sometimes last up to 2 h. It is sometimes accompanied by a prickly or itching sensation, in particular, in areas covered by clothing.

A small study has evaluated the efficacy of topically applied niacin derivatives (octyl nicotinate and tetradecyl nicotinate) for treatment of female pattern alopecia, and found increase in hair fullness compared to placebo on blinded 35 mm photographic analysis [138].

Pantothenic acid (vitamin B5) is required in order to synthesize coenzyme-A (CoA) that is essential in the energy metabolism, as well as to synthesize and metabolize proteins, carbohydrates, and fats. Its name derives from the Greek pántothen, meaning "from all sides," referring to both the vitamin's widespread functions in the body and its widespread availability in foods of all types. The anion is called pantothenate. It is commonly found as its alcohol analogue, the provitamin panthenol (pantothenol), and as calcium pantothenate.

Given its ubiquitous natural occurrence, pantothenic acid deficiency is unlikely, but may include symptoms such as fatigue, insomnia, depression, irritability, and burning feet.

Although pantothenic acid supplementation is used for a variety of conditions (recovery of bowel function after surgery, burning feet, hair loss, and others) by virtue of the vitamin's protean functions and lack of significant toxicity, there is low evidence to date as to its true efficacy. Specifically, pantothenic acid and calcium pantothenate are popularly included in a wide range of nutritionals for hair health, usually in combination with other active ingredients. In one study, injectable pantothenol in combination with biotin has been alleged to be effective for treatment of chronic telogen effluvium [139]. In this study, the intravenous route of administration seemed to be superior to oral or intramuscular application. Finally, dexpanthenol is a widely used natural humectant in hair care products, especially for thinning hair and hair loss [139, 140].

Toxicity of pantothenic acid is unlikely. In fact, no tolerable upper level intake (UL) has been established. Large doses of the vitamin, when ingested, have no reported side effects, and massive doses (10 g/day) may only result in mild diarrhea. There are no adverse reactions known following injected application of the vitamin (either intramuscular or intravenous), while allergic contact dermatitis caused by dexpanthenol has been reported with a frequency of 1.2% of patient patch tested in

one center, and more commonly related to the use of Bepanthen cream than shampoo [141], and one case of contact urticaria from panthenol in a hair conditioner [142].

Vitamin B6 (pyridoxine) refers to a group of chemically similar compounds
which can be interconverted in biological systems, while its active, pyridoxal
5′-phosphate (PLP), serves as a coenzyme in some 100 enzyme reactions in amino
acid, glucose, and lipid metabolism. It is also involved in neurotransmitter synthesis, and participates in ATP production, synthesis of the heme portion of hemoglobin, and niacin formation from tryptophan. In particular, PLP is a coenzyme needed
for the proper function of the enzymes cystathionine synthase and cystathionase.
These enzymes catalyze reactions in the catabolism of methionine. Part of this pathway also produces cysteine that is relevant to the hair. Specifically, vitamin B6 deficiency can result in impaired transsulfuration of methionine to cysteine.

One study compared orally administered calcium pantothenate twice daily in
doses of 100 mg for 4–5 months and vitamin B6 injected every day intramuscularly
for the period of 20–30 days and repeated again after 6 months [143]. The authors
found that vitamin B6 administered parenterally induced improvement in the hair
condition in a number of women and it reduced hair loss especially from telogen
effluvium, whereas calcium pantothenate did not show clearly the positive effect.
Also, treatment of seborrheic dermatitis and hair loss with vitamin B6 has been
reported [144]. Vitamin B6 is used for treatment of homocystinuria [145], including
induction of hair pigmentation [146].

Deficiency of vitamin B6 alone is relatively uncommon, because more vitamin is
available in a typical diet than is required. It often occurs in association with other
vitamins of the B complex, usually in the elderly and alcoholics. Use of oral contraceptives [147], levodopa [148], treatment with certain anticonvulsants [149], and
isoniazid [150] may negatively impact vitamin B6 status.

Foods that contain large amounts of vitamin B6 include fortified breakfast cereals, pork, turkey, beef, bananas, chickpeas, potatoes, and pistachios.

The classic clinical presentation of vitamin B6 deficiency is a seborrheic
dermatitis-like eruption, atrophic glossitis, angular cheilitis, conjunctivitis, intertriginous dermatitis [151], somnolence, confusion, neuropathy, and sideroblastic anemia.

Adverse effects have been documented from high doses of vitamin B6 to prevent
or treat certain health conditions, including premenstrual syndrome, age-related
macular degeneration, hyperemesis gravidarum, seizures, sideroblastic anemia,
depression, Alzheimer's disease, and hair loss. Although vitamin B6 is a water-
soluble vitamin and is excreted in the urine, doses of vitamin B6 in excess of the
dietary upper limit (UL) of 100 mg/day over long periods cause painful and ultimately irreversible nerve damage. Evidence as to whether a lower dosage range of
vitamin B6 (<50 mg/day) can also induce neuropathy is scarce [152]. Vrolijik et al.
have demonstrated that high concentrations of pyridoxine levels lead to decreased
vitamin B6 function due to competitive inhibition of active pyridoxal-5′-phosphate
by the inactive form of pyridoxine. Consequently, symptoms of vitamin B6 supplementation are similar to those of vitamin B6 deficiency [153].

Biotin (vitamin B7) is a water-soluble vitamin that helps the body metabolize proteins and process glucose. It is a coenzyme involved in the metabolism of fatty acids, and the essential amino acid leucine, and gluconeogenesis, the synthesis of glucose from amino and fatty acids. In this function, biotin contributes to the metabolism of nutrients, energy-producing metabolism, maintaining healthy skin and hair, hence also the designation as vitamin H from German "Haut und Haare" (skin and hair), and nervous system function.

Since biotin contributes to healthy nails, skin, and hair, it features in many cosmetic products. The percutaneous application of biotin-containing ointment has been shown to cause a significant increase in the serum biotin concentration in both healthy subjects and atopic dermatitis patients [154]. There has been an understanding that there were no known natural dietary deficiencies of biotin, since the vitamin is widely distributed in natural food, and the bacteria that normally inhabit the intestine synthesize biotin, which is available for intestinal cell absorption. However, biotin is not equally absorbed from all foods [155]. For example, the biotin in corn and soy meal is completely bioavailable while almost none of the biotin in wheat is. Moreover, disruption of the intestinal flora [156] through prolonged use of oral antibiotics, ingestion of uncooked egg whites containing the protein avidin that binds biotin, and medications that interfere with biotin metabolism, such as valproic acid [157] and isotretinoin [158], may negatively affect the body's supply with biotin. Biotin deficiency is characterized by alopecia in association with a peculiar periorificial dermatitis in the form of a scaly red rash, and neurological symptoms. Deficiencies can be caused by consuming raw egg whites over a period of months to years. When cooked, avidin in egg white is partially denatured and binding to biotin is reduced. However, one study showed that 30–40% of the avidin activity was still present in the white after frying or boiling [159].

No toxicity from the consumption of high doses of biotin is known.

Vitamin B12 (cobalamin) is involved in the metabolism of every cell of the human body, since it is essential for DNA synthesis and cell division. Of the B vitamins, it is the largest and most structurally complex vitamin, and contains the biochemically rare element cobalt positioned in the center of a corrin ring. The role of vitamin B12 in nucleic acid production may suggest that it may play a role in the highly proliferative hair follicle, and yet few studies to date have addressed the relationship between vitamin B12 and hair loss, apart from the association with alopecia areata and white hair due to autoimmunity.

The cutaneous manifestations of cobalamin deficiency include hyperpigmentation (most commonly) and oral changes, specifically glossitis (Hunter's glossitis). Additionally, several dermatologic conditions, including vitiligo, aphthous stomatitis, atopic dermatitis, and acne, have been related to cobalamin excess or deficiency. The cutaneous complications of cobalamin therapy include acne, and allergic site reactions, or anaphylaxis with cobalamin injections. As cobalt is a component of cobalamin, patients with cobalt sensitivity have been reported to have cutaneous manifestations when receiving cobalamin replacement therapy [160].

Vitamin B12 deficiency in infants is uncommonly reported from developed countries and generally lacks dermatologic manifestations. On the contrary, infantile vitamin B12 deficiency is common in India and cutaneous manifestations are a constant feature, although often overshadowed by neurologic and hematological manifestations. Kaur and Goraya examined 43 infants aged 4–27 months, with vitamin B12 deficiency in India. Skin hyperpigmentation was present in 41 infants, localized to the dorsa of hands and feet in 26 and generalized in 15, with a reticulate pattern in 10, and a homogenous pattern in 5. The scalp hair was sparse and brown in all. The skin pigmentation and mucosal changes resolved completely by 3–4 weeks of vitamin B12 treatment, but hair changes were slower to reverse [161]. In another study of infants with vitamin B12 deficiency brittle and matt hair was found in 92.3% of patients [162]. Noppakun and Swasdikul reported reversible cutaneous hyperpigmentation and white hair due to vitamin B12 deficiency [163]. Carmel reported two Latin American patients suffering from pernicious anemia with reddish hair. With treatment, the new hair growth assumed its normal premorbid dark brown color [164].

The richest dietary sources of vitamin B12 are beef liver, lean meat, clams, oysters, herring, and crab.

Folic acid or *folate* represents yet another B vitamin involved in DNA synthesis and cell division. Therefore, folate deficiency impairs DNA and RNA synthesis, affecting rapidly dividing cells. When the division of red blood cells is impaired, the result is large, immature erythrocytes (megaloblastic macrocytic anemia). Also, the vitamin is also involved in the synthesis of the amino acid glycine, which is required for heme and hemoglobin synthesis. Pregnant and lactating women are particularly prone to diminished folate concentrations and anemia as a result of higher needs. In addition, as a result of the role of folic acid in cell division during embryogenesis, adequate preconception and pregnancy intakes are linked to reduced neural tube defect (spina bifida and anencephaly) occurrences [165].

The given name folate comes from the Latin word folium, meaning "leaf," because the vitamin was originally discovered in dark green, leafy vegetables. In the plasma it exists as 5-methyl-tetrahydrofolate. Folate is a carrier of C1 groups (methyl, methylene, formyl), and in this function may act as a methyl donor with the capacity of changing the methylation patterns of genes. This has strikingly been demonstrated in rodents, where lack of methylation at the agouti gene locus promotes yellow coat color. When pregnant mice are fed the respective dietary supplement, folate promotes the methylation of the agouti locus with a resultant shift in the coat color phenotype [166]. Ultimately, the question arises whether epigenetic modifications have any possible impact on hair loss. On the scalp, there is a well-recognized intraindividual difference in the expression of the androgen receptor gene (AR) between balding and non-balding areas of the scalp, with AR expression being higher in balding scalp follicles, leading to the assumption that AR expression is protective. While these two closely lying tissue regions have the same genetic makeup, it may be that AR is more highly methylated in hair follicles protected from balding, downregulating the expression of the respective phenotype [167]. However, as yet research establishing folic acid as a hair growth-promoting nutrient is lacking.

No negative effects have been observed from the consumption of folate from foods; however excessive folic acid intake from supplements may mask the biochemical indicators of vitamin B12 deficiency and therefore risk permanent nerve damage from prolonged vitamin B12 deficiency [168]. An additional concern is that low increased AR expression is important in the development of alopecia, while decreased vitamin B12 status in combination with high folic acid intake appears to increase the risk of cognitive impairment in the elderly [169].

Essential fatty acids is the term applied to the fatty acids according to their necessity in the diet. In 1929, Burr and Burr [170] originally discovered that the exclusion of fat from the diet resulted in a new deficiency disease with reduced growth rate, reproductive failure, scaling of the skin, and impaired barrier function. This laid the foundation to the concept of the essential fatty acids (EFAs). The only fatty acids recognized to be essential for complete human nutrition are the unsaturated fatty acids linoleic acid (LA) and alpha-linolenic acid (ALA). The unsaturated fatty acids are also classified according to the location of the first double bond on the third or the sixth carbon from the methyl end or omega end into the *omega-3 fatty acids* and the *omega-6 fatty acids*. The terms omega-3 and omega-6 fatty acids are often erroneously used synonymously with ALA and LA, respectively. However, there are several omega-3 and omega-6 fatty acids. Other examples of omega-3 fatty acids are *eicosapentaenoic acid* (EPA) and *docosahexaenoic acid* (DHA). An important property of omega-3 fatty acids is their ability to competitively inhibit the metabolism of omega-6 fatty acid by cyclooxygenase and lipoxygenase enzymes, resulting in decrease of lipid-derived mediators on inflammation. Therefore, in addition to EFA deficiency, the ratio of omega-6 to omega-3 fatty acids is of importance, with higher omega-6 fatty acid levels generally associated with detrimental effects. Typically, the Paleolithic diet was low in saturated fats and with approximately equal amounts of omega-6 to omega-3 fatty acids (1–2:1) [171], while modern agriculture where animals are fed on omega-6-rich grains results in meat produce with higher omega-6 fatty acid content [172]. This is also the case in some farmed fish [173]. In humans, dietary supplementation with omega-3 fatty acids decreases the production of pro-inflammatory cytokines [174–176] and inhibits T-cell mitogenesis [177].

Since epidemiological studies demonstrate that 79–95% of adolescents in Westernized societies suffer from acne vulgaris, while there is a considerably lower incidence in non-Westernized societies, specifically Inuit populations living traditionally and consuming a large amount of fish, it has been hypothesized that diet may be a contributory factor [178].

Deficiency of EFAs may cause skin and hair changes [179, 180] resembling to those due to biotin and zinc deficiency; it is not clear though whether a minimum daily intake is important for hair health in otherwise well-nourished individuals.

However, essential fatty acid supplementation significantly improves the hair coat in dogs [181].

Munkhbayar et al. [182] assessed the role of the polyunsaturated fatty acid arachidonic acid (AA) on hair growth by using in vivo and in vitro models. AA was found to enhance the viability of human dermal papilla cells (hDPCs) and promote the expression of several factors responsible for hair growth, including fibroblast growth factor-7 (FGF-7) and FGF-10. Western blotting identified the role of AA in the phosphorylation of various transcription factors (ERK, CREB, and AKT) and increased expression of Bcl-2 in hDPCs. In addition, AA significantly promoted hair shaft elongation, with increased proliferation of matrix keratinocytes, during ex vivo hair follicle culture. It was also found to promote hair growth by induction and prolongation of anagen phase in telogen-stage C57BL/6 mice.

Phytochemicals represent yet another group of bioactive molecules with multi-faceted health benefits beyond vitamins. By definition, they are chemical compounds produced by plants that play a role in plant growth or defense against competitors, pathogens, or predators. They have a wide variety of actions, including antioxidant, hormonal, and antibacterial activity. As yet, the phytochemicals are largely deemed as research compounds rather than essential nutrients because corroboration of their health effects has not been established. What prompted the investigation into them were the health differences observed in people eating whole foods compared to those eating micronutrient-deficient refined foods and relying on dietary supplements [183]. The beneficial effects of phytochemicals are understood to result from the synergistic actions of multiple constituents as opposed to the actions of isolated compounds. In general, the use of dietary supplements is a common practice in the United States with about half of the population regularly taking a dietary supplement of the multivitamin or multimineral variety. Of interest is that the use of dietary supplements is most prevalent among the healthiest of people rather than among those who are in need of supplementation the most.

The phytochemicals under research have been classified into major categories, such as carotenoids and polyphenols, which include phenolic acids, flavonoids, and stilbenes/lignans. Flavonoids are further divided into groups based on their similar chemical structure, such as anthocyanins, flavones, flavanones, isoflavones, and flavanols. Flavanols further are classified as catechins, epicatechins, and proanthocyanidins.

There are no established dietary recommendations for specific phytochemicals; however, color is one prominent indicator that a significant quantity of the specified phytochemical or phytochemical class is present in a food. Foods of animal sources and those that have been processed and refined are virtually devoid of phytochemicals. The main cause of phytochemical loss from cooking is thermal decomposition [184]. An exception exists in the case of lycopene present in tomatoes, which remains stable or may increase in content from cooking due to liberation from cellular membranes in the cooked food [185]. In fact, food processing techniques like mechanical processing can also free carotenoids from the food matrix, increasing dietary intake [184].

The *mineral* elements are single atoms and simple compared with the vitamins, which represent large, complex, organic compounds. And yet, they are not less important in performing a variety of metabolic tasks that are essential to life. Over the Earth's geological history, with the breakup of tectonic plates and the shifting of oceans, minerals have deposited throughout the Earth's crust, and have moved from rocks to the soil, and from the soil to the plants, to the animals, and to the human

Table 4.5 Major minerals and trace minerals in human nutrition

Major minerals (required intake of more than 100 mg/day)	
Calcium (Ca)	Chloride (Cl)
Phosphorus (P)	Magnesium (Mg)
Sodium(Na)	Sulfur (S)
Potassium (K)	
Trace minerals (required intake of less than 100 mg/day	
Iron (Fe)	Cobalt (Co)
Iodine (I)	Boron (B)
Zinc (Zn)	Vanadium (V)
Selenium (Se)	Nickel (Ni)
Fluoride (Fl)	Silicon (Si)*
Copper (Cu)	Tin (Sn)*
Manganese (Mn)	Cadmium (Cd)*
Chromium (Cr)	Arsenic (As)*
Molybdenum (Mo)	Aluminium (Al)*

ᵃEssentiality unclear

species. Therefore, it is not surprising that the mineral content of the human body is quite similar to that of the Earth's crust.

Of the 118 elements on the periodic table of elements, 25 are essential to human life. These vary in amounts in the body, and perform a variety of metabolic functions. Depending on the amount of the individual mineral in the body, the minerals have been classified into the *major minerals* with a recommended intake of more than 100 mg/day, and the *trace minerals* with a recommended intake of less than 100 mg/day. Table 4.5 provides a list of the minerals that are essential to human nutrition, classified into the major minerals and trace minerals.

How much of a mineral is absorbed into the body from the gastrointestinal tract is determined by the following factors:

- **Food form.** Minerals from animal sources are usually more readily absorbed than those from plant sources. Moreover, some compounds found in foods may also affect the absorptive efficiency; specifically the presence of fiber, phytate, or oxalate (all of which again can be found in whole grains, fruits, and vegetables) can bind certain minerals in the gastrointestinal tract, thereby inhibiting their absorption.
- **Body need.** More is absorbed if the body is deficient than if the body has sufficient quantities of the respective minerals.
- **Tissue health.** If the absorbing intestinal surface is affected by disease, such as in Crohn's disease and in gluten-sensitive enteropathy, its absorptive capacity may be significantly diminished.

The two basic forms in which minerals occur in the body are as free ions in body fluids or as covalently bound minerals that are combined either with other minerals, such as calcium and phosphorus, or with organic substances, such as iron that is bound to heme and globin to form hemoglobin.

The uptake of some minerals into their target tissues is controlled by hormones, such as of calcium and of iodine: the interaction of vitamin D, parathyroid hormone, and calcitonin controls calcium's intestinal absorption and use, while thyroid-stimulating hormone (TSH) controls the uptake of iodine from the blood into the thyroid gland to produce the hormone thyroxine. Excess minerals are excreted into the urine.

Minerals with relevance to healthy hair are sulfur, iron, iodine, zinc, selenium, and copper. The relevance of silica is currently under review.

Sulfur (S) is an essential component of protein structure as part of the amino acids cysteine and methionine. Disulfide bonds between cysteine residues in the protein keratin are essential to the structure of the hair, skin, and nails. The disulfide bonding of cysteine residues is also necessary for collagen superhelix formation, and therefore it is important in the building of connective tissue. Sulfur is also a component of the vitamins thiamine and biotin, which act as coenzymes in cell metabolism.

Dietary requirements for sulfur are not stated as such, since sulfur is supplied by protein foods that contain the respective sulfur-containing amino acids. Therefore, isolated sulfur-deficiency states have not been reported, and they rather relate to general protein malnutrition. Animal protein foods are the main dietary source of sulfur.

Trichothiodystrophy is an autosomal recessive inherited disorder characterized by sulfur-deficient brittle hair associated with a range of symptoms including photosensitivity, ichthyosis, intellectual impairment, decreased fertility, and short stature [186]. The acronyms PIBIDS, IBIDS, BIDS, and PBIDS reflect the initials of the symptoms involved in the affected individual [187]. Light microscopic examination of the hair reveals evidence of breakage in the form of trichoschisis and trichorrhexis nodosa that is associated with reduction in the content of high-sulfur protein in hair, and a cystine content of about half the normal [188]. The hair displays a diagnostic alternating light-and-dark banding pattern, called tiger-tail banding, under polarizing microscopy [189].

Iron (Fe) has the longest standing and most comprehensive record of all of the micronutrients. Iron is the fourth most abundant element in the Earth's crust, composing about 5% (Fig. 4.13). Iron is essential for life, and the iron needs vary throughout life depending on the growth and development. The human body contains approximately 45 mg of iron per kilogram of body weight. Approximately 70% of the body's iron is in hemoglobin within the red blood cells; it is also part of the myoglobin in the muscle cells, and necessary for glucose metabolism, antibody production, drug detoxification in the liver, collagen and purine synthesis, and conversion of β-carotene to active vitamin A.

Women need more iron to cover the losses that occur during menstruation, throughout pregnancy and lactation. It is also noteworthy that iron need is also

Fig. 4.13 Iron ore
(origin: Brazil)

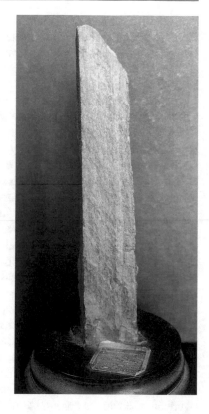

higher for vegetarians and vegans to compensate for the lower bioavailability of iron
from plant-based food sources [190].

The major condition that indicates a deficiency of iron is a hypochromic microcytic anemia due to the essential role of iron in hemoglobin synthesis. Iron is a
component of heme, which is the nonprotein part of hemoglobin. Iron-deficiency
anemia is the most prevalent nutritional problem in the world today with a frequency of 24.8% of the population worldwide according to estimates of the World
Health Organization. Major causes of iron-deficiency anemia are (1) inadequate
dietary intake in relation to the need; (2) excessive blood loss from menstruation or
hemorrhage; (3) a lack of gastric hydrochloric acid; (4) dietary inhibitors of iron
absorption, such as phytate, phosphate, tannin, and oxalate; and (5) intestinal mucosal disease that affects the absorptive surface area.

The association of telogen effluvium with non-anemic, low serum ferritin levels
has remained a subject of ongoing debate [191]. Moreover, convincing evidence for
the efficacy of iron supplementation on the outcome of telogen effluvium in non-
anemic women with low serum ferritin levels is still lacking.

Heme iron from animal food sources is the most efficiently absorbed form of
dietary iron, while nonheme iron from plant food sources is less easily absorbed,
because it is more tightly bound in foods. The body absorbs iron more efficiently
when it is taken along with vitamin C [192]. The role of the amino acid L-lysine on

iron uptake has been the objective of one study: women who only achieved a modest increase in serum ferritin level after supplementation with elemental iron 50 mg twice daily demonstrated a significant ($p < 0.001$) increase in the mean serum ferritin concentration after adding L-lysine (1.5–2 g/day) to their ongoing iron supplementation regimen [193].

Finally, a comment should be made on iron toxicity. A single large dose of 20–60 mg per kilogram of body weight results in clinical manifestations that can be lethal. Iron toxicity causes free radical damage that overwhelms the body's ability to neutralize the oxidative stress by its antioxidative defense mechanisms.

Primary hemochromatosis is an autosomal recessive genetic disorder that results in iron overload even with iron intake with the normal range. Affected individuals absorb excessive amounts of dietary iron. Over time, the iron accumulates and causes widespread organ damage, including heart and liver failure, diabetes, and arthritis, that usually presents between the ages of 40 and 60 years. Skin manifestations of the disease include clinical skin pigmentation, ichthyosis-like states, and koilonychia. By skin biopsy, the location of siderosis in eccrine sweat glands is specific for hemochromatosis providing a strong basis for a probable diagnosis of the condition. There are correlations between the skin and other manifestations of the disease [194]. Causes of secondary hemochromatosis are severe chronic hemolysis, multiple and frequent blood transfusions in individuals with hereditary anemias or severe acquired anemias such as with the myelodysplastic syndromes, excess parenteral iron supplements, or excess dietary iron.

African iron-overload disease, also known as Bantu siderosis, is an iron-overload disorder originally observed in Southern Africa and Central Africa [195]. Dietary iron overload is due to the consumption of large amounts of home-brewed beer prepared in iron pots with a high amount of iron content. The iron content in home-brewed beer is around 46–82 mg/L compared to 0.5 mg/L in commercial beer. Studies have shown that a genetic background may play a role in this disorder. Combination of excess iron and functional changes in ferroportin seems to be the probable cause [196]. Ferroportin is a transmembrane protein that transports iron from the inside of a cell to the outside of the cell. Ferroportin is the only known iron exporter [197].

Iodine's (I) essential function is as a component of the thyroid hormones triiodothyronine (T3) and thyroxine (T4). The thyroid hormones have influence on the growth and differentiation of many tissues and total energy expenditure of the organism, and on the turnover of many substrates, vitamins, and other hormones. Thyroid activity affects oxygen consumption, protein synthesis, and mitosis, and is therefore essential for the formation and growth of hair. Schell et al. [198] originally demonstrated by means of DNA flow cytometry the influence of thyroid hormones on in vivo cell cycle kinetics of human scalp hair bulbs. Expression of the thyroid hormone receptor beta 1 was demonstrated in the human hair follicle, and it was shown that T3 significantly enhances human hair survival in vitro [199]. The impact of thyroid hormone activity on the hair is most notable during deficient states (hypothyroidism).

The amount of iodine in natural food sources varies considerably depending on the iodine content in the soil from which the food was harvested. Iodine deficiency is generally found in geographic locations with mountains or frequent flooding that result in a poor iodine content of the soil. Seafood consistently provides a good amount of iodine. Actually, the most reliable source of iodine is iodized table salt.

The iodine-deficiency disorders (goiter, cretinism, and hypothyroidism) are the easiest and least expensive of nutrient disorders to prevent. While attempting to correct for iodine deficiency, practitioners must be cautious of over-supplementing, since excess iodine may lead to iodine-induced hyperthyroidism and thyrotoxicosis. Although the risk of iodine toxicity exists with a UL of 1100 mcg/day iodine in healthy adults, the sustained use of iodized salts is recommended and widely practiced in several countries, since the risk of iodine-deficiency disorders far outweighs the small potential for iodine toxicity.

Dermatitis herpetiformis Duhring is an autoimmune blistering disease associated with gluten sensitivity that can be triggered by iodine and related compounds [200]. Accordingly, potassium iodide, when applied topically to uninvolved dermatitis herpetiformis skin, will elicit vesicular lesions (Fig. 4.14) with perivascular

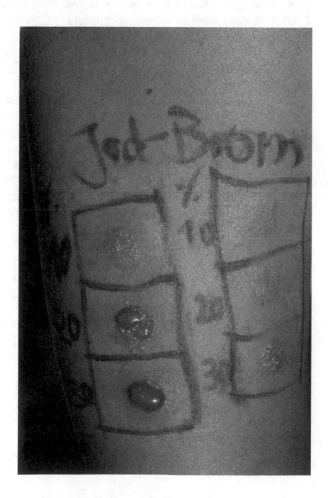

Fig. 4.14 Positive patch test in dermatitis herpetiformis Duhring

cellular infiltrates similar to those that occur in spontaneously occurring lesions [201]. One study demonstrated that the potassium iodide patch test in dermatitis herpetiformis became negative in the majority of patients treated with either gluten-free diet or dapsone [202].

Zinc (Zn) is a chemical element with the atomic number 30 and the first element of group 12 of the periodic table. Zinc is the 24th most abundant element in Earth's crust. The element was probably named by the Swiss-born German alchemist (Philippus Aureolus Theophrastus) Paracelsus (Bombastus von Hohenheim) (1493–1541), who referred to the metal as "zincum" or "zinken" in his book "Liber Mineralium II" in the sixteenth century. The word is probably derived from the German zinke, and it is supposedly meant "toothlike, pointed or jagged," since metallic zinc crystals have a needlelike appearance. Paracelsus pioneered the use of chemicals and minerals in medicine, and was one of the first to recognize that physicians required a solid academic knowledge in the natural sciences, especially chemistry. He is also a famous revolutionary for utilizing observations of nature, rather than referring to ancient texts, something of radical defiance in his age [203]. Finally, German chemist Andreas Sigismund Marggraf (1709–1782) is credited with isolation of pure metallic zinc in 1746 by heating calamine and carbon in a closed vessel without copper. Though not the first to do so, Marggraf is credited with carefully describing the process and establishing its basic theory. The procedure became commercially practical by 1752.

Zinc is an efficient Lewis acid, making it a useful catalytic agent in hydroxylation and other enzymatic reactions. The metal also has a flexible coordination geometry, which allows proteins using it to rapidly shift conformations to perform biological reactions. Therefore, enzymes with a zinc atom in the reactive center are widespread in biochemistry. In fact, zinc is required for the function of more than 300 enzymes. These metalloenzymes are active in all major metabolic pathways. Zinc serves a structural role in zinc finger proteins that form parts of some DNA transcription factors. In addition, all aspects of the immune system are dependent on adequate zinc availability.

Zinc is essential for skin biology and hair growth. Of all tissues, the skin has the third highest abundance of zinc in the body. In the skin, the zinc concentration is higher in the epidermis than in the dermis, owing to a zinc requirement for the active proliferation and differentiation of epidermal keratinocytes. Among skin disorders associated with zinc deficiency, acrodermatitis enteropathica is a disorder caused by mutations in the ZIP4 transporter and subsequent zinc deficiency, and is characterized by alopecia, diarrhea, and skin lesions. Moreover, there is accumulating evidence of a role of zinc deficiency in alopecia and in necrolytic migratory erythema, which is typically associated with glucagonoma [204].

Among food sources, oysters, lobster, and red meats, especially beef, lamb, and liver, have some of the highest concentrations of zinc. The concentration of zinc in plants varies based on levels of the element in the soil. When there is adequate zinc in the soil, the food plants that contain the most zinc are wheat (germ and bran) and various seeds (sesame, poppy, alfalfa, celery, mustard). Zinc is also found in beans, nuts, almonds, whole grains, pumpkin seeds, sunflower seeds, and black currant.

Due to a lower bioavailability of zinc from plant-based foods, it is estimated that the dietary need for zinc in vegan populations may be as high as 50% greater than their respective dietary requirements in the general population [205].

As with other minerals, zinc toxicity from food sources is uncommon. Rather, prolonged supplementations that exceed the recommended intake of zinc can have adverse effects, and cause nausea, vomiting, and epigastric pain. The upper limit for zinc of 40 mg/day was established on the basis of the negative effects of excess zinc supplementation on copper metabolism. Excessive zinc intake inhibits copper absorption, resulting in zinc-induced copper deficiency [206].

Selenium (Se) is a chemical element with the atomic number 34 in the periodic table of elements. It was discovered in 1817 by Swedish chemist Jöns Jacob Berzelius (1779–1848), who began his career as a physician, but eventually his researches in physical chemistry were of lasting significance in the development of the subject. Selenium is an element with properties that are intermediate between the elements above and below in the periodic table, sulfur and tellurium, and also has similarities to arsenic. It rarely occurs in its elemental state or as pure ore compounds in the Earth's crust, and is found in metal sulfide ores, where it partially replaces the sulfur. Although selenium salts are toxic in large amounts, trace amounts are necessary for cellular function.

In biological systems, selenium is covalently bound to cysteine, thereby substituting sulfur in the sulfhydryl groups. It is an essential component of the antioxidant enzymes glutathione peroxidase and thioredoxin reductase. In addition, selenium is also found in three deiodinase enzymes involved in thyroid hormone metabolism. It is therefore necessary for the conversion of the thyroid hormone thyroxine (T4) into its more active counterpart, triiodothyronine (T3). Such a deficiency can cause symptoms of hypothyroidism, including fatigue, mental slowing, goiter, and hair loss. Selenium supplementation has also been shown to inhibit Hashimoto's disease, with reduction of 21% on TPO antibodies reported with dietary intake of 0.2 mg of selenium [207].

The selenium content in the human body is believed to be in the 13–20 mg range. Selenium deficiency, defined by low (<60% of normal) selenoenzyme activity levels in brain and endocrine tissues, occurs only when a low selenium level is linked with an additional stress, such as high exposure to mercury [208] or increased oxidant stress such as from vitamin E deficiency. Increased dietary selenium may reduce the effects of mercury toxicity [209–212], since the molecular mechanisms of mercury toxicity include irreversible inhibition of selenoenzymes required to protect the brain and endocrine tissues from oxidative damage [208, 213].

Dietary selenium comes from nuts (Brazil nuts are an exceptionally good source of selenium), cereals, and mushrooms.

Selenium toxicity or hyperselenosis is found in isolated regions of the world where the soil bares extremely high levels of selenium, or it may occur from excess or misformulated dietary supplements [214], and rarely from poisoning with seleniferous plants (*Lecythis ollaria*, *Astragalus pectinatus*, and *Stanleya pinnata*). The most prevalent signs of selenium toxicity are gastrointestinal symptoms (nausea, vomiting, and diarrhea), hair loss, and nail discoloration.

Fig. 4.15 Natural native copper ore (origin: USA)

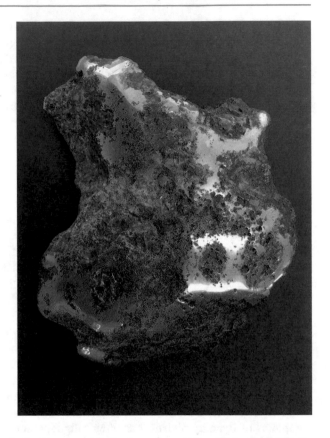

Copper (Cu) is a chemical element with the atomic number 29 in the periodic table of elements. It is present in the Earth's crust in a proportion of approximately 50 parts per million (ppm), and is one of the few metals that naturally occur in a directly usable metallic form (Fig. 4.15). This led to very early human use of copper from ca. 8000 BC to ca. 5000 BC. It was the first metal to be smelted from sulfide ores, and the first metal to be cast into a shape in a mold. In the Roman era, copper was principally mined on Cyprus, the origin of the name of the metal, from aes cyprium (metal of Cyprus), later corrupted to cuprum (Latin), from which derived the words coper (Old English) and copper, first used around 1530. Since copper occurs naturally as native metallic copper it has been known to some of the oldest civilizations on record. The Iceman Ötzi, a male dated from 3300–3200 BC, found in 1991 in the Ötztal Alps, on the border between Austria and Italy, carried an axe with a 99.7% pure copper head. Detection of high levels of arsenic in his hair suggests an involvement in copper smelting. Ultimately, experience with copper has aided the development of other metals; in particular, copper smelting led to the later discovery of iron smelting.

Copper is biostatic, meaning that bacteria and many other forms of life will not grow on it. For this purpose, it has been used to line immersed parts of ships to protect against barnacles and mussels. Similarly, copper alloys have become important netting materials in the aquaculture industry because they are antimicrobial and prevent biofouling while having strong structural and corrosion-resistant properties in marine environments. Copper alloy touch surfaces have natural properties that destroy a wide range of microorganisms, including *E. coli* O157:H7, methicillin-resistant *Staphylococcus aureus* (MRSA), *Staphylococcus*, *Clostridium difficile*, influenza A virus, adenovirus, and fungi. Some 355 copper alloys were shown to kill more than 99.9% of disease-causing bacteria within just 2 h when cleaned regularly. The United States Environmental Protection Agency (EPA) has approved the registrations of these copper alloys as antimicrobial materials with public health benefits, thus allowing manufacturers to make legal claims to the public health benefits of products made of registered alloys. Finally, textile fibers are blended with copper to create antimicrobial protective fabrics.

In folk medicine, copper is popularly used as jewelry, and according to folklore, copper bracelets relieve arthritis symptoms. In one trial for osteoarthritis and another for rheumatoid arthritis no differences were found between copper bracelet and control (non-copper) bracelet [215, 216].

Copper is essential to all living organisms as a trace dietary mineral. Copper proteins have diverse roles in biological electron transport and oxygen transportation, processes that exploit the easy interconversion of Cu(I) and Cu(II). Copper is essential in aerobic respiration. In mitochondria, it is found in cytochrome c oxidase, which is the last protein in oxidative phosphorylation. Cytochrome c oxidase is the protein that binds the O_2 between a copper and an iron; the protein transfers eight electrons to the O_2 molecule to reduce it to two molecules of water. Copper is also found in many superoxide dismutases, proteins that catalyze the decomposition of superoxides by converting it (by disproportionation) to oxygen and hydrogen peroxide.

Copper in hair is essential for oxidation of thiol groups to dithio cross-links essential for resilient properties of keratin fibers. Sheep fed on copper-deficient pastures produce wool that is weak, shows abnormal dyeing and processing qualities, and lacks grip [217].

Copper toxicity, also called copperiedus, is a metal poisoning caused by an excess of copper in the body. Symptoms include vomiting, hematemesis, hypotension, melena, coma, jaundice, and gastrointestinal distress. A significant portion of the toxicity of copper comes from its ability to accept and donate single electrons as it changes oxidation state. This catalyzes the production of very reactive radical ions, such as hydroxyl radical in a manner similar to Fenton chemistry. This catalytic activity of copper is used by the enzymes with which it is associated, and thus it is only toxic when unsequestered and unmediated. This increase in unmediated reactive radicals is generally termed oxidative stress, and is an active area of research in a variety of diseases, where copper may play an important but more subtle role than in acute toxicity [218].

Chronic copper toxicity does not normally occur in humans because of transport systems that regulate absorption and excretion. Nevertheless, excess copper in the body may result from eating acidic foods cooked in uncoated copper cookware, or from exposure to excess copper in drinking water or other environmental sources.

A study conducted in 1979 by Piérard in Belgium reported diffuse alopecia related to ingestion of toxic metals in 36 of 78 patients with diffuse alopecia. Toxic metals in abnormal amount in blood and urine were observed only when >10% of hair bulbs in the trichogram were dystrophic. Copper was involved in 17/36 alopecias related to ingestion of toxic metal. Copper intoxication was found to be related to ingestion of tap water containing a high concentration of copper salts, presumably from low pH, presence of chelating agents, or connection of electrical ground wires to copper water pipes, which caused sufficient flow of electrical current to ionize the metal [10].

Copper intrauterine devices (IUDs) have been questioned anecdotally, with claims of possible copper toxicity, but there is currently no scientific evidence to substantiate this claim [219].

Hair loss related to IUDs is related to blood loss either from heavy menstrual bleeding in women carrying copper IUDs or from the pro-androgenic action of the levonorgestrel in the hormonal IUDs [220].

Deposition of copper from exogenous sources on usually predamaged hair may cause a green discoloration of hair (chlorotrichosis) (Fig. 4.16). It has been reported

Fig. 4.16 Green hair (chlorotrichosis)

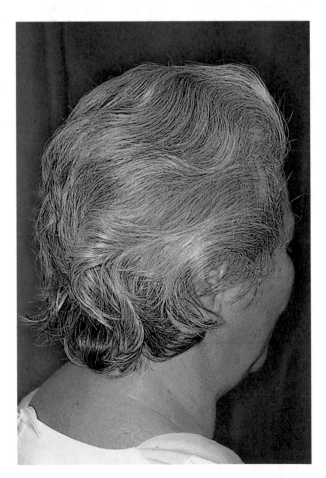

from increased concentrations of copper in domestic tap water and swimming pool water, either from corrosion of copper plumbing or from addition of copper-based algicides to the swimming pool water [221], and from copper present in cosmetic plant extracts (*Cassia obovata*) [222]. Thresholds of concentration beyond which discoloration of the hair appears are not known. However, hair discoloration has been reported after exposition to a pool containing a very low concentration of copper (0.9 ppm) [223]. Greening of the hair does not occur after systemic absorption of copper.

Finally, Marsh et al. [224] identified for the first time in hair the role of exogenous copper in increasing UV damage while elaborating on strategies to reduce copper levels in hair using chelating agents with specificity for copper, such as N,N'-ethylenediamine disuccinic acid (EDDS). The role of copper in increasing the level of damage from UV exposure was confirmed with an increase in the level of protein loss. The mechanism of action is complex, and copper can participate in a number of radical pathways including decomposition of hydrogen peroxide to hydroxyl radicals and decomposition of alkyl peroxides to alkoxy radicals.

In cases of suspected copper poisoning, penicillamine is the drug of choice, or dimercaprol, a heavy metal chelating agent, is administered. There is evidence that alpha-lipoic acid (ALA) may work as a milder chelator of tissue-bound copper [225].

Finally, elevated free copper levels have been detected in Alzheimer's disease [226] which has been hypothesized to be associated with inorganic copper consumption [227]. Copper and iron are known to bind to amyloid beta proteins in Alzheimer's disease [228]. This bound form is suspected to mediate the production of reactive oxygen species in the brain [229].

As for safety, the IOM also sets tolerable upper intake levels (ULs) for vitamins and minerals when evidence is sufficient. In the case of copper the UL is set at 10 mg/day. Collectively the EARs, RDAs, Ais, and ULs are referred to as Dietary Reference Intakes. The European Food Safety Authority reviewed the same safety question and set its UL at 5 mg/day, which is half the US value.

Silicon (Si) is the eighth most common chemical element in the universe by mass, but rarely occurs as the pure element in the Earth's crust. It is most widely distributed as various forms of silicon dioxide (silica) or silicates. More than 90% of the Earth's crust is composed of silicate minerals, making silicon the second most abundant element in the Earth's crust (about 28% by mass) after oxygen. Silicon is an essential element in biology, though only traces are required by animals. Diatoms, radiolaria, and siliceous sponges use biogenic silica as a structural material for their skeletons. In more advanced plants, the silica phytoliths are rigid microscopic bodies occurring in the cell. Silicon has been shown to improve plant cell wall strength and structural integrity [230].

Silicon is currently under consideration for elevation to the status of a plant beneficial substance by the Association of American Plant Food Control Officials (AAPFCO). There has been some evidence that silicon may be important to human health for the nails, hair, bone, and skin tissues [231].

Silicon dioxide, also known as silica, is an oxide of silicon with the chemical formula SiO_2. Even though it is poorly soluble, silica occurs in many plants. Silica phytoliths exist in the cells of many plants, particularly *Equisetaceae*, and practically all grasses. Crystalline minerals formed in the physiological environment often show exceptional physical properties, specifically strength, hardness, and fracture resilience. It is unclear in what ways silica is important in the nutrition of animals. This field of research is challenging because silica is ubiquitous and in most circumstances dissolves in trace quantities only. The current consensus is that it seems important in the growth, strength, and management of many connective tissues. Silicon is needed for synthesis of elastin and collagen, and has therefore been considered an essential element [232]. Ultimately, its essentiality to human health is difficult to prove, because silicon is very common, and therefore deficiency conditions are unknown.

Equisetum, also referred to as horsetail, is the only living genus of the *Equisetaceae* family of plants that reproduce by spores rather than seeds. *Equisetum* is a "living fossil," the only living genus of the entire class, which for over 100 million years was much more diverse and dominated the understory of late Paleozoic forests. The name "horsetail" arose from the resemblance of the branched species that somewhat resembles a horse's tail. Extracts and other preparations, specifically of *Equisetum arvense*, have served as herbal remedies, with records dating over centuries. In 2009, the European Food Safety Authority concluded that there was no evidence for the supposed health benefits of *E. arvense*, such as for invigoration, weight control, skin care, hair health, or bone health. As of 2018, there remained insufficient scientific evidence for its effectiveness as a medicine to treat any specific human condition.

Silica ingested orally is essentially nontoxic, with an LD50 of 5000 mg/kg (5 g/kg). *E. arvense* contains thiaminase, which metabolizes the B vitamin thiamine, potentially causing thiamine deficiency and liver damage, if taken chronically [233]. Further, its safety for oral consumption has not been sufficiently evaluated, especially in children and during pregnancy.

Micronutrients relevant to healthy hair and their recommended daily intake are listed in Table 4.6.

4.2.3 Life Cycle Needs

It appears that on a typical Western diet, people are not subject to nutritional deficiencies. Nevertheless, genetic diversity in nutrient requirements, inappropriate food selection or preparation, intensive physical exertion, comorbidities, and use of drugs may lead to deficiency symptoms. In fact, nutritional needs fluctuate with age and with situations that occur throughout the life cycle: infancy, childhood, adolescence, pregnancy, lactation, old age, lifestyle (restricted diets, smoking, alcohol consumption), and health status (chronic disease, medications). Specifically, nutritional deficiencies relevant to the condition of the hair are not uncommonly observed in adolescents feeding on junk food, young women with eating disorders (anorexia and bulimia), people on fad diets, alcoholics, and the chronically ill, and are especially common in the elderly population.

Table 4.6 Micronutrients relevant to healthy hair with recommended daily intake (adults)

Vitamins:
B-Vitamins:
• Thiamin (Vitamin B1) –men: 1.2 mg, women: 1.1 mg
• Riboflavin (Vitamin B2) –men: 1.3 mg, women: 1.1 mg
• Niacin (VItamin B3) –men: 16 mg, women: 14 mg
• Pantothenic acid (Vitamin B5) –5 mg
• Pyridoxine (Vitamin B6) –between 19 and 50 years: 1.3 mg, men 50 years or older: 1.7 mg, women 50 years or older: 1.5 mg
• Biotin (Vitamin B7 or H) –30 micrograms
• Folic acid (Vitamin B9 or 11) –400 mcg
• Cyanocobolamin (Vitamin B12) –2.4 mcg
Antioxidants:
• Vitamin A/Beta-carotene –men: 900 mcg, women 700 mcg
• Vitamin C –men: 90 mg, women: 75 mg, smokers: an additional 35 mg
• Alpha-tocopherol (Vitamin E) –15 mg
Others:
• Vitamin D –between 1 and 70 years: 600 U, 70 years or older: 800 U
• Vitamin K –men: 120 mcg, women: 90 mcg
Minerals:
• Sulphur –Diets that are adequate in protein contain adequate sulphur
• Iron - men and women 50 years or older: 8mg, women between 19-50 years: 18 mg
• Zinc –men: 11 mg, women: 8 mg
• Iodine –150 mcg
• Selenium –55 mcg
• Copper –900 mcg
• Silica -Essentiality unclear

In instances of protein and calorie malnutrition, deficiency of essential amino acids, of vitamins, and of minerals, hair growth and pigmentation may be impaired.

As yet, there is little evidence to support nutritional supplement as an effective prevention of chronic diseases or hair loss. However, for patients with certain medical conditions, dietary supplements may be justified to help avert specific nutrient deficiencies resulting from the disease and causing hair loss, specifically in states of malabsorption, debilitation, or hypermetabolic demand.

The human life cycle spans four stages of growth and development: infancy, childhood, adolescence, and adulthood, with the nutritional needs and patterns depending on the age group.

4.2.3.1 Infancy

Growth is rapid during the first year of life, with most infants doubling their birth weight by the time they are 6 months old, and tripling it by the time they reach 12–15 months of age. Infants generally increase their birth length by 50% during the first year, and double it by 4 years of age. Growth requires an ample supply of macronutrients and micronutrients. Specifically, during the first 3 years of life, children require between 80 and 120 kcal/kg/day to support normal growth [234]. Carbohydrates are the preferred energy source, and also spare proteins for the critical task of growth instead of burned energy. Protein is the fundamental tissue-building substrate for the body. For the first 6 months of life, the protein requirements of an infant are 1.52 g/kg/day, while the protein needs of a fully grown adult are 0.8 g/kg/day [230]. As the growth rate slows with age, the protein requirements decline. All minerals and vitamins have an essential role in tissue growth and maintenance as well as in overall energy metabolism. There has been much debate over the need of dietary supplements for infants and children, while the American Academy of Pediatrics has come to the conclusion that only two vitamins are potentially needed in supplemental form: vitamins K and D [235]. In fact, excessive supplementation is not uncommon, and toxicity is a danger. Excess amounts of vitamin A and D are of special concern in children. Finally, the fortification of cereals and breads with iron has significantly reduced the frequency of iron-deficiency anemia.

4.2.3.2 Childhood

Between infancy and adolescence, the childhood growth rate slows and becomes irregular. The children form patterns, attitudes, and basic eating habits as a result of social and emotional experiences involving eating. Parental eating habits have the most influence on a child's eating behavior, though peer food habits and the school environment eventually introduce other stimuli that impact food choices as the child is moving towards independence.

4.2.3.3 Adolescence

The onset of puberty introduces the second phase of rapid growth, which continues until adult maturity. Levels of growth and sex hormones rise, with multiple body changes, including the hair. During this stage, the long bones grow quickly, sex characteristics develop, and fat and muscle mass increase significantly with the distinct patterns of female and male body composition. Teenagers' eating habits are considerably influenced by their rapid growth, increasing self-consciousness, and peer pressure. Due to their larger appetite and the amounts of food consumed, boys usually fare better than girls with regard to their overall nutrition. In contrast, girls may tend to restrict their food and have an inadequate nutrient intake because they are under a greater social pressure for thinness. Ultimately, the eating disorders involve a distorted body image with an irrational pursuit of thinness resulting in morbidity.

4.2.3.4 Adulthood

After physical maturity is established, energy requirements decrease. Beginning at about the age of 30 years, a gradual loss of functioning cells occurs, resulting in a reduced cell metabolism and changes in body composition. This change in metabolic rate reflects in lean muscle mass loss and as a loss of high metabolically active organ tissues such as the brain, liver, heart, and kidney [236, 237]. In addition, hormonal changes during the aging process have influence: a decline in insulin production or sensitivity, decrease in the levels of melatonin, and decrease in the levels of growth hormone and sex hormones estrogen and testosterone all have their repercussions for the general health status, and for the condition of the hair.

4.2.3.5 Pregnancy and Lactation

The growth and development of a baby from the moment of conception to the time of birth depend entirely on the nourishment of the mother. The metabolic expenditure of pregnancy is significant over the course of gestation. Especially during the second and third trimesters of pregnancy, there is an increased need of protein and energy. As the total energy intake increases, so do the nutrients contained in the foods consumed, specifically the vitamins and minerals. Women require additional copper, iodine, iron, magnesium, manganese, molybdenum, selenium, zinc, and chromium. A good supply of calcium, along with phosphorus, magnesium, and vitamin D, is essential for the fetal development of bones and teeth. Special attention is given to iron intake due to increased hemoglobin synthesis, and folate is essential for both the mother and the fetus throughout pregnancy due to its role in DNA synthesis, cell division, and hemoglobin synthesis. Folate is particularly important during the early periconceptional period from approximately 2 months before conception to 6 weeks of gestation to ensure adequate availability during the critical period of fetal neural tube formation from 21 to 28 days of gestation.

During the second half of pregnancy, the percentage of anagen hairs increases from the normal 85 to 95%. At this time also the percentage of hairs of large shaft diameter is higher than in nonpregnant women of the same age [238]. After parturition, the follicles in which anagen has been prolonged rapidly enter catagen and then telogen, with an increased shedding of hair evident after 3–4 months in the form of postpartum effluvium (Fig. 4.17). Most women will return to their usual hair growth cycle between 6 and 12 months after birth. Postpartum hair loss usually returns the hair to prepregnancy thickness, unless it leads over to female androgenetic alopecia. In case of postpartum effluvium persisting over 12 months, excessive

Fig. 4.17 Postpartum effluvium

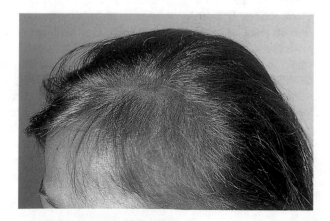

hair loss may be caused by common conditions, such as female androgenetic alopecia, iron deficiency, or hypothyroidism. Lesser common conditions include persistent hyperprolactinemia (Chiari-Frommel syndrome [239]) and postpartum hypopituitarism caused by pituitary necrosis due to blood loss and hypovolemic shock during childbirth (Sheehan's syndrome [240]).

The Dietary Reference Intakes (DRIs) recommend an increased need of 340 kcal/ day of energy during the second trimester, and approximately 452 kcal/day during the third trimester of pregnancy, and an increase of 25 g/day of protein more than the average woman's protein requirement. The current DRIs recommend a daily iron intake of 27 mg/day during pregnancy, which is significantly above the nonpregnant woman's DRI of 18 mg/day. The current DRIs recommend a daily folate intake of 400 mcg/day for nonpregnant women during their childbearing years, and 600 mcg/day during pregnancy. Finally, the current DRIs recommend pregnant women consume 600 IU/day of vitamin D.

In general, the basic requirements of protein and energy recommended for the mother during pregnancy, as well as the prenatal supplements, should be continued during the lactation period.

4.2.3.6 Smoking

Besides being the single most preventable cause of significant cardiovascular and pulmonary morbidity and an important cause of death in the general population, tobacco smoking has been associated with various adverse effects on the skin and hair. Premature skin aging has attracted the attention of the medical community only since the 1960s [241], although a relation between smoking and skin complexion was first suggested as early as 1856 [242]. In 1996, Mosley and Gibbs [243] originally reported a significant relationship between smoking, premature gray hair, and baldness in patients visiting a general surgical outpatient clinic in the United Kingdom. Subsequently, the observation of strikingly dissimilar androgenetic alopecia in a 52-year-old monozygotic male twin pair led to further speculations on the possibility of an association between smoking and hair loss [244], since studies on the degree of alopecia among monozygotic twins aged over 50 have shown that intrapair differences are negligible in 92%, slight in 8%, and striking in none [245]. A salient feature differing the twin brothers in their personal histories was that the balding brother admitted to long-standing, heavy cigarette smoking, while the other was a nonsmoker. Eventually, a population-based cross-sectional survey among Asian men 40 years or older showed statistically significant positive associations between moderate or severe androgenetic alopecia and smoking status, current cigarette smoking of 20 cigarettes or more per day, and smoking intensity [246]: The odds ratio of early-onset history for androgenetic alopecia grades increased in a dose–response pattern. Risk for moderate or severe androgenetic increased for family history of first-degree and second-degree relatives, as well as for paternal relatives.

The mechanisms by which smoking accelerates hair loss have not been fully examined, but are believed to be multifactorial, and related to effects of cigarette smoke on the microvasculature [247], cutaneous collagen [248], and elastic tissue [249]; to prooxidant effects of smoking; and to increased hydroxylation of estradiol, as well as inhibition of the enzyme aromatase [250], which converts androgens to estrogens, creating a relative hypoestrogenic state. Evidence of the consequence of impaired circulation and wound healing is a higher complication rate of hair restoration surgery in smokers versus nonsmokers [251]. Besides inducing local ischemia, the decreased capillary blood flow in the dermal papilla of the hair follicles may focally shunt more toxic substances. Cigarette smoke contains over 4800 chemicals, many of which are known to be toxic to cells and 69 are known to cause cancer. Both nicotine and cotinine are detected in hair samples of smokers [252]. Smoke genotoxicants metabolized in hair follicle cells may cause DNA damage through the production of DNA adducts, and smoking-associated mitochondrial DNA mutations have been shown in human hair follicles [253], though the relevance of these for hair follicle pathology is as yet unknown. Since substantial extracellular matrix remodeling is involved in the hair follicle growth cycle, especially during catagen-associated hair follicle regression, it is conceivable that cigarette smoke-induced imbalance in the intra- and perifollicular protease/antiprotease systems controlling tissue remodeling may also affect the hair follicle growth cycle [254]. Finally, smoking-induced oxidative stress and a disequilibrium of antioxidant systems may lead to the release of pro-inflammatory cytokines from follicular keratinocytes, which by themselves have been shown to inhibit the growth of isolated hair follicles in culture [255].

The fact that cigarette smoke-associated hair loss is of the androgenetic type indicates that genetic factors contribute. On the other hand, recent studies on the evolution of androgenetic hair loss have focused on oxidative stress: Naito et al. [256] analyzed the effect of the lipid peroxides on hair follicles, and observed that the topical application of linolein hydroperoxides, one of the lipid peroxides, leads to the early onset of the catagen phase in murine hair cycles. Furthermore, they found that lipid peroxides induced apoptosis of hair follicle cells. They also induced apoptosis in human epidermal keratinocytes by upregulating apoptosis-related genes. These results indicate that lipid peroxides, which can cause free radicals, induce the apoptosis of hair follicle cells, and this is followed by early onset of the catagen phase.

Bahta et al. [257] cultured dermal hair papilla cells (DPC) from balding and non-balding scalp and demonstrated that balding DPCs grow slower in vitro than non-balding DPCs. Loss of proliferative capacity of balding DPCs was associated with changes in cell morphology, expression of senescence-associated beta-galactosidase, decreased expression of proliferating cell nuclear antigen and Bmi-1, upregulation of p16(INK4a)/pRb, and nuclear expression of markers of oxidative stress and DNA damage including heat-shock protein-27, superoxide dismutase catalase, ataxia-telangiectasia-mutated kinase (ATM), and ATM- and Rad3-related protein. The finding of premature senescence of balding DPC in vitro in association with the expression of markers of oxidative stress and DNA damage suggests that balding DPCs are particularly sensitive to environmental stress.

Upton et al. [258] further investigated the effects of oxidative stress on balding and occipital scalp DPCs. Patient-matched DPCs from balding and occipital scalp were cultured at atmospheric (21%) or physiologically normal (2%) O_2. At 21% O_2,

DPCs showed flattened morphology and a significant reduction in mobility, population doubling, increased levels of reactive oxygen species and senescence-associated β-Gal activity, and increased expression of p16(INK4a) and pRB. Balding DPCs secreted higher levels of the negative hair growth regulators TGF beta 1 and 2 in response to H_2O_2 but not cell culture-associated oxidative stress. Balding DPCs had higher levels of catalase and total glutathione but appeared to be less able to handle oxidative stress compared with occipital DPCs. These in vitro findings suggest that there may be a role for oxidative stress in the pathogenesis of androgenetic alopecia, in relation to both cell senescence and migration, but also secretion of known hair follicle inhibitory factors, at the same time offering new opportunities for treatment of androgenetic alopecia beyond minoxidil and 5α-reductase inhibitors.

Interestingly, an experiment performed on C57BL/6 mice that developed hair loss when exposed to cigarette smoke [259] demonstrated that this effect could be prevented by the oral administration of N-acetylcysteine, an analogue and precursor of cysteine and reduced glutathione, as well as cystine, the oxidized form of cysteine. The effect was interpreted as to be possibly related to the glutathione-related detoxification system [260].

4.2.3.7 Medications

There is evidence that drugs may produce deficiencies in vitamins, minerals, fatty acids, and/or amino acids. Some cause specific, and others multiple, deficiencies. Medications have the potential to impact nutritional needs by altering the way the body absorbs, metabolizes, or excretes nutrients. In addition, some medications may disrupt the balance of intestinal bacteria that can impact the overall nutritional status. Medications interact with minerals either by blocking absorption or by inducing renal excretion; examples are the antacids, chelating agents, and diuretics, respectively. The acidic environment of the stomach is essential for the proper absorption of many nutrients, including the minerals. Chelating agents, such as penicillamine, are used to remove excess metals from the body, such as in Wilson's disease. The drug also attaches to zinc, thereby potentially leading to its depletion. Finally, the diuretics that are usually required on a long-term base for treatment of arterial hypertension lead to an excretion of sodium, potassium, magnesium, and zinc with excess water. Finally, nutrients may also interact with each other, often cooperatively, but sometimes in competition with each other. An example is zinc-induced copper deficiency.

The depletion of nutrients can contribute to some of the adverse reactions that people experience while taking drugs. An example is isotretinoin-induced hair loss related to biotin deficiency from suppression of hepatic biotinidase activity [158].

Short course of drugs is usually less of a risk than long-term courses. Polypharmacy may cause increased problems. Finally, people whose nutritional status is marginal, or who are already deficient, are at a particular risk.

As yet, research on drug-nutrient interactions is very limited, and where studies have only been carried out on laboratory animals, these need to be followed up in humans. Examples are the effect of paracetamol (acetaminophen) on sulfur amino acids in mice [261], and that of the lipase inhibitor orlistat on the availability of the essential fatty acids EPA and DHA in rat tissues [262].

Nutrients relevant to healthy hair that may be affected by medications include iron, zinc, copper, selenium, biotin, vitamin B12, niacin, and vitamin D, and possibly the sulfur amino acids, and essential fatty acids (Table 4.7).

Table 4.7 Exemplary selection of drugs that may interact with absorption or activity of nutrients of potential relevance to hair health

Drug or type of drug	Possible deficiency or interference
ACE inhibitors	Zinc
Antacids	Iron
	Zinc
	Biotin
	Vitamin B12
Antibiotics	Beneficial intestinal bacteria
	Biotin
	Vitamin K
Aspirin and NSAR	Iron
Diuretics	Zinc
Isoniazid	Niacin
	Vitamin B6
Isotretinoin	Biotin
Levodopa	Vitamin B6
Metformin	Vitamin B12
Methotrexate	Folic acid
Oral contraceptives	Vitamin B1
	Vitamin B6
	Vitamin B12
	Folic acid
	Vitamin C
Orlistat	Essential fatty acids (in rats)
Paracetamol (acetaminophen)	Sulphur amino acids (in mice)
Penicillamine	Copper
	Zink
Statins	Selenium
	Coenzyme Q10
Valproic acid (anticonvulsant)	Biotin
Zinc	Copper

A way to deal with the problem of drug–nutrient interaction is to prescribe smaller quantities of drugs, together with the relevant nutrient supplements where these act synergistically; to promote further research into the deficiencies caused by medications; and ultimately to require medical schools and residency programs to teach nutrition in greater depth to include nutritional deficiencies which may be related to drugs [263].

Finally, women on contraceptive agents are a special concern considering their nutritional status. While most physicians are concerned with the major risks of oral contraceptives, such as venous thromboembolism, cardiovascular risk, and breast cancer, the potential side effects related to nutritional depletion in oral contraceptive users are often ignored, specifically the following: (1) vitamin B6, which is linked to depression and tryptophan-level abnormalities in pill users and may be associated with nausea and weight gain: studies show a daily need 10–30 times greater than that for women not on the pill; (2) folic acid, common among women, but a 25% deficiency rate has been noted in pill users: this has been associated with cell malformation and may be a reason for the high spontaneous abortion rate in women who conceive immediately after discontinuing the pill; (3) vitamins B1 and B12, the vitamins affecting energy, skin, and hair; and (4) vitamin C. Full vitamin supplementation is therefore recommended for women taking oral contraceptives, including these vitamins as well as vitamin E and bioflavonoids. Vitamin supplements are routine for pregnancy. They should also be routine for the pseudopregnant state of oral contraception [264].

References

1. Trüeb RM. From hair in India to hair India. Int J Trichol. 2017;9:1–6.
2. Paus R. Control of the hair cycle and hair diseases as cycling disorders. Curr Opin Dermatol. 1996;3:248–58.
3. Paus R, Cotsarelis G. The biology of hair follicles. N Engl J Med. 1999;341:491–7.
4. Guarrera M, Rebora A. Anagen hairs may fail to replace telogen hairs in early androgenic female alopecia. Dermatology. 1996;192:28–31.
5. Rebora A, Guarrera M. Kenogen. A new phase of the hair cycle? Dermatology. 2002;205:108–10.
6. Guarrera M, Rebora A. Kenogen in female androgenetic alopecia. A longitudinal study. Dermatology. 2005;210:18–20.
7. Stenn K. Exogen is an active, separately controlled phase of the hair growth cycle. J Am Acad Dermatol. 2005;52:374–5.
8. Rathman-Josserand M, Genty G, Lecardonnel J, Chabane S, Cousson A, François Michelet J, Bernard BA. Human hair follicle stem/progenitor cells express hypoxia markers. J Invest Dermatol. 2013;133:2094–7.
9. Saleh D, Cook C. Anagen effluvium. SourceStatPearls [Internet]. Treasure Island, FL: StatPearls Publishing; 2019; 2020–2019 Jul 31.
10. Piérard GE. Toxic effects of metals from the environment on hair growth and structure. J Cutan Pathol. 1979;6:237–42.
11. Liu J, Lu Y, Wu Q, Goyer RA, Waalkes MP. Mineral arsenicals in traditional medicines: orpiment, realgar, and arsenolite. J Pharmacol Exp Ther. 2008;326:363–8.

12. Arsenic in drinking water threatens up to 60 million in Pakistan. Science | AAAS; 23 August 2017.Accessed 11 Sep 2017.
13. Talhout R, Schulz T, Florek E, Van Benthem J, Wester P, Antoon O. Hazardous compounds in tobacco smoke. Int J Environ Res Public Health. 2011;8:613–28.
14. The Tox guide for arsenic. The US Agency for Toxic Substances and Disease Registry; 2007.
15. Sharma S, Gupta A, Deshmukh A, Puri V. Arsenic poisoning and Mees' lines. QJM. 2016;109:565–6.
16. Stillman JM. Story of alchemy and early chemistry. Whitefish: Kessinger Publishing; 2003. p. 7–9. ISBN: 978-0-7661-3230-6.
17. Mayell H. Did mercury in "little blue pills" make Abraham Lincoln Erratic? National Geographic News; 2007. Archived from the original on 22 May 2008. Accessed 15 June 2008.
18. What happened to Mercurochrome? 23 July 2004. Archived from the original on 11 April 2009. Accessed 7 July 2009.
19. Czarnetzki A, Ehrhardt S. Re-dating the Chinese amalgam-filling of teeth in Europe. Int J Anthropol. 1990;5(4):325–32.
20. Bharti R, Wadhwani KK, Tikku AP, Chandra A. Dental amalgam: an update. J Conserv Dent. 2010;13(4):204–8.
21. About Dental Amalgam Fillings. Food and Drug Administration. Accessed 19 April 2015.
22. Final opinion on dental amalgam. European Commission; 2 June 2015. Accessed 17 Jan 2016.
23. Dental amalgam: what others say. American Dental Association; May 2015. Accessed 17 Jan 2016.
24. Bratel J, Haraldson T, Meding B, et al. Potential side effects of dental amalgam restorations. An oral and medical investigation. Eur J Oral Sci. 1997;105:234–43.
25. Furhoff AK, Tomson Y, Ilie M, Bågedahl-Strindlund M, Larsson KS, Sandborgh-Englund G, Torstenson B, Wretlind K. A multidisciplinary clinical study of patients suffering from illness associated with release of mercury from dental restorations. Medical and odontological aspects. Scand J Prim Health Care. 1998;16:247–52.
26. Langworth S, Björkman L, Elinder CG, Järup L, Savlin P. Multidisciplinary examination of patients with illness attributed to dental fillings. J Oral Rehabil. 2002;29:705–13.
27. Lindberg NE, Lindberg E, Larsson G. Psychologic factors in the etiology of amalgam illness. Acta Odontol Scand. 1994;52:219–28.
28. Bailer J, Rist F, Rudolf A, Staehle HJ, Eickholz P, Triebig G, Bader M, Pfeifer U. Adverse health effects related to mercury exposure from dental amalgam fillings: toxicological or psychological causes? Psychol Med. 2001;31:255–63.
29. Sundström A, Bergdahl J, Nyberg L, Bergdahl M, Nilsson LG. Stressful negative life events and amalgam-related complaints. Community Dent Oral Epidemiol. 2011;39:12–8.
30. Bågedahl-Strindlund M, Ilie M, Furhoff AK, Tomson Y, Larsson KS, Sandborgh-Englund G, Torstenson B, Wretlind K. A multidisciplinary clinical study of patients suffering from illness associated with mercury release from dental restorations: psychiatric aspects. Acta Psychiatr Scand. 1997;96:475–82.
31. Cocoros G, Cahn PH, Siler W. Mercury concentrations in fish, plankton and water from three Western Atlantic estuaries. J Fish Biol. 1973;5:641–7.
32. Bose-O'Reilly S, McCart KM, Steckling N, Lettmeier B. Mercury exposure and children's health. Curr Probl Pediatr Adolesc Health Care. 2010;40:186–215.
33. Clarkson TW, Magos L. The toxicology of mercury and its chemical compounds. Crit Rev Toxicol. 2006;36(8):609–62.
34. Bray M. SKIN DEEP: dying to be white. CNN; 2002. Archived from the original on 2010-04-08. Accessed 12 May 2010.
35. Wüstner H, Orfanos CE, Steinbach H, Käferstein H, Herpers H. Nail changes and loss of hair: cardinal signs of mercury poisoning from hair bleaches [article in German]. Dtsch Med Wochenschr. 1975;100(1694–7)
36. Peters JB, Warren MP. Reversible alopecia associated with high blood mercury levels and early menopause: a report of two cases. Menopause. 2019;26:915–8.
37. Bjørklund G. Mercury and acrodynia. J Orthomol Med. 1995;10(3 & 4):145–6.

38. Stoica A, Katzenellenbogen BS, Martin MB. Activation of estrogen receptor-alpha by the heavy metal cadmium. Mol Endocrinol (Baltimore, MD). 2000;14:545–53.
39. Ali I, Penttinen-Damdimopoulou PE, Mäkelä SI, Berglund M, Stenius U, Akesson A, Håkansson H, Halldin K. Estrogen-like effects of cadmium in vivo do not appear to be mediated via the classical estrogen receptor transcriptional pathway. Environ Health Perspect. 2010;118(10):1389–94.
40. Ali I, Damdimopoulou P, Stenius U, Adamsson A, Mäkelä SI, Åkesson A, Berglund M, Håkansson H, Halldi K. Cadmium-induced effects on cellular signaling pathways in the liver of transgenic estrogen reporter mice. Toxicol Sci. 2012;127:66–75.
41. Johnson MD, Kenney N, Stoica A, Hilakivi-Clarke L, Singh B, Chepko G, Clarke R, Sholler PF, Lirio AA, Foss C, Reiter R, Trock B, Paik S, Martin MB. Cadmium mimics the in vivo effects of estrogen in the uterus and mammary gland. Nat Med. 2003;9:1081–4.
42. Maret W, Moulis JM. The bioinorganic chemistry of cadmium in the context of its toxicity. cadmium: from toxicity to essentiality. Met Ions Life Sci. 2013;11:1–29.
43. Wallin M, Barregard L, Sallsten G, Lundh T, Karlsson MK, Lorentzon M, Ohlsson C, Mellström D. Low-level cadmium exposure is associated with decreased bone mineral density and increased risk of incident fractures in elderly men: the MrOS Sweden study. J Bone Miner Res. 2016;31:732–41.
44. Bachanek T, Staroslawska E, Wolanska E, Jarmolinska K. Heavy metal poisoning in glass worker characterised by severe. Ann Agric Environ Med. 2000;7:51–3.
45. Dias F, Bonsucesso JS, Oliveira LC, Dos Santos WNL. Preconcentration and determination of copper in tobacco leaves samples by using a minicolumn of sisal fiber (Agave sisalana) loaded with Alizarin fluorine blue by FAAS. Talanta. 2012;89:276–9.
46. Järup L, Berglund M, Elinder CG, Nordberg G, Vahter M. Health effects of cadmium exposure—a review of the literature and a risk estimate. Scand J Work Environ Health. 1998;24(Suppl 1):1–51.
47. Li H, Wallin M, Barregard L, Sallsten G, Lundh T, Ohlsson C, Mellström D, Andersson EM. Smoking-induced risk of osteoporosis is partly mediated by cadmium from tobacco smoke: the MrOS Sweden study. J Bone Miner Res. 2020; https://doi.org/10.1002/jbmr.4014. [Epub ahead of print].
48. Dowling GB. Ringworm of the scalp treated by thallium acetate epilation. Proc R Soc Med. 1927;20:1055–6.
49. Gross P, Runne E, Wilson JW. Studies on the effect of thallium poisoning of the rat: the influence of cystine and methionine on alopecia and survival periods. J Invest Dermatol. 1948;10:119–34.
50. Lu CI, Huang CC, Chang YC, Tsai YT, Kuo HC, Chuang YH, Shih TS. Short-term thallium intoxication: dermatological findings correlated with thallium concentration. Arch Dermatol. 2007;143(1):93–8.
51. Campbell C, Bahrami S, Owen C. Anagen effluvium caused by thallium poisoning. JAMA Dermatol. 2016;152:724–6.
52. Saha A, Sadhu HG, Karnik AB, Patel TS, Sinha SN, Saiyed HN. Erosion of nails following thallium poisoning: a case report. Occup Environ Med. 2004;61:640–2.
53. Feldman J, Levisohn DR. Acute alopecia: clue to thallium toxicity. Pediatr Dermatol. 1993;10:29–31.
54. Daniel CR 3rd, Piraccini BM, Tosti A. The nail and hair in forensic science. J Am Acad Dermatol. 2004;50(2):258–61.
55. Gross M. Beethoven's ringlets—from a medical point of view [article in German]. Dtsch Med Wochenschr. 2013;138:2633–8.
56. Kintz P, Ginet M, Cirimele V. Multi-element screening by ICP-MS of two specimens of Napoleon's hair. J Anal Toxicol. 2006;30:621–3.
57. Kerdel-Vegas F. Generalized hair loss due to the ingestion of "coco dem mono". J Invest Dermatol. 1964;42:91–4.
58. Aronow L, Kerdel-Vegas F. Seleno-cystathionine, a pharmacologically active factor in the seeds of Lecythis ollaria. Nature. 1965;205:1185–7.

59. Müller D, Desel H. Acute selenium poisoning by paradise nuts (Lecythis ollaria). Hum Exp Toxicol. 2010;29:431–4.
60. Crounse RG, Maxwell JD, Blank H. Inhibition of growth of hair by mimosine. Nature. 1962;194:694–5.
61. Montagna W, Yun JS. The effects of the seeds of *Leucaena glauca* on the hair follicles of the mouse. J Invest Dermatol. 1963;40:325–32.
62. Nerlekar N, Beale A, Harper RW. Colchicine—a short history of an ancient drug. Med J Aust. 2014;201:687–8.
63. Finkelstein Y, Aks SE, Hutson JR, Juurlink DN, Nguyen P, Dubnov-Raz G, Pollak U, Koren G, Bentur Y. Colchicine poisoning: the dark side of an ancient drug. Clin Toxicol. 2010;48(5):407–14.
64. Malkinson FD, Lynfield YL. Colchicine alopecia. J Invest Dermatol. 1959;33:371.
65. Combalia A, Baliu-Piqué C, Fortea A, Ferrando J. Anagen effluvium following acute colchicine poisoning. Int J Trichol. 2016;8:171–2.
66. Kande Vidanalage CJ, Ekanayeka R, Wijewardane DK. Case report: a rare case of attempted homicide with Gloriosa superba seeds. BMC Pharmacol Toxicol. 2016;17:26.
67. Bains A, Verma GK, Vedant D, Negi A. Anagen effluvium secondary to Gloriosa superba ingestion. Indian J Dermatol Venereol Leprol. 2016;82:677–80.
68. Gooneratne BWM. Massive generalized alopecia after poisoning by Gloriosa superba. Br Med J. 1966;1:1023–4.
69. Assouly P. Hair loss associated with cucurbit poisoning. JAMA Dermatol. 2018;154:617–8.
70. Headington JT. Telogen effluvium. New concepts and review. Arch Dermatol. 1993;129:356–63.
71. Trüeb RM. Telogen effluvium: is there a need for a new classification? Skin Appendage Disord. 2016;2:39–44.
72. Barraud-Klenovsek MM, Trüeb RM. Congenital hypotrichosis due to short anagen. Br J Dermatol. 2000;143:612–7.
73. Van Scott EJ, Reinertson RP, Steinmuller R. The growing hair roots of the human scalp and morphologic changes therein following amethopterin therapy. J Invest Dermatol. 1957;29:197–204.
74. Van Scott EJ, Reinertson RP. Detection of radiation effects on hair roots of the human scalp. J Invest Dermatol. 1957;29:205–12.
75. Pecoraro V, Astore I, Barman J, Ignacioaraujo C. The normal trichogram in the child before the age of puberty. Invest Dermatol. 1964;42:427–30.
76. Braun-Falco O, Heilgemeir GP. The trichogram. Structural and functional basis, performance, and interpretation. Sem Dermatol. 1985;4:40–52.
77. Blume-Peytavi U, Orfanos CE. Microscopy of the hair—the trichogram. In: Derup J, Jemec GBE, editors. Handbook of non-invasive methods and the skin. London: CRC Press; 1995. p. 549–54.
78. Galliker NA, Trüeb RM. Value of trichoscopy versus trichogram for diagnosis of female androgenetic alopecia. Int J Trichol. 2012;4:19–22.
79. Trüeb RM, Reis Gavazzoni Dias MF. A comment on trichoscopy. Int J Trichol. 2018;10(4):147–9.
80. Tosti A, Peluso AM, Misciali C, et al. Loose anagen hair. Arch Dermatol. 1997;133:1089–93.
81. Hambidge KM. Hair analyses: worthless for vitamins, limited for minerals. Am J Clin Nutr. 1982;36:943–9.
82. Sherertz E. Misuse of hair analysis as a diagnostic tool. Arch Dermatol. 1985;121:1504–5.
83. Zlotken SH. Hair analysis. A useful tool or a waste of money? Int J Dermatol. 1985;24:161–4.
84. Seidel S, Kreutzer R, Smith D, McNeel S, Gilliss D. Assessment of commercial laboratories performing hair mineral analysis. JAMA. 2001;285:67–72.
85. Drasch G, Roider G. Assessment of hair mineral analysis commercially offered in Germany. J Trace Elem Med Biol. 2002;16(1):27–31.
86. Gummer CL. Diet and hair loss. Semin Dermatol. 1985;4:35–9.
87. Finner AM. Nutrition and hair: deficiencies and supplements. Dermatol Clin. 2013;31:167–72.

88. Wolfe RR, Miller SL. The recommended dietary allowance of protein: a misunderstood concept. JAMA. 2008;299:2891–3.
89. Estimated calorie needs per day, by age, sex, and physical activity level—2015–2020 Dietary guidelines. Office of Disease Prevention and Health Promotion. U.S. Department of Health and Human Services and U.S. Department of Agriculture; December 2015.
90. Kealey T, Williams R, Philpott MP. The human hair follicle engages in glutaminolysis and aerobic glycolysis: implications for skin, splanchnic and neoplastic metabolism. Skin Pharmacol. 1994;7:41–6.
91. Philpott MP, Kealey T. Metabolic studies on isolated hair follicles: hair follicles engage in aerobic glycolysis and do not demonstrate the glucose fatty acid cycle. J Invest Dermatol. 1991;96:875–9.
92. Cottle DJ, editor. Australian sheep and wool handbook. Christchurch: Inkata Press; 1991. p. 202.
93. Tanumihardjo SA. Vitamin A: biomarkers of nutrition for development. Am J Clin Nutr. 2011;94:658S–65S.
94. Fuchs E, Green H. Regulation of terminal differentiation of cultured human keratinocytes by vitamin A. Cell. 1981;25(3):617–25.
95. Combs GF. The vitamins: fundamental aspects in nutrition and health. 3rd ed. Burlington, MA: Elsevier Academic Press; 2008.
96. Nelson AM, Zhao W, Gilliland KL, Zaenglein AL, Liu W, Thiboutot DM. Neutrophil gelatinase-associated lipocalin mediates 13-cis retinoic acid-induced apoptosis of human sebaceous gland cells. J Clin Invest. 2008;118(4):1468–78.
97. McClean FC, Budy AM. Vitamin A, vitamin D, cartilage, bones, and teeth. Vitamins and hormones, vol. 21. New York: Academic Press; 1964. p. 51–2.
98. Bolland MJ, Grey A, Gamble GD, Reid IR. The effect of vitamin D supplementation on skeletal, vascular, or cancer outcomes: a trial sequential meta-analysis. Lancet Diabetes Endocrinol. 2014;2:307–20.
99. Khan SU, Khan MU, Riaz H, Valavoor S, Zhao D, Vaughan L, et al. Effects of nutritional supplements and dietary interventions on cardiovascular outcomes. Ann Intern Med. 2019;171:190–8.
100. Spiro A, Buttriss JL. Vitamin D: an overview of vitamin D status and intake in Europe. Nutr Bull. 2014;39(4):322–50.
101. Evans HM, Bishop KS. On the existence of a hitherto unrecognized dietary factor essential for reproduction. Science. 1922;56:650–1.
102. Sidgwick GP, McGeorge D, Bayat A. A comprehensive evidence-based review on the role of topicals and dressings in the management of skin scarring. Arch Dermatol Res. 2015;307:461–77.
103. Tanaydin V, Conings J, Malyar M, van der Hulst R, van der Lei B. The role of topical vitamin E in scar management: a systematic review. Aesthet Surg J. 2016;36:959–65.
104. Tilburt JC, Emanuel EJ, Miller FG. Does the evidence make a difference in consumer behavior? Sales of supplements before and after publication of negative research results. J Gen Intern Med. 2008;23:1495–8.
105. Miller ER, Pastor-Barriuso R, Dalal D, Riemersma RA, Appel LJ, Guallar E. Meta-analysis: high-dosage vitamin E supplementation may increase all-cause mortality. Ann Intern Med. 2005;142:37–46.
106. Poppe H, Poppe LM, Goebeler M, Trautmann A. Treatment of disseminated granuloma annulare with oral vitamin E: 'primum nil nocere'. Dermatology. 2013;227:83–8.
107. Ayres S Jr, Mihan R. Lupus erythematosus and vitamin E: an effective and nontoxic therapy. Cutis. 1979;23:49–52, 54.
108. Shirakata Y, Shiraishi S, Sayama K, Shinmori H, Miki Y. High-dose tocopherol acetate therapy in epidermolysis bullosa siblings of the Cockayne-Touraine type. J Dermatol. 1993;20:723–5.
109. Ayres S Jr, Mihan R. Yellow nail syndrome: response to vitamin E. Arch Dermatol. 1973;108:267–8.

110. Prussick R, Ali MA, Rosenthal D, Guyatt G. The protective effect of vitamin E on the hemolysis associated with dapsone treatment in patients with dermatitis herpetiformis. Arch Dermatol. 1992;128:210–3.
111. Cox NH. Vitamin E for dapsone-induced headache. Br J Dermatol. 2002;146:174.
112. Martin-Jimenez M, Diaz-Rubio E, Gonzalez Larriba JL, Sangro B. Failure of high-dose tocopherol to prevent alopecia induced by doxorubicin. N Engl J Med. 1986;315:894–5.
113. Furie B, Bouchard BA, Furie BC. Vitamin K-dependent biosynthesis of gamma-carboxyglutamic acid. Blood. 1999;93:1798–808.
114. Maresz K. Proper calcium use: vitamin K2 as a promoter of bone and cardiovascular health. Integr Med. 2015;14:34–9.
115. Whitlon DS, Sadowski JA, Suttie JW. Mechanism of coumarin action: significance of vitamin K epoxide reductase inhibition. Biochemistry. 1978;17:1371–7.
116. Akella P, Jindal V, Maradana S, Siddiqui AD. Dying to be ill: Munchausen meets warfarin overdose. J Family Med Prim Care. 2019;8:2741–3.
117. Groszek B, Piszczek P. Vitamin K antagonists overdose [article in Polish]. Przegl Lek. 2015;72:468–71.
118. Shirai K, Obara K, Tohgi N, Yamazaki A, Aki R, Hamada Y, Arakawa N, Singh SR, Hoffman RM, Amoh Y. Expression of anti-aging type-XVII collagen (COL17A1/BP180) in hair follicle-associated pluripotent (HAP) stem cells during differentiation. Tissue Cell. 2019;59:33–8.
119. Pullar JM, Carr AV, Vissers MCM. The roles of vitamin C in skin health. Nutrients. 2017;9:866.
120. Sung YK, Hwang SY, Cha SY, Kim SR, Park SY, Kim MK, Kim JC. The hair growth promoting effect of ascorbic acid 2-phosphate, a long-acting vitamin C derivative. J Dermatol Sci. 2006;4:150–2.
121. Kwack MH, Shin SH, Kim SR, Im SU, Han IS, Kim MK, Kim JC, Sung YK. l-Ascorbic acid 2-phosphate promotes elongation of hair shafts via the secretion of insulin-like growth factor-1 from dermal papilla cells through phosphatidylinositol 3-kinase. Br J Dermatol. 2009;160:1157–62.
122. Granger M, Eck P. Dietary vitamin C in human health. Adv Food Nutr Res. 2018;83:281–310.
123. Hirschmann JV, Raugi GJ. Adult scurvy. J Am Acad Dermatol. 1999;41:895–906.
124. Edsall JT. Linus Pauling and vitamin C. Science. 1972;178:696.
125. Moritsugu KP. The 2006 report of the surgeon general: the health consequence of involuntary exposure to tobacco smoke. Am J Prev Med. 2007;32:542–3.
126. Goodwin JS, Tangum MR. Battling quackery: attitudes about micronutrient supplements in American academic medicine. Arch Intern Med. 1998;158:2187–9.
127. Naidu KA. Vitamin C in human health and disease is still a mystery? An overview. Nutr J. 2003;2:7.
128. Thomas LD, Elinder CG, Tiselius HG, Wolk A, Akesson A. Ascorbic acid supplements and kidney stone incidence among men: a prospective study. JAMA Intern Med. 2013;173:386–8.
129. Almohanna HM, Ahmed AA, Tsatalis JP, Tosti A. The role of vitamins and minerals in hair loss: a review. Dermatol Ther (Heidelb). 2019;9:51–70.
130. Hengl T, Herfert J, Soliman A, Schlinzig K, Trüeb RM, Abts HF. Cystine-thiamin-containing hair-growth formulation modulates the response to UV radiation in an in vitro model for growth-limiting conditions of human keratinocytes. J Photochem Photobiol B. 2018;189:318–25.
131. Chiossi G, Neri I, Cavazzuti M, Basso G, Facchinetti F. Hyperemesis gravidarum complicated by Wernicke encephalopathy: background, case report, and review of the literature. Obstet Gynecol Surv. 2006;6:255–68.
132. Lonsdale D. A review of the biochemistry, metabolism and clinical benefits of thiamin(e) and its derivatives. Evid Based Complement Alternat Med. 2006;3:49–59.
133. Katta N, Balla S, Alpert MA. Does long-term furosemide therapy cause thiamine deficiency in patients with heart failure? A focused review. Am J Med. 2006;129:753.

134. Rybicka I, Gliszczynska-Swiglo A. Gluten-free flours from different raw materials as the source of vitamin B 1, B 2, B 3 and B 6. J Nutr Sci Vitaminol (Tokyo). 2017;63:125–32.
135. Riboflavin RR. Encyclopedia of dietary supplements. London and New York: Informa Healthcare; 2010. p. 691–9.
136. Forbat E, Al-Niaimi F, Ali FR. Use of nicotinamide in dermatology. Clin Exp Dermatol. 2017;42(2):137–44.
137. Rolfe HM. A review of nicotinamide: treatment of skin diseases and potential side effects. J Cosmet Dermatol. 2014;13:324–8.
138. Draelos ZD, Jacobson EL, Kim H, Kim M, Jacobson MK. A pilot study evaluating the efficacy of topically applied niacin derivatives for treatment of female pattern alopecia. J Cosmet Dermatol. 2005;4:258–61.
139. Dupré A, Lassère J, Christol B, et al. Traitement des alopecies diffuse chroniques par le panthenol et la D-biotin injectables. Rev Med Toulouse. 1977;123:675–7.
140. Davis MG, Thomas JH, van de Velde S, Boissy Y, Dawson TL Jr, Iveson R, Sutton K. A novel cosmetic approach to treat thinning hair. Br J Dermatol. 2011;165(Suppl 3):24–30.
141. Fernandes RA, Santiago L, Gouveia M, Gonçalo M. Allergic contact dermatitis caused by dexpanthenol-probably a frequent allergen. Contact Dermatitis. 2018;79:276–80.
142. Schalock PC, Storrs FJ, Morrison L. Contact urticaria from panthenol in hair conditioner. Contact Dermatitis. 2000;43:223.
143. Brzezińska-Wcisło L. Evaluation of vitamin B6 and calcium pantothenate effectiveness on hair growth from clinical and trichographic aspects for treatment of diffuse alopecia in women [article in Polish]. Wiad Lek. 2011;54:11–8.
144. Vialkowtisch B. The treatment of seborrheic disease picture and falling hair with vitamin B6 [article in German]. Med Welt. 1962;22:1260–2.
145. Barber GW, Spaeth GL. The successful treatment of homocystinuria with pyridoxine. J Pediatr. 1969;75:463–78.
146. Shelley WB, Rawnsley HM, Morrow G 3rd. Pyridoxine-dependent hair pigmentation in association with homocystinuria. The induction of melanotrichia. Arch Dermatol. 1972;106:228–30.
147. Reinken L, Dapunt O, Kammerlander H. Vitamin B 6 deficiency with intake of oral contraceptives [article in German]. Int J Vitam Nutr Res. 1973;43(1):20–7.
148. van der Steen W, den Heijer T, Groen J. Vitamin B6 deficiency caused by the use of levodopa [article in Dutch]. Ned Tijdschr Geneeskd. 2018;162:D2818.
149. Mintzer S, Skidmore CT, Sperling MR. B-vitamin deficiency in patients treated with antiepileptic drugs. Epilepsy Behav. 2012;24:341–4.
150. No authors listed. Vitamin B6 deficiency following isoniazid therapy. Nutr Rev 1968;26:306–8.
151. Lakdawala N, Grant-Kels JM. Acrodermatitis enteropathica and other nutritional diseases of the folds (intertriginous areas). Clin Dermatol. 2015;33:414–9.
152. van Hunsel F, van de Koppel S, Puijenbroek E, Kant A. Vitamin B6 in health supplements and neuropathy: case series assessment of spontaneously reported cases. Drug Saf. 2018;4:859–69.
153. Vrolijk MF, Opperhuizen A, Jansen EHJM, Hageman GJ, Bast A, Guido R, Haenen GRMM. The vitamin B6 paradox: supplementation with high concentrations of pyridoxine leads to decreased vitamin B6 function. Toxicol In Vitro. 2017;44:206–12.
154. Makino Y, Osada K, Sone H, Sugiyama K, Komai M, Ito M, Tsunoda K, Furukawa Y. Percutaneous absorption of biotin in healthy subjects and in atopic dermatitis patients. J Nutr Sci Vitaminol (Tokyo). 1999;45:347–52.
155. van den Berg H. Bioavailability of biotin. Eur J Clin Nutr. 1997;51(Suppl 1):S60–1.
156. Hayashi A, Mikami Y, Miyamoto K, Kamada N, Sato T, Mizuno S, Naganuma M, Teratani T, Aoki R, Fukuda S, Suda W, Hattori M, Amagai M, Ohyama M, Kanai T. Intestinal dysbiosis and biotin deprivation induce alopecia through overgrowth of Lactobacillus murinus in mice. Cell Rep. 2017;20(7):1513–24.
157. Schulpis KH, Karikas GA, Tjamouranis J, Regoutas S, Tsakiris S. Low serum biotinidase activity in children with valproic acid monotherapy. Epilepsia. 2001;42(10):1359–62.

158. Schulpis KH, Georgala S, Papakonstantinou ED, Michas T, Karikas GA. The effect of isotretinoin on biotinidase activity. Skin Pharmacol Appl Skin Physiol. 1999;12(1–2):28–33.
159. Durance TD. Residual avid in activity in cooked egg white assayed with improved sensitivity. J Food Sci. 1991;56(3):707–9.
160. Brescoll J, Daveluy S. A review of vitamin B12 in dermatology. Am J Clin Dermatol. 2015;16:27–33.
161. Kaur S, Goraya JS. Dermatologic findings of vitamin B(12) deficiency in infants. Pediatr Dermatol. 2018;35:796–9.
162. Demir N, Doğan M, Koç A, Kaba S, Bulan K, Ozkol HU, Doğan SZ. Dermatological findings of vitamin B12 deficiency and resolving time of these symptoms. Cutan Ocul Toxicol. 2014;33:70–3.
163. Noppakun N, Swasdikul D. Reversible hyperpigmentation of skin and nails with white hair due to vitamin B12 deficiency. Arch Dermatol. 1986;122:896–9.
164. Carmel R. Hair and fingernail changes in acquired and congenital pernicious anemia. Arch Intern Med. 1985;145:484–5.
165. Wald NJ, Morris JK, Blakemore C. Public health failure in the prevention of neural tube defects: time to abandon the tolerable upper intake level of folate. Public Health Rev. 2018;39:2.
166. Jirtle RL, Skinner MK. Environmental epigenomics and disease susceptibility. Nat Rev Genet. 2007;8:253–62.
167. Ellis JA. Future directions: gene polymorphism diagnostics relevant to hair. In: Trüeb RM, Tobin DJ, editors. Aging hair. Berlin Heidelberg: Springer; 2010. p. 221.
168. Smelt HJM, Pouwels S, Said M, Smulders JF. Neuropathy by folic acid supplementation in a patient with anaemia and an untreated cobalamin deficiency: a case report. Clin Obes. 2018;8:300–4.
169. Smith AD. Folic acid fortification: the good, the bad, and the puzzle of vitamin B-12. Am J Clin Nutr. 2007;85:3–5.
170. Burr GO, Burr MM. A new deficiency disease produced by the rigid exclusion of fat from the diet. J Biol Chem. 1929;82:35–367.
171. Simopoulos A. Omega 3 fatty acids in wild plants, nuts and seeds. Asia Pac J Cin Nutr. 2002;11:163–73.
172. Gale MM, Crawford MA, Woodford MH. The fatty acid composition of adipose and muscle tissue in domestic and free-living ruminants. Biochem J. 1969;113:6P.
173. van Vliet T, Katan MB. Lower ratio of n-3 to n-6 fatty acids in cultured than in wild fish. Am J Clin Nutr. 1990;51:1–2.
174. Endres S, Ghorbani R, Kelley VE, Georgilis K, Lonnemann G, van der Meer JW, Cannon JG, Rogers TS, Klempner MS, Weber PC, et al. The effect of dietary supplementation with n-3 polyunsaturated fatty acids on the synthesis of interleukin-1 and tumor necrosis factor by mononuclear cells. N Engl J Med. 1989;320:265–71.
175. Caughey GE, Mantzioris E, Gibson RA, Cleland LG, James MJ. The effect on human tumor necrosis factor alpha and interleukin 1 beta production of diets enriched in n-3 fatty acids from vegetable oil or fish oil. Am J Clin Nutr. 1996;63:116–22.
176. Trebble T, Arden NK, Stroud MA, Wootton SA, Burdge GC, Miles EA, Ballinger AB, Thompson RL, Calder PC. Inhibition of tumour necrosis factor-alpha and interleukin 6 production by mononuclear cells following dietary fish-oil supplementation in healthy men and response to antioxidant co-supplementation. Br J Nutr. 2003;90:405–12.
177. Meydani SN, Endres S, Woods MM, Goldin BR, Soo C, Morrill-Labrode A, Dinarello CA, Gorbach SL. Oral (n-3) fatty acid supplementation suppresses cytokine production and lymphocyte proliferation: comparison between young and older women. J Nutr. 1991;121:547–55.
178. Cordain L, Lindeberg S, Hurtado M, et al. Acne vulgaris: a disease of Western civilization. Arch Dermatol. 2002;138:1584–90.
179. Truchetet E, Brändle I, Grosshans E. Skin changes, pathophysiology and therapy in deficiency of essential fatty acids. Z Hautkr. 1988;63:290–301.
180. Schroeter AL, Tucker SB. Essential fatty acid deficiency. Arch Dermatol. 1978;114:800–1.

181. Kirby NA, Hester SL, Bauer JE. Dietary fats and the skin and coat of dogs. J Am Vet Med Assoc. 2007;230:1641–4.
182. Munkhbayar S, Jang S, Cho A, Choi S, Yup Shin C, Chul Eun H, Han Kim K, Kwon O. Role of arachidonic acid in promoting hair growth. Ann Dermatol. 2016;28:55–64.
183. van Breda SG, de Kok TM, van Delft JH. Mechanisms of colorectal and lung cancer prevention by vegetables: a genomic approach. J Nutr Biochem. 2008;19:139–57.
184. Palermo M, Pellegrini N, Fogliano V. The effect of cooking on the phytochemical content of vegetables. J Sci Food Agric. 2014;94:1057–70.
185. Dewanto V, Wu X, Adom KK, Liu RH. Thermal processing enhances the nutritional value of tomatoes by increasing total antioxidant activity. J Agric Food Chem. 2002;50(10):3010–4.
186. Lambert WC, Gagna CE, Lambert MW. Trichothiodystrophy: photosensitive, TTD-P, TTD, Tay syndrome. Adv Exp Med Biol. 2010;685:106–10.
187. Itin PH, Sarasin A, Pittelkow MR. Trichothiodystrophy: update on the sulfur-deficient brittle hair syndromes. J Am Acad Dermatol. 2001;44:891–920.
188. Liang C, Morris A, Schlücker S, Imoto K, Price VH, Menefee E, Wincovitch SM, Levin IW, Tamura D, Strehle KR, Kraemer KH, DiGiovanna JJ. Structural and molecular hair abnormalities in trichothiodystrophy. J Invest Dermatol. 2006;126:2210–6.
189. Liang C, Kraemer KH, Morris A, Schiffmann R, Price VH, Menefee E, DiGiovanna JJ. Characterization of tiger-tail banding and hair shaft abnormalities in trichothiodystrophy. J Am Acad Dermatol. 2005;52:224–32.
190. Haider LM, Schwingshackl L, Hoffmann G, Ekmekcioglu C. The effect of vegetarian diets on iron status in adults: a systematic review and meta-analysis. Crit Rev Food Sci Nutr. 2018;58:1359–74.
191. Bregy A, Trueb RM. No association between serum ferritin levels >10 microg/l and hair loss activity in women. Dermatology. 2008;217:1–6.
192. Lynch SR, Cook JD. Interaction of vitamin C and iron. Ann N Y Acad Sci. 1980;355:32–44.
193. Rushton DH. Nutritional factors and hair loss. Clin Exp Dermatol. 2002;27:396–404.
194. Chevrant-Breton J, Simon M, Bourel M, Ferrand B. Cutaneous manifestations of idiopathic hemochromatosis. Study of 100 cases. Arch Dermatol. 1977;113:161–5.
195. Kew MC, Asare GA. Dietary iron overload in the African and hepatocellular carcinoma. Liver Int. 2007;27(6):735–41.
196. Fleming RE, Ponka P. Iron overload in human disease. N Engl J Med. 2012;366:348–59.
197. Ward DM, Kaplan J. Ferroportin-mediated iron transport: expression and regulation. Biochim Biophys Acta. 2012;1823:1426–33.
198. Schell H, Kiesewetter F, Seidel C, von Hintzenstern J. Cell cycle kinetics of human anagen scalp hair bulbs in thyroid disorders determined by DNA flow cytometry. Dermatologica. 1991;182:23–6.
199. Billoni N, Buan B, Gautier B, Gaillard O, Mahé YF, Bernard BA. Thyroid hormone receptor beta1 is expressed in the human hair follicle. Br J Dermatol. 2000;142:645–52.
200. Thomsen K. Dermatitis herpetiformis. A case provoked by iodine. Br J Dermatol. 1974;91:221–4.
201. Reitamo S, Reunala T, Konttinen YT, Saksela O, Salo OP. Inflammatory cells, IgA, C3, fibrin and fibronectin in skin lesions in dermatitis herpetiformis. Br J Dermatol. 1981;105:167–77.
202. Haffenden GP, Blenkinsopp WK, Ring NP, Wojnarowska F, Fry L. The potassium iodide patch test in the dermatitis herpetiformis in relation to treatment with a gluten-free diet and dapsone. Br J Dermatol. 1980;103:313–7.
203. Senn HJ. Paracelsus, scientific research and supportive care—500 years after! Support Care Cancer. 1993;1:230–2.
204. Ogawa Y, Kawamura T, Shimada S. Zinc and skin biology. Arch Biochem Biophys. 2016;611:113–9.
205. Foster M, Chu A, Petocz P, Samman S. Effect of vegetarian diets on zinc status: a systematic review and meta-analysis of studies in humans. J Sci Food Agric. 2013;93:2362–71.
206. Maret W, Sandstead HH. Zinc requirements and the risks and benefits of zinc supplementation. J Trace Elem Med Biol. 2006;20:3–18.

207. Mazokopakis EE, Papadakis JA, Papadomanolaki MG, et al. Effects of 12 months treatment with L-selenomethionine on serum anti-TPO levels in patients with Hashimoto's thyroiditis. Thyroid. 2007;17:609–12.
208. Ralston NVC, Raymond LJ. Dietary selenium's protective effects against methylmercury toxicity. Toxicology. 2010;278:112–23.
209. Ralston NV, Ralston CR, Blackwell JL III, Raymond LJ. Dietary and tissue selenium in relation to methylmercury toxicity. Neurotoxicology. 2008;29:802–11.
210. Penglase S, Hamre K, Ellingsen S. Selenium prevents downregulation of antioxidant selenoprotein genes by methylmercury. Free Radic Biol Med. 2014;75:95–104.
211. Usuki F, Yamashita A, Fujimura M. Post-transcriptional defects of antioxidant selenoenzymes cause oxidative stress under methylmercury exposure. J Biol Chem. 2011;286:6641–9.
212. Ohi G, Seki H, Maeda H, Yagyu H. Protective effect of selenite against methylmercury toxicity: observations concerning time, dose and route factors in the development of selenium attenuation. Ind Health. 1975;13(3):93–9.
213. Carvalho CML, Chew Hashemy SI, Hashemy J, et al. Inhibition of the human thioredoxin system: a molecular mechanism of mercury toxicity. J Biol Chem. 2008;283(18):11,913–23.
214. Mac Farquhar JK, Broussard DL, Melstrom P, Hutchinson R, Wolkin A, Martin C, Burk RF, Dunn JR, Green AL, Hammond R, Schaffner W, Jones TF. Acute selenium toxicity associated with a dietary supplement. Arch Intern Med. 2010;170:256–61.
215. Richmond SJ, Gunadasa S, Bland M, Macpherson H. Copper bracelets and magnetic wrist straps for rheumatoid arthritis—analgesic and anti-inflammatory effects: a randomised double-blind placebo controlled crossover trial. PLoS One. 2013;8(9):e71529.
216. Richmond SJ, Brown SR, Campion PD, Porter AJL, Moffett JAK, Jackson DA, Featherstone VA, Taylor AJ. Therapeutic effects of magnetic and copper bracelets in osteoarthritis: a randomised placebo-controlled crossover trial. Complement Ther Med. 2009;17(5–6):249–56.
217. Myers Hill G, Carlson SM. Copper and zinc nutritional issues for agricultural animal production. Biol Trace Elem Res. 2019;188:148–59.
218. Valko M, Morris H, Cronin MT. Metals, toxicity and oxidative stress. Curr Med Chem. 2005;12:1161–208.
219. Kaneshiro B, Aeby T. Long-term safety, efficacy, and patient acceptability of the intrauterine Copper T-380A contraceptive device. Int J Womens Health. 2010;2:211–20.
220. Hardeman J, Weiss BD. Intrauterine devices: an update. Am Fam Physician. 2014;89:445–50.
221. Melnik BC, Plewig G, Daldrup T, Borchard F, Pfeiffer B, Zahn H. Green hair: guidelines for diagnosis and therapy. J Am Acad Dermatol. 1986;15(5 Pt 1):1065–8.
222. Tosti A, Mattioli D, Misciali C. Green hair caused by copper present in cosmetic plant extracts. Dermatologica. 1991;182:204–5.
223. Lampe RM, Henderson AL, Hansen GH. Green hair. JAMA. 1977;237:2092.
224. Marsh JM, Iveson R, Flagler MJ, Davis MG, Newland AB, Greis KD, Sun Y, Chaudhary T, Aistrup ER. Role of copper in photochemical damage to hair. Int J Cosmet Sci. 2014;36:32–8.
225. Marangon K, Devaraj S, Tirosh O, Packer L, Jialal I. Comparison of the effect of α-lipoic acid and α-tocopherol supplementation on measures of oxidative stress. Free Radic Biol Med. 1999;27:1114–21.
226. Brewer GJ. Copper excess, zinc deficiency, and cognition loss in Alzheimer's disease. Biofactors. 2012;38:107–13.
227. Brewer GJ. The risk of copper toxicity contributing to cognitive decline in the aging population and to Alzheimer's disease. J Am Coll Nutr. 2009;28:238–42.
228. Faller P. Copper and zinc binding to amyloid-beta: coordination, dynamics, aggregation, reactivity and metal-ion transfer. Chembiochem. 2009;10:2837–45.
229. Hureau C, Faller P. A beta-mediated ROS production by Cu ions: structural insights, mechanisms and relevance to Alzheimer's disease. Biochimie. 2009;91:1212–7.
230. Kim SG, Kim KW, Park EW, Choi D. Silicon-induced cell wall fortification of rice leaves: a possible cellular mechanism of enhanced host resistance to blast. Phytopathology. 2002;92:1095–103.

231. Martin KR. Chapter 14. Silicon: the health benefits of a metalloid. In: Sigel A, Sigel H, Sigel RKO, editors. Interrelations between essential metal ions and human diseases, Metal Ions in Life Sciences, vol. 13. New York: Springer; 2013. p. 451–73. https://doi. org/10.1007/978-94-007-7500-8_14. ISBN: 978-94-007-7499-5.
232. Barel A, Calomme M, Timchenko A, De Paepe K, Demeester N, Rogiers V, Clarys P, Vanden BD. Effect of oral intake of choline-stabilized orthosilicic acid on skin, nails and hair in women with photodamaged skin. Arch Dermatol Res. 2005;297:147–53.
233. Fabre B, Geay B, Beaufils P. Thiaminase activity in Equisetum arvense and its extracts. Plant Med Phytother. 1993;26:190–7.
234. Food and Nutrition Board, Institute of Medicine. Dietary reference intakes for energy, carbohydrates, fiber, fat, fatty acids, cholesterol, protein, and amino acids. Washington DC: National Academies Press; 2002.
235. American Academy of Pediatrics Committee on Nutrition. Breastfeeding and the use of human milk. Pediatrics. 2012;129:e827–41.
236. St-Onge MP, Gallagher D. Body composition changes with aging: the cause or the result of alterations in metabolic rate and macronutrient oxidation? Nutrition. 2010;26:152–5.
237. Javed F, He Q, Davidson LE, Thornton JC, Albu J, Boxt L, Krasnow N, Elia M, Kang P, Heshka S, Gallagher D. Brain and high metabolic rate organ mass: contributions to resting energy expenditure beyond fat-free mass. Am J Clin Nutr. 2010;91:907–12.
238. Lynfield YL. Effect of pregnancy on the human hair cycle. J Invest Dermatol. 1960;35:323–7.
239. Barzilai D, Paldi E. A critical review of the Chiari-Frommel syndrome. Gynaecologia. 1966;162:216–24.
240. Matsuzaki S, Endo M, Ueda Y, Mimura K, Kakigano A, Egawa-Takata T, Kumasawa K, Yoshino K, Kimura T. A case of acute Sheehan's syndrome and literature review: a rare but life-threatening complication of postpartum hemorrhage. BMC Pregnancy Childbirth. 2017;17:188.
241. Ippen M, Ippen H. Approaches to a prophylaxis of skin ageing. J Soc Cosmet Chemists. 1965;16:305–8.
242. Solly S. Clinical lectures on paralysis. Lancet. 1856;ii:641–3.
243. Mosley JG, Gibbs CC. Premature grey hair and hair loss among smokers: a new opportunity for health education? BMJ. 1996;313:1616.
244. Trüeb RM. Association between smoking and hair loss: another opportunity for health education against smoking? Dermatology. 2003;206:189–91.
245. Hayakawa K, Shimizu T, Ohba Y, et al. Intrapair differences of physical aging and longevity in identical twins. Acta Genet Med Gemellol (Roma). 1992;41:177–85.
246. Su L-S, Chen TH-H. Association of androgenetic alopecia with smoking and its prevalence among Asian men. Arch Dermatol. 2007;143:1401–6.
247. Tur E, Yosipovitch G, Oren-Vulfs S. Chronic and acute effects of cigarette smoking on skin blood flow. Angiology. 1992;43:328–35.
248. Raitio A, Risteli J, Väjäkangas K, Oikarinen A. Evidence of disturbed collagen metabolism in smokers—a possible etiologic factor for accelerated skin aging. J Invest Dermatol. 2000;114:822.
249. Laurent P, Janoff A, Kagan HM. Cigarette smoke blocks cross-linking of elastin in vitro. Annu Rev Respir Dis. 1983;127:189–94.
250. Osawa Y, Tochigi B, Tochigi M, et al. Aromatase inhibitors in cigarette smoke, tobacco leaves and other plants. J Enzyme Inhib. 1990;4:187–200.
251. Dardour JC, Pugash E, Aziza R. The one-stage preauricular flap for male pattern baldness: long-term results and risk factors. Plast Reconstr Surg. 1988;81:907–12.
252. Haley NJ, Hoffmann D. Analysis for nicotine and cotinine in hair to determine cigarette smoker status. Clin Chem. 1985;31:1598–600.
253. Liu CS, Kao SH, Wei YH. Smoking-associated mitochondrial DNA mutations in human hair follicles. Environ Mol Mutagen. 1997;30:47–55.
254. Yin L, Morita A, Tsuji T. Alterations of extracellular matrix induced by tobacco smoke extract. Arch Dermatol Res. 2000;292:188–94.

255. Philpott MP, Sander DA, Bowen J, Kealey T. Effects of interleukins, colony stimulating factor and tumour necrosis factor on human hair follicle growth in vitro: a possible role for interleukin-1 and tumour necrosis factor-α in alopecia areata. Br J Dermatol. 1996;135:942–8.

256. Naito A, Midorikawa T, Yoshino T, Ohdera M. Lipid peroxides induce early onset of catagen phase in murine hair cycles. Int J Mol Med. 2008;22:725–9.

257. Bahta AW, Farjo N, Farjo B, Philpott M. Premature senescence of balding dermal papilla cells in vitro is associated with p16(INK4a) expression. J Invest Dermatol. 2008;128(5):1088–94.

258. Upton JH, Hannen RF, Bahta AW, Farjo N, Farjo B, Philpott MP. Oxidative stress-associated senescence in dermal papilla cells of men with androgenetic alopecia. J Invest Dermatol. 2015;135:1244–52.

259. D'Agostini F, Balansky R, Pesce C, et al. Induction of alopecia in mice exposed to cigarette smoking. Toxicol Lett. 2000;114:117–23.

260. D'Agostini F, Fiallo P, Pennisi TM, De Flora S. Chemoprevention of smoke-induced alopecia in mice by oral administration of L-cystine and vitamin B6. J Dermatol Sci. 2007;46:189–98.

261. Reicks M, Calvert RJ, Hathcock JN. Effects of prolonged acetaminophen ingestion and dietary methionine on mouse liver glutathione. Drug Nutr Interact. 1988;5:351–63.

262. Cruz-Hernandez C, Oliveira M, Pescia G, Moulin J, Masserey-Elmelegy I, Dionisi F, Destaillats F. Lipase inhibitor orlistat decreases incorporation of eicosapentaenoic and docosahexaenoic acids in rat tissues. Nutr Res. 2010;30:134–40.

263. Moss M. Drugs as anti-nutrients. J Nutr Environ Med. 2007;16:149–66.

264. Henley S. Women on the pill are opening up a small case of side effects every morning. Body Forum. 1977;2:20.

Nutritional Disorders of the Hair and Their Management

5

5.1 Inborn Errors of Metabolism

In the year of his death, English physician William Harvey (1578–1657) made the statement, "Nature is nowhere accustomed more openly to display her secret mysteries than in cases where she shows tracings of her workings apart from the beaten paths; nor is there any better way to advance the proper practice of medicine than to give our minds to the discovery of the usual law of nature, by careful investigation of cases of rarer forms of disease." (Letter IX, to John Vlackveld, April 24 1657).

Harvey was among the league of physicians, who—starting in the sixteenth century—used experimental research to challenge the prevailing medical theories from ancient Greece, dogmatically followed in Europe and the Middle East since they were laid down by Galen 1400 years earlier. Harvey himself is credited with the first known detailed description of the systemic circulation and properties of blood being pumped to the brain and body by the heart [1].

Particularly among the genetic disorders, Harvey's paradigm holds true for the observations on the rare inborn errors of metabolism of copper, zinc, biotin, and amino acids, establishing our understanding of their role in hair growth and pigmentation.

At the turn of the century, English physician Sir Archibald Garrod (1857–1936) introduced the term of inborn errors of metabolism, while he discovered alkaptonuria, recognizing its inheritance [2]. Inborn errors of metabolism occur when some enzyme involved in metabolism is abnormal due to a mutation in the gene encoding the respective enzyme. The affected enzyme may be either deficient or totally absent.

The inborn errors of metabolism often represent serious health disorders that necessitate early recognition and rigorous treatment. For some, newborn testing is routinely performed within the respective screening programs, since they are clinically only detectable after irreversible usually central nervous system damage has occurred, e.g., phenylketonuria (Guthrie test). For others, the associated hair abnormality may serve as a marker of disease, e.g., Menkes kinky hair. Finally, genetic counseling is recommended to assess risk and to identify other affected family members.

© Springer Nature Switzerland AG 2020
R. M. Trüeb, *Nutrition for Healthy Hair*,
https://doi.org/10.1007/978-3-030-59920-1_5

5.1.1 Copper (Menkes Kinky Hair Syndrome and Wilson's Disease)

Menkes kinky hair syndrome, also known as *Menkes disease*, is named after its original describer, Austrian-born American pediatric neurologist and author of fictional novels and plays ("The Last Inquisitor," "After the Tempest," "The Angry Puppet Syndrome") John Hans Menkes (1928–2008) in 1962 [3].

The condition represents a rare X-linked recessive disorder caused by mutations in genes coding for the copper-transport protein ATP7A resulting in copper deficiency [4]. The ATP7A gene encodes a transmembrane protein that transports copper across the cell membranes. As the result of a mutation in the ATP7A gene, copper is poorly distributed to cells in the body, and rather accumulates in some tissues, such as the small intestine and kidneys, while the brain and other tissues have unusually low levels. The decreased supply of copper affects the activity of numerous copper-containing enzymes necessary for the structure and function of bone, skin, hair, blood vessels, and nervous system, such as ascorbic acid oxidase, tyrosinase, and lysyl oxidase [5].

Affected infants may be born prematurely, with symptoms usually appearing in infancy, typically after a 2- to 3-month period of normal or slightly retarded development that is followed by developmental delay. Patients exhibit weak muscle tone, failure to thrive, hypothermia, sagging facial features with plump cheeks, pale and lax skin, and seizures. Arteries in the brain are twisted with frayed and split inner walls and the risk of rupture or blockage of the respective arteries. Osteoporosis may result in fractures, and there can be extensive degeneration of the gray matter of the brain with subsequent nervous system deterioration.

The hair appears strikingly peculiar: kinky, colorless or silvery, and brittle. Therefore, Menkes syndrome can be suspected upon optical microscopic examination of the hair to view characteristic abnormalities, and further corroborated by blood tests of the copper and ceruloplasmin levels. X-rays of the skull and skeleton are conducted to detect respective abnormalities in bone formation.

The occipital horn syndrome is considered a mild form of Menkes syndrome [6] that begins in early to middle childhood, and is characterized by calcium deposits at the base of the skull, coarse hair, and loose skin and joints, and therefore sometimes it is also called X-linked cutis laxa or Ehlers-Danlos syndrome type 9.

Like all X-linked recessive conditions, Menkes disease is more common in males than in females. About 30% of cases are due to new mutations, and 70% are inherited, almost always maternally. One European study reported a frequency of 1 in 254,000 [7].

There is no cure for Menkes disease. Early treatment with injections of copper supplements in the form of acetate salts may be of some benefit. The earlier the treatment is given, the better the prognosis [8]. Management is otherwise symptomatic and supportive with the aim of helping to relieve symptoms, including pain medication, anti-seizure medication, tube feeding, and physical and occupational therapy. Since 70% of cases are inherited, genetic testing of the mother can be performed to search for a mutation in the ATP7A gene. Pili torti (Fig. 5.1) was observed in all affected males and in 43% of the females studied. The presence of pili torti

Fig. 5.1 Pili torti
(scanning electron
microscopy)

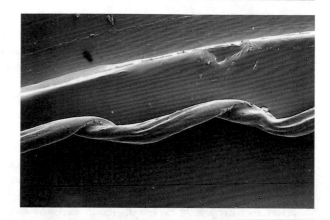

may be considered a reliable diagnostic feature of the carrier state. Suggestions are given for evaluation of the hair in individuals in Menkes pedigrees [9].

The counterpart of Menkes disease is *Wilson's disease* that represents a genetic disorder in which excess copper builds up in the body. It is inherited in an autosomal recessive manner and is due to a mutation in the Wilson's disease protein (ATP7B) gene. The respective gene codes for a P-type (cation transport enzyme) ATPase that transports copper into bile and incorporates it into ceruloplasmin. The net result is that copper accumulates in the liver tissue, while ceruloplasmin is secreted in a form that lacks copper (termed apoceruloplasmin) and is rapidly degraded in the bloodstream. When the amount of copper in the liver overwhelms the proteins that bind it, it causes oxidative damage through a process known as Fenton chemistry that eventually leads to chronic active hepatitis, fibrosis, and cirrhosis of the liver. At the same time, the liver releases copper into the bloodstream that is not bound to ceruloplasmin. The free copper precipitates throughout the body and particularly in the kidneys, eyes, and brain. In the brain, most copper is deposited in the basal ganglia. These areas normally participate in the coordination of movement as well as play a role in neurocognitive processes. Damage to these areas, again by Fenton chemistry, produces the neuropsychiatric symptoms of Wilson's disease [4].

Fenton's reagent is a solution of hydrogen peroxide with ferrous iron as a catalyst that is used to oxidize contaminants or wastewaters. Fenton's reagent can be used to destroy organic compounds, and was originally developed in the 1890s by the British chemist Henry John Horstman Fenton (1854–1929) as an analytical reagent. The Fenton's reaction has importance in biology because it involves the creation of free radicals by chemicals that are present in vivo. Transition metal ions such as iron and copper donate or accept free electrons via intracellular reactions and help in creating free radicals. Most intracellular iron is in ferric (+3 ion) form and must be reduced to the ferrous (+2) form to take part in Fenton's reaction. Superoxide ions and transition metals act in a synergistic manner in the creation of free radical damage [10]. Although the clinical significance is as yet not fully elucidated, it is one of the viable reasons to avoid iron supplementation in patients with active infections [11].

Symptoms of Wilson's disease are typically related to the brain and liver. Liver-related symptoms include vomiting, weakness, ascites, peripheral edema, jaundice, and pruritus. Brain-related symptoms include tremors, muscle stiffness, trouble speaking, and personality changes. Symptoms usually begin between the ages of 5 and 35 years. People with liver problems tend to come to medical attention earlier, usually in childhood or in teenage, and then those with neurological and psychiatric symptoms, who tend to be in their 20s or older [12].

Deposits of copper in a ring around the cornea, so-called Kayser–Fleischer rings, represent a pathognomonic sign, and may be seen either directly or on slit-lamp examination.

There is no totally reliable diagnostic test for Wilson's disease, but levels of ceruloplasmin and copper in the blood, as well as of the amount of copper excreted in urine during a 24-h period, are together used to form an approximation of the amount of copper in the body. The gold standard remains a liver biopsy that is assessed microscopically for the degree of steatosis and cirrhosis, and with histochemistry and quantification of copper [13]. If there are neurological symptoms, magnetic resonance imaging (MRI) of the brain is usually performed; this shows hyperintensities in the basal ganglia in the T2 setting [14]. MRI may also demonstrate the characteristic "face of the giant panda" pattern [15].

No hair abnormalities have been noted in Wilson's disease.

For management of the condition, a diet low in copper-containing foods is recommended with avoidance of mushrooms, nuts, chocolate, dried fruit, liver, sesame products, and shellfish. Cookware in which copper is the main structural element is sometimes manufactured without a lining when intended to be used for any of number of specific culinary tasks, such as preparing preserves or meringues. Otherwise, copper cookware is lined with a nonreactive metal to prevent contact between acidic foods and structural copper element of the cookware. Continuous, small exposures of acidic foods to copper may result in toxicity in cases where either surface area interaction potentials are significant or pH is exceptionally low and concentrated in the case of cooking for example with vinegar or wine.

Copper is also a constituent of tobacco smoke [16]. The tobacco plant readily absorbs and accumulates heavy metals, such as copper from the surrounding soil into its leaves. These are readily absorbed into the user's body following smoke inhalation [17].

Medical treatments available for Wilson's disease either increase the removal of copper from the body or prevent the absorption of copper from the diet. Generally, penicillamine or trientine hydrochloride is used as a chelating agent to bind copper and lead to its excretion in the urine. Once all results have returned to normal, zinc acetate may be used instead of chelators to maintain stable copper levels in the body. Zinc stimulates metallothionein, an intestinal protein that binds copper and prevents its absorption and transport to the liver [14].

5.1.2   Zinc (Acrodermatitis Enteropathica)

Acrodermatitis enteropathica is a rare autosomal recessive metabolic disorder affecting the uptake of zinc through the inner lining of the duodenum and jejunum and resulting in severe zinc deficiency. It is caused by mutations in the SLC39A4 (solute carrier family 39 member 4) gene, which determines a congenital deficiency of the zinc transporter protein zinc ligand-binding protein 4 (ZIP4). This can only be corrected by a high dietary intake of zinc that allows for a small fraction of zinc to be absorbed paracellularly, without the aid of ZIP4 [18].

Since zinc is involved in the function of approximately 100 enzymes in the human body, deficiency results in multiple signs and symptoms, including growth retardation, impaired immune function, and multiple skin and gastrointestinal lesions. Zinc is an essential cofactor of numerous metal enzymes and an important structural component of gene regulatory proteins [19].

The clinical manifestations of acrodermatitis enteropathica and acquired zinc deficiency are similar, and consist of the three essential symptoms, periorificial and acral dermatitis, alopecia, and diarrhea, and in acrodermatitis enteropathica they usually manifest during childhood after weaning from breast milk. The disease begins with symmetrical erythematous, squamous, or eczematous lesions, sometimes vesiculobullous or pustular lesions, located around perioral, anogenital, and acral areas. Other signs of cutaneous, mucous membrane and skin appendage involvement include glossitis, gingivitis, stomatitis, diffuse alopecia, loss of eyelashes and eyebrows, onychodystrophy, onycholysis, and pachyonychia. Secondary bacterial infections or candidiasis are common [20].

The diagnosis is based on clinical suspicion, and is confirmed by low plasma zinc levels, light microscopy of skin biopsy, and rapid clinical response to zinc supplementation. Low serum alkaline phosphatase value, a zinc-dependent metal protease, has an indirect role in establishing the diagnosis. Histopathologic findings are a pale psoriasiform necrolysis, by cytoplasmic vacuolization, and focal or confluent necrosis of keratinocytes in the superficial part of the epidermis with parakeratosis [20].

Without treatment, the condition is fatal. Treatment includes lifelong dietary zinc supplementation, with initial dosages of 5–10 mg/kg/day of elemental zinc, followed by maintenance doses of 1–2 mg/kg/day taken orally. Zinc may be administered as sulfate, acetate, gluconate, or amino acid chelates. Zinc and copper levels should be monitored regularly. Dosages need to be increased during periods of growth, such as adolescence and during pregnancy, when relapses can occur. With adherence to lifelong zinc substitution therapy, the prognosis is good [21]. Genetic counseling is recommended to identify other affected family members before the onset of symptoms.

5.1.3 Biotin (Biotinidase and Holocarboxylase Synthetase Deficiency)

Biotinidase deficiency is a rare autosomal recessive metabolic disorder in which the vitamin biotin, also called vitamin B7, is not released from proteins in the diet during digestion or from normal protein turnover in the cell. Biotin is a vitamin that is found in foods such as liver, egg yolks, and milk, and is chemically bound to proteins. Without biotinidase activity, biotin cannot be separated from the foods and consequently cannot be utilized by the body. It also cannot be recycled from enzymes that are important in metabolism.

Biotin is essential for the normal production and breakdown of proteins, fats, and carbohydrates in the body. When it is lacking, specific biotin-dependent enzymes called carboxylases cannot process the proteins, fats, or carbohydrates. Functionally, there is no significant difference between genetic deficiency of biotin-related enzyme activity and dietary biotin deficiency.

Symptoms of the deficiency are caused by the deficiency of biotin molecules that are needed for cell growth, production of fatty acids, and metabolism of fats and amino acids. The symptoms include seizures, hypotonia and muscle/limb weakness, ataxia, paresis, hearing loss, optic atrophy, seborrheic-like dermatitis, and alopecia.

Signs and symptoms of a biotinidase deficiency can appear several days after birth, and if untreated may lead to coma and death. Symptoms can also appear later in life as late-onset biotinidase deficiency with similar, but more mild, symptoms. If an individual survives the neonatal period there likely is some residual activity of biotin-related enzymes. Symptom severity is predictably correlated with the severity of the enzyme defect. Profound biotinidase deficiency refers to situations where enzyme activity is 10% or less. Individuals with partial biotinidase deficiency may have enzyme activity of 10–30%. Studies have noted individuals who were asymptomatic until adolescence or early adulthood [22]. One study pointed out that untreated individuals may not show symptoms until age 21 [22]. Furthermore, in rare cases, even individuals with profound deficiencies of biotinidase can be asymptomatic [23].

Individuals lacking functional biotinidase enzymes can still have normal carboxylase activity if they ingest adequate amounts of biotin. The standard treatment regimen calls for 5–10 mg of biotin per day.

Biotinidase deficiency can be found by genetic testing. This is often done at birth as part of newborn screening [24], and is considered as a very effective secondary prevention program [25]. Based on the results of worldwide screening of biotinidase deficiency in 1991, the incidence of the disorder is 5 in 137,401 for profound biotinidase deficiency, and 1 in 109,921 for partial biotinidase deficiency. Carrier frequency in the general population is approximately 1 in 120 [26].

Holocarboxylase synthetase deficiency is yet another autosomal recessive metabolic disorder in which the body is unable to utilize biotin effectively. The condition is also classified as a multiple carboxylase deficiency, a group of disorders characterized by impaired activity of biotin-dependent enzymes. Symptoms are very similar to biotinidase deficiency, and treatment with large doses of biotin is the same [27].

5.1.4 Amino Acids

Amino acids are organic compounds containing amine (–NH$_2$) and carboxyl (–COOH) functional groups, along with a side chain (R group) specific to each amino acid. The key elements of an amino acid are carbon (C), hydrogen (H), oxygen (O), and nitrogen (N), although other elements are found in the side chains of certain amino acids, such as sulfur (S). In biochemistry, amino acids having both the amine and the carboxylic acid groups attached to the first (alpha-) carbon atom have particular importance. They are known as 2-, alpha-, or α-amino acids (generic formula H2NCHRCOOH in most cases, where R is an organic substituent known as a side chain; often the term amino acid is used to refer specifically to these). They include the protein-building or proteinogenic amino acids, which combine into peptide chains (polypeptides) to form the building blocks of a vast array of proteins, and the non-proteinogenic amino acids. Both proteinogenic and non-proteinogenic amino acids have many biological functions. In the form of proteins, amino acid residues form the second largest component after water of human muscles and other tissues, while the nonprotein amino acids have important roles as metabolic intermediates and participate in a number of processes such as neurotransmitter transport and biosynthesis.

When taken up into the human body from the diet, the amino acids either are used to synthesize proteins and other biomolecules or are oxidized to urea and carbon dioxide as a source of energy. The oxidation pathway starts with the removal of the amino group by a transaminase. The amino group is then fed into the urea cycle, while the other product of transamination is a keto acid that enters the citric acid cycle. The glucogenic amino acids can also be converted into glucose for energy, through gluconeogenesis.

The dietary requirements for amino acids depend on the age and health of the individual, so it is hard to make general statements. About 500 naturally occurring amino acids are known, though only 20 are encoded directly by triplet codons in the genetic code. They are known as the standard amino acids.

Of the 20 standard amino acids, 9 (histidine, isoleucine, leucine, lysine, methionine, phenylalanine, threonine, tryptophan, and valine) are called essential amino acids because they cannot be synthesized de novo, so they must be obtained from food. In addition, six other amino acids are considered conditionally essential in the human diet, meaning their synthesis can be limited under special pathophysiological conditions, such as prematurity in the infant or individuals in severe catabolic distress. These six are arginine, cysteine, glycine, glutamine, proline, and tyrosine. Five amino acids are dispensable in humans, meaning they can be synthesized in sufficient quantities in the body. These five are alanine, aspartic acid, asparagine, glutamic acid, and serine.

If one of the essential amino acids is less than needed for an individual the utilization of other amino acids will be hindered and thus protein synthesis will be less than what it usually is. Nevertheless, essential amino acid deficiency should be distinguished from protein-energy malnutrition. The amino acids that are essential in the human diet were established in a series of trials led by American biochemist and nutritionist William Cumming Rose (1887–1985) involving diets in healthy male graduate students, consisting of corn starch, sucrose, butterfat without protein, corn oil, inorganic salts, known vitamins, liver extract, and mixtures of highly purified individual amino acids. Rose noted that the symptoms of nervousness, exhaustion, and dizziness were encountered to a greater or lesser extent whenever human subjects were deprived of an essential amino acid [28].

Finally, dietary exposure to the nonstandard amino acid β-methylamino-L-alanine (BMAA) has been linked to human neurodegenerative diseases [29, 30]. BMAA is a derivative of the amino acid alanine with a methylamino group on the side chain produced by cyanobacteria, and has been found in aquatic organisms with cyanobacterial symbionts. BMAA can cross the blood–brain barrier, where it may be disincorporated into nascent proteins in place of L-serine, possibly causing protein misfolding and aggregation, both features of Alzheimer's disease, Parkinson's disease, and amyotrophic lateral sclerosis (ALS). High concentrations of BMAA are present in shark fins [31], which is why the consumption of shark fin soup in Chinese cuisine may pose a serious health risk and should therefore be considered obsolete.

Inborn errors of metabolism occur in the metabolism of all nutrients, including amino acids. Inborn errors of amino acid metabolism are metabolic disorders which impair the synthesis and degradation of amino acids, occurring as a result of decreased synthesis of products, accumulation of intermediates, or formation of alternate metabolites. Over 50 inborn errors of amino acid metabolism are known. Many result in neurological abnormalities and mental retardation. Therefore, early diagnosis and therapy are important to prevent irreversible neurological defects. The treatment generally consists of restricted intake or exclusion of the respective amino acid from the diet.

Inborn errors of amino acid metabolism relevant to the condition of the hair are [32] homocystinuria, Hartnup disease, phenylketonuria, and methionine malabsorption syndrome (or oasthouse urine disease), and others are citrullinemia and argininosuccinic aciduria. The latter are also classified as urea cycle disorders. The urea cycle represents the sequence of reactions in the cells of the liver that process excess nitrogen, generated when protein is used by the body, to make urea that is then excreted in the urine.

The morphological hair changes associated with the inborn errors of amino acid metabolism include defective hair pigmentation in *phenylketonuria*, changes in hair texture in *Hartnup dis*ease, brittle hair (congenital trichorrhexis nodosa) in *argininosuccinic aciduria*, white hair in *methionine malabsorption syndrome*, and sparse, blond, brittle hair in *homocystinuria*. The reason for the respective hair abnormalities is not completely understood, but related in part to derangements of amino acid composition and melanogenesis of the hair, specifically deficiency of cystine in homocystinuria and of tyrosine in phenylketonuria.

5.1.4.1 Homocystinuria

Homocystinuria is an autosomal recessive inherited disorder characterized by an excess of the compound homocysteine in the urine due to a defect in the conversion of the amino acid methionine to cysteine. Usually, homocystinuria is caused by a deficiency of the enzyme cystathionine beta synthase resulting in a multisystemic disorder of the connective tissue and central nervous and cardiovascular system [33].

Affected infants may fail to thrive at the expected rate and have developmental delays. By approximately age 3, the more disease-specific symptoms become apparent. These include ocular abnormalities (partial dislocation of the lens with quivering of the iris, myopia, and others) and a particular physical appearance (tall, thin built, with a caved-in or pigeon chest, long limbs, arachnodactyly, knock knees, and high-arched feet). Although intelligence may be normal in some, children may be affected by a progressive intellectual disability, and may develop psychiatric disturbances and/or seizures. Finally, affected individuals develop arterial atheromatosis at an early age, and are at risk for the development of intravascular thrombosis potentially leading to life-threatening complications. Although less common, additional findings reported in individuals with homocystinuria have been kyphoscoliosis, spontaneous pneumothorax, and inguinal hernia.

Due to his peculiar habitus in his depictions of the Amarna period (later half of the Eighteenth Dynasty), it has been suggested that Egyptian pharaoh Akhenaten (1353–1336 BC) may have suffered from homocystinuria [34]. This revolutionary king introduced radical new concepts, both in the Egyptian arts and in religion. In art, Akhenaten broke out from the old Egyptian canon with caricature-like physical portrayals (Fig. 5.2). In religion, he abandoned the traditional Egyptian polytheism for a monotheistic worship of the solar deity Aten, and with this probably laid the foundation for future Abrahamic monotheism. The idea of Akhenaten as the pioneer of a monotheistic religion that later became Judaism has been proposed by various

Fig. 5.2 Egyptian pharaoh Akhenaten with features reminiscent of homocystinuria in his caricature-like physical portrayals during the Amarna period (replica from the Egyptian Museum, Berlin, Germany, private collection)

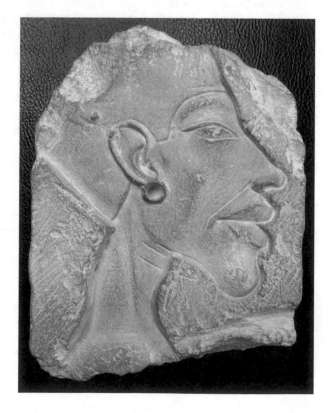

scholars, pioneered by Austrian psychoanalyst Sigmund Freud (1856–1939) [35]. Most stunning are the strong stylistic similarities between Akhenaten's "Great Hymn to the Aten" and the Biblical Psalm 104 that led Freud to argue that Moses may have been an Atenist priest forced to leave Egypt following Akhenaten's death in 1336 BC (*"¹Praise the Lord, my soul. Lord my God, you are very great; you are clothed with splendor and majesty. ²The Lord wraps himself in light as with a garment; he stretches out the heavens like a tent ³and lays the beams of his upper chambers on their waters"*; etc.). While Akhenaten was striving to promote monotheism, only Moses was able to achieve the task. Rabbinic Judaism calculated a life span of Moses corresponding to 1391–1271 BC, while other scholars consider that the figure of Moses is legendary, and not historical [36], though a Moses-like figure may have existed in the mid-late thirteenth century BC [37], possibly a priest of the Aten cult. In fact, neither Egyptian sources mention Moses and the events of Exodus-Deuteronomy, nor is there any archaeological evidence to support the Biblical account of Moses.

Cutaneous features of homocystinuria may be abnormally thin and fragile skin, hypopigmentation, and malar flushes, and the hair may be sparse, blond, and brittle.

Deficiency of the enzyme cystathionine beta synthase leads to increased levels of methionine and of homocysteine in body fluids, while concentrations of cysteine are reduced. In untreated homocystinuria, reduced levels of cystine have been demonstrated in the hair that normalized after treatment with vitamin B6 [38].

The treatment of homocystinuria is directed towards preventing or reducing the symptoms associated with the disorder by controlling plasma levels of homocysteine. Treatment may include supplementation with vitamin B6 (pyridoxine), a diet that restricts protein and methionine, betaine therapy, and supplementation with folate. Slightly less than 50% respond to vitamin B6, and need to take supplemental vitamin B6 for the rest of their lives. Affected individuals therefore first undergo a pyridoxine response assessment. In order to determine whether an individual is responsive to pyridoxine therapy, folate levels must be normal, and some individuals may require folate supplementation. A normal dose of folic acid supplement and adding cysteine to the diet can be helpful, as glutathione is synthesized from cysteine which can be important to reduce the oxidative stress. Individuals who do not respond to therapy with vitamin B6 require a restricted diet that is low in protein and methionine, combined with cysteine supplementation. Betaine (N,N,N-trimethylglycine) is used to reduce concentrations of homocysteine by promoting the conversion of homocysteine back to methionine [39].

The life expectancy of patients with homocystinuria is reduced if left untreated, with almost one-quarter of patients dying as a result of thrombotic complications.

Homocystinuria may be diagnosed by routine metabolic biochemistry. In the first instance, plasma or urine amino acid analysis will frequently show an elevation of methionine and the presence of homocysteine. Many neonatal screening programs include methionine as a metabolite. Again, as with other serious inborn errors of metabolism, genetic counseling is recommended for affected individuals and their families.

5.1.4.2 Hartnup Disease

Hartnup disease (pellagra-cerebellar ataxia-renal aminoaciduria syndrome) is a rare autosomal recessive inborn error of metabolism that affects the absorption of non-polar amino acids, particularly tryptophan. Tryptophan is, in turn, converted into serotonin, melatonin, and niacin which is a precursor to nicotamide, a necessary component of nicotinamide adenine dinucleotide (NAD+), hence the clinical resemblance to pellagra. In metabolism, NAD+ is involved in redox reactions, carrying electrons from one reaction to another. Pellagra is the acquired condition caused by deficiency of nicotinamide and resulting in dermatitis, diarrhea, and dementia (3 Ds). Telogen effluvium may be an additional, though unspecific and multifactorial trichological, symptom.

Hartnup disease is named after the indicator family Hartnup, who suffered from the disease. The failure of amino acid transport was originally reported in 1960 from the increased presence of tryptophan and indoles (bacterial metabolites of tryptophan) in the urine of patients as part of a generalized aminoaciduria of the disease [40]. The excessive loss of tryptophan from malabsorption is the cause of the pellagra-like symptoms.

The disorder is characterized by a distinctive pellagra-like skin rash and sometimes neurological involvement that can include ataxia, nystagmus, and cognitive delays. The symptoms of the disease vary greatly from one individual to another. The majority of affected individuals are asymptomatic. When symptoms do develop, they most often occur between the ages of 3 and 9 years, and are often triggered by sunlight, fever, drugs, and emotional or physical stress. A period of poor nutrition nearly always precedes an attack.

Due to the variability of symptoms, definite diagnosis can only be made through urine analysis. With urine chromatography, increased levels of neutral amino acids (glutamine, valine, phenylalanine, leucine, asparagine, citrulline, isoleucine, threonine, alanine, serine, histidine, tyrosine, tryptophan) and indican are found. Low levels of B complex have been demonstrated in the hair of pellagrous subjects [41]. Molecular genetic testing for alterations in the underlying SLC19A6 gene known to cause the disorder can confirm a diagnosis of Hartnup disease, but usually is not necessary.

A high-protein diet can overcome the deficient transport of neutral amino acids in most patients. Poor nutrition leads to more frequent and more severe attacks of the disease, which is otherwise asymptomatic. All patients who are symptomatic are advised to practice protection from sunlight: avoid excessive exposure to sunlight, wear protective clothing, and use chemical sunscreens with a SPF of 15 or greater. In patients with niacin deficiency, additional daily supplementation with nicotinic acid or nicotinamide is advised [42].

5.1.4.3 Phenylketonuria

Phenylketonuria is an autosomal recessive inborn error of metabolism due to mutations in the phenylalanine hydroxylase gene, which results in decreased metabolism of the amino acid phenylalanine and buildup of dietary phenylalanine to potentially toxic levels. Phenylalanine is converted into phenylpyruvate, also known as phenyl-ketone, which can be detected in the urine, hence the name phenylketonuria.

Untreated, the condition leads to intellectual disability, seizures, behavioral problems, and mental disorders. The disease was discovered in 1934 by Norwegian physician and biochemist Ivar Asbjørn Følling (1888–1973) [43], with the importance of diet determined in 1953.

Treatment is with a diet low in foods that contain phenylalanine and special supplements. The diet should begin as soon as possible after birth and be continued for at least 10 years, if not lifelong. People who are diagnosed early and maintain a strict diet can have normal health and a normal life span. The diet requires restricting or eliminating foods high in phenylalanine, such as soybeans, egg whites, shrimp, chicken breast, spirulina, watercress, fish, nuts, crayfish, lobster, tuna, turkey, legumes, and low-fat cottage cheese. The sweetener aspartame, present in many diet foods and soft drinks, must also be avoided, as aspartame is metabolized into phenylalanine. Effectiveness may be monitored through periodic blood tests [44].

Tetrahydrobiopterin, also known as sapropterin dihydrochloride, may be useful in some patients. It is a cofactor of the aromatic amino acid hydroxylase enzymes used in the degradation of phenylalanine and in the biosynthesis of the neurotransmitters serotonin (5-hydroxytryptamine), melatonin, dopamine, norepinephrine, and epinephrine [45].

Cutaneous symptoms of phenylketonuria are a particularly fair skin and hair, with a musty smell.

Phenylketonuria is included in the newborn screening panel of developed countries [46].

Before the causes of phenylketonuria and its treatment were understood, the condition caused severe disability in most people who inherited the relevant mutations of the respective gene. It is the most common amino acid metabolic problem in the United Kingdom. Many untreated phenylketonuria patients born before widespread newborn screening are still alive, largely in dependent living homes/institutions. Nobel and Pulitzer Prize-winning American writer and novelist Pearl S. Buck (1892–1973) had a daughter named Carol who lived with phenylketonuria before treatment was available, and wrote a moving account on it in a book called "The Child Who Never Grew: A Memoir" [47]. What many do not acknowledge is that she wrote that masterpiece of literary art with the motivation of financing a special school for her child. What was called mental retardation at the time was a disability that could cause great suffering for the affected and their parents. There was little awareness of how to deal with such children, and as a result they were considered a source of shame and simply hidden away. In her remarkable account, Buck helped bring the issue to light, while candidly discussing her own experience as a mother, from her struggle to accept Carol's diagnosis of phenylketonuria to her determination to give her child as happy and fulfilled a life as possible, including a top-quality education designed around her needs and abilities. "The Child Who Never Grew" provides a perspective on just how much progress has been made since, while offering at the same time common sense and timeless wisdom for the challenges still faced today by family of those in special need.

5.1.4.4 Methionine Malabsorption Syndrome (Oasthouse Urine Disease)

Methionine malabsorption syndrome is a rare autosomal recessive disorder of the absorption of the amino acid methionine from the small intestine. Unabsorbed methionine is degraded by colonic bacteria to alpha-hydroxybutyric acid, which causes the characteristic unpleasant odor in the patients and their excreta that is reminiscent of the interior of a room where tobacco, hops, and malt are dried (oasthouse). Smith and Strang originally described the disorder in 1958 and gave it its name [48]. Characteristic features of the disorder include mental retardation, convulsions, hyper/tachypnea, and strikingly white hair. In methionine malabsorption syndrome there is no amino aciduria, and the specific defect of intestinal methionine absorption is detectable only from stool chromatograms [49].

5.1.4.5 Citrullinemia and Argininosuccinic Aciduria

Trichorrhexis nodosa refers to white knots with transverse fracturing along the hair shaft. Patients complain that the hair is not growing. Microscopic examination, either by dermoscopy or light and electron microscopy reveals brushlike hair fractures (Fig. 5.3). In general, trichorrhexis nodosa represents an unspecific finding related to excess stress of hair in relation to its fragility. It can be observed in diverse hair shaft abnormalities with increased fragility, or more frequently as a consequence of cumulative physical and chemical trauma and hair weathering.

Congenital trichorrhexis nodosa, albeit unspecific, is a trichological marker of citrullinemia [50] and argininosuccinic aciduria. In addition, pili torti has been associated with both [51, 52].

Citrullinemia is an autosomal recessive urea cycle disorder that causes ammonia and other toxic substances to accumulate in the blood. The urea cycle is a sequence of chemical reactions taking place in the liver to process excess nitrogen that is generated when protein is used for energy, to make urea, which is excreted by the kidneys. Mutations in the argininosuccinate synthetase gene are the cause of the condition. Reduction in the activity of the respective enzyme disrupts the urea cycle and prevents the body from processing nitrogen effectively. Excess nitrogen, in the

Fig. 5.3 Trichorrhexis nodosa (scanning electron microscopy)

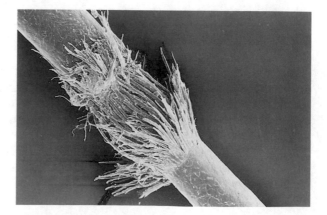

form of ammonia, and other by-products of the urea cycle accumulate in the bloodstream, leading to the characteristic features of the condition.

Infants affected with citrullinemia typically appear normal at birth, but as ammonia builds up in the body, they develop lethargy, poor feeding, vomiting, seizures, and loss of consciousness. Low-protein diets are intended to minimize production of ammonia. Arginine, sodium benzoate, and sodium phenylacetate help to remove ammonia from the blood. Dialysis may be used to remove ammonia from the blood when it reaches critical levels. In some cases, liver transplant has been successful [53].

Argininosuccinic aciduria represents yet another autosomal recessive urea cycle disorder that causes the accumulation of argininosuccinic acid in the blood and urine and is associated with brittle hair [54]. The underlying enzymatic defect affects argininosuccinate lyase that is involved in the conversion of argininosuccinate to arginine within the urea cycle. The urea cycle cannot proceed normally, and nitrogen accumulates in the bloodstream in the form of ammonia.

Argininosuccinic aciduria may become evident in the first few days of life because of high blood ammonia, or later in life presenting with sparse and brittle hair, developmental delay, and tremors. During an acute hyperammonemic episode, oral proteins must be avoided and intravenous lipids, glucose, and insulin (if needed) should be given to promote anabolism. Intravenous nitrogen-scavenging therapy with sodium benzoate and/or sodium phenylacetate should normalize ammonia levels, but if unsuccessful, hemodialysis is recommended. Long-term management involves dietary protein restriction as well as arginine supplementation.

Diagnosis is based mainly on clinical findings and laboratory test results. Plasma concentrations of ammonia (>150 μmol/L), citrulline (200–300 μmol/L), and argininosuccinic acid (5–110 μmol/L) in the plasma or urine, respectively, are elevated.

Due to the paucity of the urea cycle disorders, an estimate of life expectancy or mortality rates is difficult to make. One 2003 study which followed 88 cases receiving two different kinds of treatment found that very few persons lived beyond age 20 and none beyond age 30 [55].

5.2   Acquired Deficiency Disorders

Nutritional deficiency results from an inadequate supply of essential nutrients in the diet resulting in malnutrition or disease. There are a number of conditions that are caused by nutritional deficiency, the most prevalent of which are anemia, beriberi, osteoporosis, pellagra, and rickets. All vitamins were identified by 1948, ushering in a half century of discovery focused on single-nutrient-deficiency diseases. The first half of the twentieth century witnessed the identification and synthesis of many of the known essential vitamins and minerals and their use to prevent and treat nutritional deficiency-related diseases.

Acquired deficiency disorders that may affect the condition of the hair are protein-calorie malnutrition, biotin deficiency, vitamin C deficiency (scurvy), vitamin B12 deficiency (pernicious anemia), niacin deficiency (pellagra), deficiency of essential fatty acids, iron deficiency, zinc deficiency, copper deficiency, selenium deficiency, and vitamin D deficiency. The study of the inborn errors of metabolism has shed some light on the clinical features of the respective deficiency disorders, specifically biotinidase and holocarboxylase synthetase deficiency (biotin), Hartnup disease (niacin), acrodermatitis enteropathica (zinc), Menkes kinky hair syndrome (copper), and possibly vitamin D-dependent rickets with alopecia (vitamin D).

5.2.1   Protein-Calorie Malnutrition

Protein-calorie or protein-energy malnutrition is a form of malnutrition that is defined as a range of pathological conditions arising from coincidental lack of dietary protein and/or calories in varying proportions.

Protein-calorie malnutrition is probably the best studied of possible forms of undernutrition in man. It occurs commonly in developing countries; in developed countries it predominantly affects chronically ill and hospitalized patients: children on protein-restricted diets for management of urea cycle disorders, such as argininosuccinic aciduria; infants on milk-restricted diets because of suspected lactose intolerance or milk protein allergy [56]; children and adolescents with gastrointestinal disease, cystic fibrosis, and anorexia nervosa; and patients with chronic renal failure, severe neurologic impairment, or malignancy.

By definition, kwashiorkor is a predominant protein malnutrition, marasmus is deficiency in calorie intake, and marasmic kwashiorkor is combined protein and calorie deficiency. The prognosis of marasmus is better than it is for kwashiorkor [57] but half of severely malnourished children finally succumb due to unavailability of adequate treatment.

5.2.1.1   Kwashiorkor

Jamaican pediatrician Cicely Williams (1893–1992) originally introduced the term kwashiorkor into the medical community 2 years after publishing the first formal description of the condition in the Western medical literature in 1933 [58]. The name comes from coastal Ghana language meaning "the sickness the baby gets when the new baby comes" [59] reflecting on the development of the condition in an older child who has been weaned from the breast when a younger sibling follows. In at-risk populations, kwashiorkor may develop after a mother weans her child from breast milk, replacing it with a diet high in carbohydrates, while breast milk contains proteins vital to a child's growth and development.

The clinical hallmark of kwashiorkor in a malnourished child is pitting edema of the hands and feet; other signs include a distended abdomen, hypopigmentation of the skin, and a peculiar dermatitis with dry, fissured areas and cracked appearance that has been compared to flaky paint [60].

Alterations of hair are a change of texture and color with a rusty-brown to reddish hair color [61], increased pluckability of hair [62], and alterations in hair root morphology [63].

The flag sign is a peculiar change in hair color resulting from periods of severe malnutrition from kwashiorkor, in which the hair becomes discolored (reddish, blond, or gray, depending on original color) in a band perpendicular to its long axis. The presence of sharply demarcated alternating bands of pigmented and depigmented as well as thicker and thinner hair is evidence of intermittent malnutrition [64]. It indicates periods of severe malnutrition in kwashiorkor.

Williams was one of the few colonial physicians who gave attention to the traditional knowledge of the locals, despite risking to be at odds with her peers. The repeated observation of young children with swollen bellies and stick-thin limbs who died in thousands despite treatment, together with the account of the local women calling the condition kwashiorkor, led Williams to disagree with the then prevalent opinion that it was pellagra. Her findings that the condition was due to a lack of protein in the diets of weanlings after the arrival of a new baby were originally published in the Archives of Disease in Childhood in 1933 [65]. Her colleagues in the colonies were quick to alienate her claims, and despite a follow-up paper on the subject, more directly contrasting kwashiorkor and pellagra, published in The Lancet in 1935 [66], colonial physicians continued to avoid the term kwashiorkor, or even acknowledge the distinction from pellagra, despite the death of children who continued to be treated for pellagra. Ultimately, in 2005 a UK-trained Ghanaian physician wrote in praise of Dr Williams' ability to identify and acknowledge the social context of kwashiorkor, and commended her for her respect for local traditions, as evidenced by her referring to the condition by its local name [67].

5.2.1.2 Marasmus

The word marasmus comes from the Greek μαρασμός (marasmus) for withering. While kwashiorkor is protein deficiency with adequate energy intake, marasmus is inadequate energy intake that exceeds the deficit of protein. The amino acids are utilized to maintain body function. The result is an atrophy of most organs.

Accordingly, the clinical presentation of marasmus is that of a shrunken, wasted appearance, with loss of muscle mass and subcutaneous fat tissue. The buttocks and upper limb muscle groups are usually more affected than others. Other symptoms include pathological body temperature with either hypothermia or pyrexia, anemia, dehydration, hypovolemic shock with weak radial pulse, cold extremities, decreased consciousness, tachypnea from heart failure or pneumonia, corneal lesions associated with vitamin A deficiency, and dermal manifestations associated with other vitamin deficiencies with frequent evidence of infection [68].

The hair is thin, sparse, and easily plucked [69].

Marasmic kwashiorkor is a severe protein-calorie malnutrition disease resulting from the deficiency of both calories and protein [70]. It is characterized by extreme weight loss, weakness, and features of kwashiorkor, specifically peripheral edema.

5.2.2 Deficiency of Essential Fatty Acids

In addition to the carbohydrate, fats serve as a fuel for energy. They compose a concentrated fuel source for the energy system. With the adipose tissue, as compared with the carbohydrates that are stored as glycogen, a large amount of energy can be stored in fat within a relatively small space. The bulk of dietary fats are glycerides, which consist of fatty acids attached to glycerol. The fatty acids are classified by their length, and according to their saturation. Fatty acids are saturated or unsaturated according to whether each carbon is filled with hydrogen.

The saturated fats are filled in all of their available carbon bonds with hydrogen, thus making the fat harder and more solid at room temperature. Saturated fats are generally from animal sources.

The unsaturated fats are not completely filled with all of the hydrogen they could hold. As a result, they are less heavy and less dense and therefore liquid at room temperature, such as in the vegetable oils. The fats from fish and plant sources are mostly unsaturated.

Noteworthy exceptions are palm and coconut oils, which are predominantly saturated.

The unsaturated fatty acids are again classified according to the location of the first double bond on the third or the sixth carbon, respectively, from the methyl end or omega end into the *omega-3 fatty acids* and the *omega-6 fatty acids*.

Food with a high content of fat is generally also a good source of fat-soluble vitamins, with the fat aiding in the absorption of those vitamins.

Furthermore, fat in the diet adds flavor to the food and contributes to the feeling of satiety from a given meal.

The essential fatty acids *linoleic acid* (LA) and *alpha-linolenic* acid (ALA) represent essential nutrients, according to the definition for their necessity in the diet: their absence will create a specific deficiency disorder, and the body cannot synthesize them in sufficient amounts and therefore must obtain them from diet. Both serve important functions related to tissue strength, cholesterol metabolism, muscle tone, blood clotting, and heart action. Thus, they are also named *vitamin F*.

The biological effects of the omega-3 and omega-6 fatty acids are mediated by their mutual interactions, but it is as yet unresolved to what extent the dietary ratio of omega-3 and omega-6 fatty acids is important for human health. In 1964, it was discovered in sheep that omega-6 arachidonic acid (AA) may be enzymatically converted into the pro-inflammatory agent, prostaglandin E2 (PGE2) [71]. Later, additional fatty acid metabolites collectively termed eicosanoids were identified, including thromboxanes, prostacyclins, and leukotrienes [72].

The eicosanoids typically have a short period of activity in the body, from the synthesis of fatty acids to the metabolism by enzymes. If the rate of synthesis exceeds the rate of metabolism, an excess of eicosanoids may be detrimental [72]. Researchers found that omega-3 fatty acids are also converted to eicosanoids and docosanoids [73], but at a slower rate. If both omega-3 and omega-6 fatty acids are present, they will compete to be transformed [72], so the ratio of omega-3 to omega-6 fatty acids directly may affect the type of eicosanoids that are produced and the degree of tissue inflammation.

Deficiency of the long-chain polyunsaturated fatty acids LA and ALA may be due to impaired fat absorption in children with biliary atresia, cystic fibrosis, or intestinal lymphangiectasia; dietary supplements consisting primarily of medium-chain triglycerides in short bowel syndrome; and inadequately supplemented parenteral alimentation.

Cutaneous manifestations of deficiency of essential fatty acids are severe dryness and scaling of skin (Fig. 5.4), redness and scaling of scalp and eyebrows, and weeping intertriginous lesions [74]. The hair is dry, unruly, and lighter in color, and there is significant telogen hair shedding [75].

With an adequate dietary supply of essential fatty acids, the body is capable of producing saturated, monounsaturated, and polyunsaturated fatty acids, as well as cholesterol. Therefore, no Dietary Reference Intake (DRI) exists for fat compounds other than for LA and ALA (Table 5.1).

Fig. 5.4 Deficiency of essential fatty acids: severe dryness, redness, and scaling of skin with alopecia

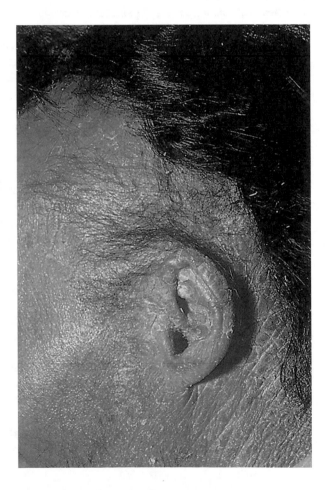

Table 5.1   AIs (adequate intakes) for linoleic acid and alpha-linolenic acid

Life stage group	Linoleic acid (g/dl)	Alpha-linolenic acid (g/dl)
Infants		
Birth to 6 months	4.4	0.5
6–12 months	4.6	0.5
Children		
1–3 years	7	0.7
4–8 years	10	09
Males		
9–13 years	12	1.2
14–18 years	16	1.6
19–30 years	17	1.6
31–50 years	17	1.6
51–70 years	14	1.6
>70 years	14	1.6
Females		
9–13 years	10	1.0
14–18 years	11	1.1
19–30 years	12	1.1
31–50 years	12	1.1
51–70 years	11	1.1
>70 years	11	1.1
Pregnancy		
14–18 years	13	1.4
19–30 years	13	1.4
31–50 years	13	1.4
Lactation		
14–18 years	13	1.3
19–30 years	13	1.3
31–50 years	13	1.3

Source: Dietary Reference Intakes for energy, carbohydrates, fiber, fat, fatty acids, cholesterol, protein, and amino acids (2002/2005). The report may be accessed via www.nap.edu

Since good sources of the long-chain omega-3 fatty acids, EPA and DHA, include cold-water fish and seafood, vegans might be at risk for inadequate intake since their diets do not include animal-origin foods. Typically, omnivores obtain enough dietary EPA and DHA, but unless vegans consume algal omega-3 supplements, they rely on endogenous production of long-chain fatty acids. Vegan diets have several possible concerns: (1) Vegans have high intakes of LA as compared to nonvegetarian diets. (2) High intakes of LA competitively interfere with the endogenous conversion of ALA to EPA and DHA. (3) High somatic levels of LA/low ALA indicate a decreased ALA conversion to EPA and DHA. (4) Some, not all, vegans meet the Dietary Reference Intake-Adequate Intake (DRI-AI) for dietary ALA. (5) Vegan diets are high in fiber, which possibly interferes with fat absorption. Consequently, health professionals and registered dietitians/registered dietitian nutritionists working with vegans need specific essential fatty acid diet guidelines [76].

While results from a trial utilizing a supplement of fatty acids to evaluate the effect on hair loss were reported, limited conclusions may be drawn, as this supplement combined multiple fatty acids with antioxidants [77].

5.2.3   Biotin Deficiency

Biotin, also known as vitamin H (the H represents Haar und Haut, German words for "hair and skin") or vitamin B7, is a water-soluble vitamin of the B complex. Biotin is a coenzyme for carboxylase enzymes that assist in various metabolic reactions involved in the transfer of carbon dioxide. Biotin is important in fatty acid synthesis, branched-chain amino acid catabolism, and gluconeogenesis.

Biotin is often recommended as a dietary supplement for strengthening hair and nails. While response of splitting brittle nails (onychoschizia, onychoschisis) to daily biotin supplementation (in a magnitude of 5–10 mg daily), irrespective of serum biotin levels, has been demonstrated [78–81], there is little data on the frequency of biotin deficiency in the general population, or on the value of oral biotin for hair growth and quality [82–84]. Shelley and Shelley reported on response of uncombable hair syndrome (Fig. 5.5) to biotin in siblings with ectodermal dysplasia [85]. However, differentiation of cultured human follicular keratinocytes has been demonstrated not to be influenced by biotin [86].

The only human health condition for which there is strong evidence of biotin's potential benefit as treatment is biotin deficiency that is either due to the inborn errors of biotin metabolism or acquired [87].

Acquired biotin deficiency is generally believed to be infrequent, because intestinal bacteria produce biotin in excess of the body's daily requirements. However, the extent to which biotin is absorbed from the large intestine and contributes to biotin requirements is uncertain.

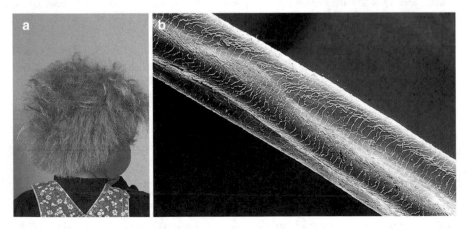

Fig. 5.5 (**a**, **b**) Uncombable hair syndrome. (**a**) Unruly hair. (**b**) Longitudinal grooving of hair shaft (scanning electron microscopy)

Finally, biotin is consumed from a wide range of food sources in the diet, though few are particularly rich sources. Biotin content in different food sources is listed in Table 5.2.

The average dietary biotin intake in Western populations has been estimated to be 35–70 µg/day. For that reason, statutory agencies in many countries do not prescribe a recommended daily intake of biotin. However, a number of metabolic disorders and conditions exist in which an individual's metabolism or uptake of biotin may be abnormal.

Since endogenous biotin production occurs in the intestine, dysbacteriosis of the gastrointestinal tract due to inflammatory bowel disease or broad-spectrum antibiotic treatment may impair the body to generate biotin on its own.

The first demonstration of acquired biotin deficiency in animals was observed in rats fed raw egg white. The rats were found to develop dermatitis, alopecia, and neuromuscular dysfunction. The syndrome, called "egg white injury" [88], was found to be caused by a glycoprotein found in egg white, avidin, that binds extremely well with biotin, making it unavailable for use in enzymatic reactions. Avidin in egg white denatures upon heating (cooking).

The frequency of marginal biotin status in the general population is not known. Nevertheless, the incidence of low-circulating biotin levels has been found to be greater in alcoholics than in the general population [89]. Smoking may further accelerate biotin catabolism in women [90]. Also, relatively low levels of biotin

Table 5.2 Biotin content in different food sources

Food source	Biotin in µg/100g
Egg yolk	53.0
(Egg, total)	(25.0)
Pork liver	27.0
Oat flakes	20.0
Wheat germ	17.0
White mushrooms	16.0
Unpolished rice	12.0
(Polished rice)	(3.0)
Spinach	6.9
Milk and milk products:	
Cheese (Brie)	6.2
Curd	6.0
Cow milk	3.5
Wheat, whole grain	6.0
Pork	5.0
Carrot	5.0
Apple	4.5
Tomato	4.0
Beef	3.0
Chicken	2.0
Lettuce	1.9
Potato	0.4

have been reported in patients on parenteral nutrition [91], who have had a partial gastrectomy or other causes of achlorhydria [92]; patients on antiepileptics [93, 94]; patients on oral isotretinoin therapy for acne [95]; elderly individuals; and athletes. Pregnancy [96] and lactation may be associated with an increased demand for biotin. In pregnancy, this may be due to a possible acceleration of biotin catabolism, whereas in lactation, the higher demand has yet to be elucidated.

Symptoms of biotin deficiency include alopecia; conjunctivitis; dermatitis in the form of a scaly, red rash around the eyes, nose, and mouth that has been termed the biotin-deficient face by some experts [97]; and neurological symptoms, such as depression, lethargy, hallucination, and numbness and tingling of the extremities. Coulter et al. [98] have proposed the term "neurotrichosis" for conditions in which hair abnormalities, albeit unspecific and not pathognomonic, may indicate a group of neurological disorders including potentially treatable inborn errors of metabolism. Nevertheless, the neurological and psychological symptoms of biotin deficiency can occur with only mild deficiencies, while dermatitis, conjunctivitis, and hair loss generally occur only when deficiency becomes more severe. Individuals with hereditary disorders of biotin deficiency additionally have evidence of impaired immune system function, including increased susceptibility to bacterial and fungal infections [99].

Regardless of the cause, biotin deficiency can usually be addressed directly with nutritional supplementation. Due to its availability, affordability, and effective marketing for this purpose, biotin is a popular nutritional supplement for treatment of hair loss. Moreover, there is no known toxicity of biotin in an order of magnitude greater than that of the nutritional requirements. Finally, efficacy of oral biotin for treatment of brittle nails has additionally contributed to the popularity of the supplement.

Blood levels of biotin show a wide variability ranging from 400 to 1200 ng/L with daily fluctuations in the magnitude of up to 100%, which is why at least two determinations on two different days are recommended. Ultimately, the most reliable detection method of biotin deficiency is elevated excretion of 3-hydroxyisovaleric acid in the urine (>195 µmol/24 h). Using this method it has been demonstrated that a daily allowance of 30 µg is sufficient to provide normal excretion levels of 3-hydroxyisovaleric acid in the adult.

Nevertheless, a practical approach to determine biotin status in relation to serum levels is to classify into optimal levels (>400 ng/L), suboptimal levels (100–400 ng/L), and deficiency (<100 ng/L).

A retrospective study of serum biotin levels was performed on 541 female patients aged between 9 and 92 years (mean: 45.9 years) with the complaint of hair loss [100]. Of the women complaining of hair loss assessed for serum biotin levels, 38% had values consistent with biotin deficiency (<100 ng/L), and 13% optimal (>400 ng/L). In the women in whom trichograms were performed, both groups (biotin deficiency, and optimal levels) demonstrated diffuse telogen effluvium at 24%. Therefore, the trichogram was not helpful in detecting hair loss relating to biotin deficiency, since it is neither sensitive nor specific, with telogen effluvium in women usually being of multifactorial origin. Rather, associated seborrheic-like dermatitis found in 35% of women with serum biotin levels <100 ng/L and telogen effluvium versus 0% of women with optimal biotin levels and telogen effluvium may point to the significance of biotin deficiency for hair loss. Finally, the patient's history may be helpful in detecting biotin deficiency, though with low sensitivity, since in the biotin deficiency group 11% versus 1.5% in the group with optimal biotin levels presented with a history of risk factors for biotin deficiency. Recognized risk factors for biotin deficiency from patients' personal history include gastrointestinal disease, specifically inflammatory bowel disease, or intake of drugs interfering with biotin metabolism or uptake, specifically antiepileptics, antibiotics, or isotretinoin.

The custom of treating women complaining of hair loss in an indiscriminate manner with oral biotin supplementation is inappropriate, unless biotin deficiency and its significance for the complaint of hair loss in the individual patient at hand have been demonstrated. In fact, treating the patient exclusively with oral biotin poses the risk of neglect or delay of appropriate treatment of hair loss of another underlying cause in the particular case. It must be kept in mind that hair loss in women may be of multifactorial origin, including female androgenetic alopecia; other nutritional deficiencies, e.g., iron deficiency; and/or endocrine disorders, e.g., thyroid disorder.

Rather, a careful patient history and clinical examination with respect to risk factors for biotin deficiency, such as gastrointestinal disease; medication with isotretinoin, antibiotics, or antiepileptics; and associated symptoms of seborrheic-like dermatitis or neurological disorder, must be performed. When biotin deficiency is suspected, the serum biotin level must be determined, and in case of biotin deficiency (<100 ng/L), the cause must be sought, unless obvious from the patient history, and treated.

Regardless of the cause, the deficiency can usually be successfully addressed directly with nutritional supplementation with usually high bioavailability of oral biotin supplements usually in a dosage of 5 mg/day (Fig. 5.6a–d).

At the same time, potential additional causes of hair loss, e.g., androgenetic alopecia, other nutritional deficiencies, and endocrine disorders, must systematically be addressed and treated as needed.

The high percentage of marginal biotin levels in the respective study may reflect that a number of other factors may contribute, such as anorexia/bulimia, alcoholism, smoking, pregnancy, lactation, athleticism, and old age.

Finally, a wide variability in biotin bioavailability from foodstuff may be due to the ability of an organism to break various biotin-protein bonds from food. Most biotin in foods is bound to protein. Gastrointestinal proteases and peptidases break down the protein-bound forms of ingested biotin from foods into biocytin and biotin-oligopeptides, which undergo further processing by biotinidase, an enzyme in the intestinal lumen, to release free biotin. Free biotin is then absorbed in the small intestine, and most biotin is stored in the liver.

Uptake of free biotin in the small intestine occurs through diffusion or active transport, depending on the present concentration of biotin. At physiological concentrations (<5 μmol/L) the carrier-mediated sodium-dependent transport by the

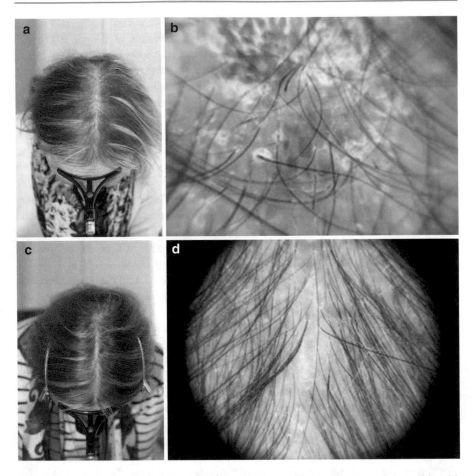

Fig. 5.6 (**a–d**) Successful treatment of biotin deficiency-related alopecia and dermatitis with 5 mg oral biotin. (**a, b**) Before treatment: (**a**) alopecia, (**b**) redness and scaling of scalp (dermoscopy). (**c, d**) Significant improvement of symptoms after 3 months of treatment

sodium-dependent multivitamin transporter predominates, whereas at pharmacological concentrations (>25 μmol/L) passive diffusion contributes to biotin uptake. Biotin uptake into the liver and the peripheral tissues occurs via a specific sodium-dependent, carrier-mediated process and by diffusion [101].

Several studies have examined the pharmacokinetics of orally administered free biotin in healthy subjects. These have demonstrated that orally administered free biotin in doses of 0.6–20 mg is taken up rapidly. Doses of biotin that exceed the normal dietary intake 60–600 times are 100% bioavailable [102–104]. Absorption efficiency of free biotin is high upon ingestion of large doses (up to 20 mg/day) due to passive diffusion.

5.2.4   Vitamin C Deficiency

Vitamin C or ascorbic acid is not synthesized in the human body; therefore dietary intake is essential. The recommended dietary allowance for adults is 60 mg per day. Vitamin C deficiency or scurvy is mainly found in alcoholics and elderly living alone. Patients with chronic disease, such as cancer or chronic renal failure, are also at risk.

Egyptians have recorded its symptoms as early as 1550 BCE, and Hippocrates documented scurvy as a disease. Hippocrates described symptoms of scurvy in book 2 of his *Prorrheticorum* and in his *Liber de internis affectionibus* [106]. Symptoms of scurvy were also described by (i) Pliny, in *Naturalis Historia*, book 3, chapter 49, and (ii) Strabo, in *Geographicorum*, book 16 [107]. The knowledge that consuming foods containing vitamin C is a cure for scurvy has been repeatedly forgotten and rediscovered only much later. Scurvy was a limiting factor in long-distance sea travel, often killing large numbers of people [108]. During the Age of Sail (1571–1862), when international trade and naval warfare were dominated by sailing ships, it was assumed that 50% of sailors would succumb to scurvy on a given trip, until James Lind proved that scurvy can be successfully treated with citrus fruit in 1753, and Scottish physician and Royal Navy health reformist Gilbert Blane (1749–1834) finally persuaded the British Royal Navy to routinely give lemon juice to its sailors [109].

Today, scurvy occurs more often in the developing world as one of the accompanying diseases of malnutrition along with beriberi and pellagra, and therefore remains existent in areas of the world depending on external food aid. Rates among refugees are reported at 5–45% [110]. Nevertheless, in the developed world, scurvy may occur in people with mental disorders, unusual eating habits, alcoholism, and older people who live alone [111]. Other risk factors include intestinal malabsorption and dialysis [112].

It takes at least a month of little to no vitamin C in the diet before symptoms occur [112]. Early symptoms of deficiency include weakness, feeling tired, and sore arms and legs [112].

Mucocutaneous symptoms of vitamin C deficiency are related to the role of vitamin C in collagen synthesis: ecchymoses (Fig. 5.7a), bleeding gums, follicular hyperkeratosis with corkscrew hairs, and perifollicular hemorrhages (Fig. 5.7b) [113]. The follicular changes are a direct consequence of decreased cross-linkage of hair keratin resulting from decreased number of reduced disulfide bonds, and curling of follicles results from altered perifollicular connective tissue [114]. Hemorrhages, poor wound healing, and infections are significant causes of morbidity and death.

Adult scurvy can be treated with 300–1000 mg of ascorbic acid per day, and improvement is generally seen in less than a week.

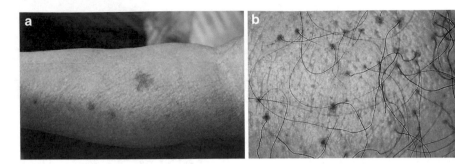

Fig. 5.7 (**a, b**) Vitamin C deficiency (scurvy). (**a**) Ecchymosis. (**b**) Perifollicular hemorrhage and corkscrew hairs

5.2.5   Vitamin B12 Deficiency

Most omnivorous people in developed countries obtain enough vitamin B12 from consuming animal products including meat, milk, eggs, and fish.

Deficiency of vitamin B12 is seen in strict vegetarianism, celiac disease, stagnant bowel syndrome, pancreatic disease with steatorrhea, infestation with fish tapeworm (*Diphyllobothrium latum*), after surgical removal of the stomach, and chronic atrophic gastritis with antibodies to intrinsic factor IF (pernicious anemia), which must be bound to food-source B12 in order for absorption to occur [115].

Because there are few common vegetable sources of vitamin B12, vegans must use a supplement or fortified foods for B12 intake or risk serious health consequences from vitamin B12 deficiency [116]. Another group at risk for vitamin B12 deficiency are those on long-term antacid therapy, using proton pump inhibitors, H2 blockers, or other antacids [117]. Also, reduced serum levels of vitamin B12 occur in up to 30% of people taking long-term antidiabetic metformin [117].

Vitamin B12 supplements are available in single-agent or multivitamin tablets, and pharmaceutical preparations may be given by intramuscular injection, inasmuch as the most common cause of vitamin B12 deficiency in developed countries is impaired absorption due to a loss of gastric intrinsic factor function from autoimmunity [118].

Deficiency is more likely after age 60 with a frequency of 20%, and increases in incidence with advancing age. Nevertheless, in the United States and the United Kingdom vitamin B12 deficiency occurs in about 6% of those under the age of 60. In underdeveloped countries, the rates are higher: across Latin America 40% are deficient, in parts of Africa 70%, and in parts of India 70–80% [119].

In mild deficiency, a person may feel tired and have a reduced number of red blood cells (anemia). In moderate deficiency, soreness of the tongue may occur (Hunter's glossitis, Fig. 5.8a), angular cheilitis (Fig. 5.8b), and beginning of neurological symptoms, including abnormal sensations such as pins and needles. Severe deficiency may include symptoms of heart insufficiency as well as more severe

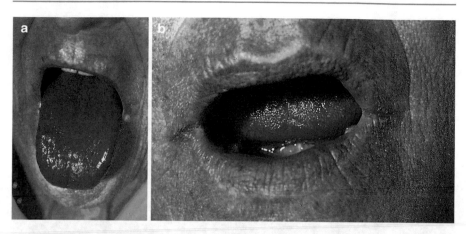

Fig. 5.8 (**a, b**) Vitamin B12 deficiency. (**a**) Hunter's glossitis. (**b**) Angular cheilitis

neurological symptoms, including changes in reflexes, poor muscle function (funicular myelosis), memory problems (dementia), decreased taste, decreased level of consciousness, and psychosis.

Vitamin B12 deficiency is frequently first suspected when a routine complete blood count shows anemia with an elevated MCV. In addition, on the peripheral blood smear, hypersegmented polymorphonuclear leukocytes may be seen. Diagnosis is confirmed based on vitamin B12 blood levels below 120–180 pmol/L (170–250 pg/mL). Decreased levels of holotranscobalamin [120], and increased levels of homocysteine, and methylmalonic acid levels, have been considered more sensitive indicators of B12 deficiency than the concentration of B12 in blood. However, more recently it has been demonstrated that in women <50 years and in men, holotranscobalamin, homocysteine, and methylmalonic acid do not appear superior to B12 for detection of B12 deficiency. For women 50 years and older, holotranscobalamin seems to be the preferred first-line marker for the detection of subclinical B12 deficiency [121].

Large amounts of folic acid can correct the megaloblastic anemia caused by vitamin B12 deficiency without correcting the neurological abnormalities, and could also worsen the anemia and the cognitive symptoms associated with vitamin B12 deficiency [122].

Vitamin B12 deficiency, besides a strong family history and hypothyroidism, has been linked to premature hair graying [123]; however it is as yet not clear whether the whitening of hair is due to the vitamin deficiency or rather of autoimmune origin, since autoimmune vitamin B12 deficiency is not infrequently associated with alopecia areata and vitiligo, the most prevalent causes of poliosis (Fig. 5.9a,b).

An association of alopecia areata with vitamin B12 deficiency has been recognized in the context of polyglandular autoimmune syndrome type III [124]. Moreover, in one study association of alopecia areata with antiparietal cell antibodies has been found in 42.3% of alopecia areata patients [125].

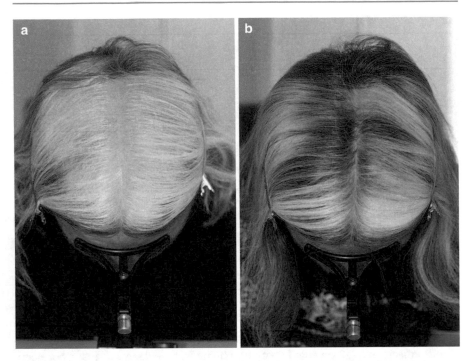

Fig. 5.9 (**a, b**) Alopecia areata with poliosis and vitamin B12 deficiency. (**a**) Before treatment. (**b**) Regrowth and partial repigmentation of hair with topical immunotherapy with diphenylcyclopropenone and intramuscular vitamin B12 supplementation

Finally, Daly and Daly suggested that a subtype of telogen effluvium with scalp dysesthesia (trichodynia) may be associated with low vitamin B12 levels and respond to vitamin B12 supplementation [126].

The recommended daily intake of vitamin B12 is 2.4 μg. Severe vitamin B12 deficiency is corrected with frequent intramuscular injections of large doses of vitamin B12, followed by maintenance doses of injections at longer intervals. One guideline specified intramuscular injections of 1000 micrograms (μg) of hydroxycobalamin three times a week for 2 weeks, followed by the same amount once every 2 or 3 months [127]. Risk of toxicity due to vitamin B12 is low. Injection side effects include skin rash, itching, chills, fever, hot flushes, nausea, and dizziness [127].

5.2.6 Niacin Deficiency

Niacin is an essential component of NADH that connects the citric acid cycle to the process of oxidative phosphorylation important for generation of ATP and therefore energy supply.

Pellagra results from a deficiency of B vitamins, most notably of niacin or vitamin B3. It occurs endemically in areas where maize and millet form the main diet [128], such as in Asia, Africa, and India, while sporadic cases are seen in Hartnup disease, with inadequate dietary intake, specifically alcoholics and individuals with anorexia nervosa [129], impaired absorption of niacin from Crohn's disease [130], drugs that interfere with niacin metabolism (isoniazid) [131], and tumors that interfere with niacin metabolism (carcinoid syndrome) [132]. Pellagra was common among Far East prisoners of World War II [133]. In addition, pellagra frequently affects populations of refugees and other displaced people due to their unique, long-term residential circumstances and dependence on food aid [134].

Pellagra was first described for its dermatological manifestations in Spain in 1735 by Catalan physician Gaspar Casal (1681–1759) remembered for describing the respective Casal collar. He originally explained that the disease causes dermatitis in exposed skin areas such as hands, feet, and neck and that the origin of the disease is poor diet and atmospheric influences. It was an endemic disease in northern Italy, where it was named, from Lombard, as "pell agra" (agra = holly-like or serum-like; pell = skin) by Francesco Frapolli (?–1733) from Milan, Italy, and later observed by German writer Johann Wolfgang von Goethe (1749–1832) during his journey through the Italian Alps [135].

Symptoms of niacin deficiency are a peculiar photosensitive dermatitis with hyperpigmentation (Fig. 5.10a,b), diarrhea, dementia, and eventually death (4 Ds [136, 137]. Initial manifestations are nonspecific and include anorexia, weakness, irritability, weight loss, mouth soreness, glossitis, and stomatitis. Alopecia has been observed in pellagra patients with steatorrhea [138].

The recommended daily intake of niacin is 6.6 mg per 1000 kcal, and at least 13 mg/day [139]. The most common adverse effects of niacin at higher dosages (50–500 mg) are flushing, headache, abdominal pain, diarrhea, dyspepsia, nausea, vomiting, rhinitis, pruritus, and rash. These can be minimized choosing lower dosages, and avoiding administration on an empty stomach.

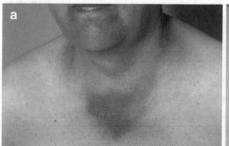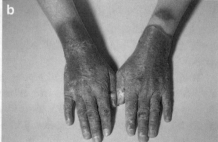

Fig. 5.10 (**a**, **b**) Niacin deficiency (pellagra). (**a**) Peculiar photosensitive dermatitis of the sun-exposed neck area (Casal's necklace). (**b**) Scaly, erythematosus, and hyperpigmented dermatitis on the dorsal hands. Note the sparing of the wristwatch area

5.2.7 Iron Deficiency

While there is no doubt that iron deficiency represents the most common nutritional deficiency, with a prevalence of 12–16% in adolescent girls and women of child-bearing age (16–49 years of age) and 6–9% in women 50 years of age and older in the United States [140], and iron deficiency is undisputedly a cause of significant morbidity, the various observational studies that evaluated the association between decreased ferritin levels and hair loss have resulted in conflicting results [141–153]. Moreover, almost all of these studies have focused exclusively on women, in whom the most common causes of iron deficiency have been menstrual blood loss, pregnancy, and lactation among the premenopausal women, while among the postmenopausal women (and men) they are decreased absorption and gastrointestinal bleeding.

Ferritin is an intracellular protein that stores iron and releases it in a controlled fashion. It acts as a buffer against both iron deficiency and iron overload. Ferritin is found in most tissues as a cytosolic protein, but small amounts are released into the circulation where it functions as an iron carrier. Serum ferritin is therefore an indirect marker of the total amount of iron stored in the body, and is used as a diagnostic test for iron-deficiency anemia [154]. The ferritin levels measured usually have a direct correlation with the total amount of iron stored in the body. However, ferritin levels may be artificially elevated in cases of anemia of chronic disease where ferritin is elevated in its capacity as an inflammatory acute-phase protein and not as a marker for iron overload [155]. Ultimately, a normal serum ferritin may not always exclude iron deficiency, and the utility is improved by taking a concurrent C-reactive protein (CRP).

The controversy over serum ferritin levels in women complaining of hair loss starts with a debate over what is the normal serum ferritin level for women [156], and is further complicated by the use of variable reference ranges in different laboratories, based on individual interpretations of the literature on this subject. A cutoff point of 10–15 microgL^{-1} is considered to yield a sensitivity of 59% and a specificity of 99% for diagnosing iron deficiency [157] and is used by many laboratories as the lower limits of normal based on reference sample groups. In women of child-bearing age, using a cutoff of 10–15 microgL^{-1} yields a sensitivity of 75% and specificity of 98% [158]. A cutoff of 30 microgL^{-1} yields a sensitivity of 92% and a specificity of 98% [157].

Total body iron is distributed among storage iron, transport iron, and functional iron. Storage iron is the body's iron reserves that are tissue bound and measured by the serum ferritin concentration, transport iron is transported to the tissues and measured by transferrin concentration and saturation, and functional iron consists of iron that is bound to hemoglobin, myoglobin, and diverse enzymes. It is measured by hemoglobin concentration.

Iron deficiency is viewed as a continuum ranging from iron depletion to iron-deficiency anemia. In the former, body iron stores are reduced, but functional and transport iron remains normal, leaving little reserves if the body requires more iron; in the latter, storage, transport, and functional iron is severely decreased and can lead to impaired function of multiple organ sites.

The symptoms of iron deficiency include fatigue and decreased exercise tolerance; signs of severe anemia include skin and conjunctival pallor, tachycardia, and low blood pressure; and dermatologic findings include hair loss (telogen effluvium), cheilosis, and koilonychia (Fig. 5.11).

It must be noted however that some patients with iron deficiency and even anemia may remain completely asymptomatic.

Although non-anemic iron deficiency as an etiologic factor for diffuse hair loss in women was first postulated by Hard in 1963 [141], it is not until more recently that the significance of iron stores as assessed by serum ferritin levels in women with hair loss has been studied systematically. Ultimately, Bregy et al. [159] evaluated the relationship between serum ferritin levels and hair loss activity determined by trichograms in a retrospective case study of 181 women with hair loss who underwent biochemical investigations and trichograms, and found no correlation between ferritin levels >10 microgL^{-1} and telogen rates (Fig. 5.12a), both in women with telogen effluvium (Fig. 5.12b) and in women with androgenetic alopecia (Fig. 5.12c), refuting at the same time the common opinion that androgenetic alopecia should have a threshold effect on sensitivity to low ferritin levels.

The authors only found a correlation between serum ferritin levels and patient age (Fig. 5.13).

Fig. 5.11 Iron deficiency: koilonychia

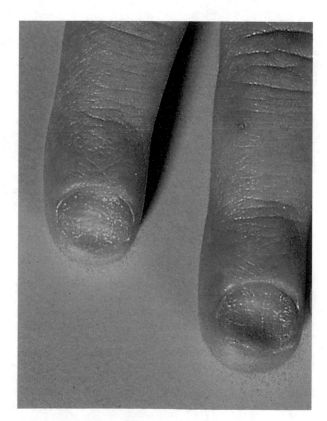

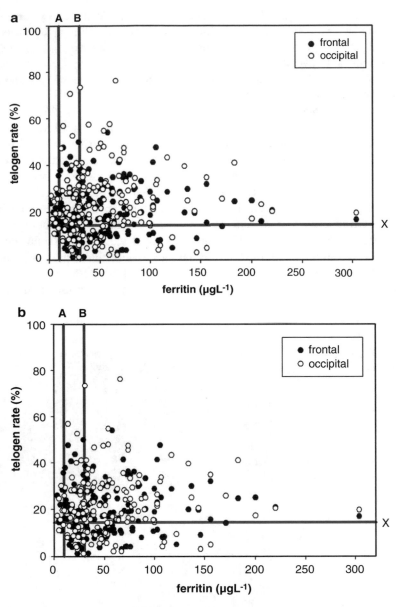

Fig. 5.12 (**a–c**) Correlation between telogen rates and ferritin levels in (**a**) all subjects (*n* = 181), (**b**) subjects with female androgenetic alopecia (*n* = 159), and (**c**) in total subjects with telogen effluvium, irrespective of combination with female androgenetic alopecia or not (*n* = 135). Diagram shows the ferritin values (μg L^{-1}) and corresponding telogen rates (%) of the frontal and occipital scalp of all patients in a linear scale. Vertical line A represents the lower reference limit of normal with 75% sensitivity and 98% specificity for diagnosing iron deficiency in women of childbearing age; vertical line B represents the cutoff point with sensitivity of 92% and specificity of 98% for diagnosing iron deficiency. Horizontal line X represents cutoff point for pathologic telogen rate (>15%) (from Bregy A, Trüeb RM. No association between serum ferritin levels >10 microg/L and hair loss activity in women. Dermatology 217:1–6 (2008))

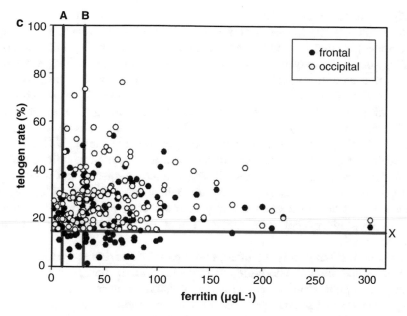

Fig. 5.12 (continued)

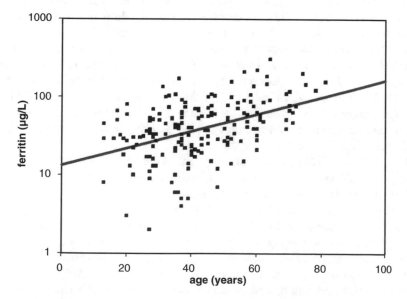

Fig. 5.13 Correlation between patient age (years) and serum ferritin values (μg L⁻¹) (from Bregy A, Trüeb RM. No association between serum ferritin levels >10 microg/L and hair loss activity in women. Dermatology 217:1–6 (2008))

Therefore, the role of tissue iron status within limits regarded as normal in women with hair loss has been overestimated. Specifically, search satisficing is the tendency to stop searching for a diagnosis once you find something [160]. Finding something may be satisfactory, but not finding everything is suboptimal. It is a natural cognitive tendency to stop searching, and therefore stop thinking, when one makes a seemingly significant finding. We value too highly information that fulfils our desires, and fail by confirming what we expect to find by selectively accepting or ignoring information. A typical example of this error is reducing treatment of hair loss in a female, especially of childbearing age, with detected low serum ferritin levels to iron supplementation, while in fact she may be suffering from female androgenetic alopecia, and is on an oral contraceptive with pro-androgenic action, which are the actual culprits. The genuine expert having learned about bias and search satisfaction consciously tries to keep his or her mind open so that he or she sees beyond these preconceptions.

Oral iron is often poorly tolerated, with up to 70% or more of patients noting gastrointestinal issues. Therefore, intravenous iron is being used more frequently to replete iron stores. True anaphylaxis is very rare, but probably complement-mediated anaphylactoid infusion reactions may be seen in up to 1 in every 200 patients [161]. Major risk factors for hypersensitivity reactions include a previous reaction to an iron infusion, a fast iron infusion rate, multiple drug allergies, severe atopy, and possibly systemic inflammatory diseases. Early pregnancy is a contraindication to iron infusions, while old age and serious comorbidity may worsen the impact of acute reactions if they occur [162]. Furthermore, cutaneous hyperpigmentation may be an issue with iron infusion, usually localized to the area of extravasation (Fig. 5.14), and rarely widespread due to increased vascular permeability in the case of an urticarial infusion reaction [163]. Skin discoloration can last from 6 months to 2 years or longer. Management of iron infusions requires meticulous observation, and, in the event of an adverse reaction, prompt recognition and appropriate interventions by well-trained medical and nursing staff.

Finally, Moltz [164] pointed in an investigation of 125 women with female androgenetic alopecia to the complexity of correlations between (1) the levels of the various androgens, prolactin, and thyroid-stimulating hormone and (2) the estradiol, sexual binding globulin, and free testosterone values. These, in turn, were correlated to (3) the occurrence of certain bleeding anomalies (amount, duration, interval) and corresponding iron deficiency. Therapy is therefore to be directed at normalizing the disturbed estrogen-androgen balance, using low-dose antiandrogens, estrogens, prolactin suppressants, or glucocorticoids depending on the underlying pathology, as well as minoxidil lotion, besides iron II preparations for effective treatment of alopecia.

Correction of iron deficiency below the level of normal together with its associated pathologies will usually lead to sustainable regrowth of hair (Fig. 5.15a,b).

Fig. 5.14 Cutaneous hyperpigmentation from iron infusion, localized to the area of extravasation

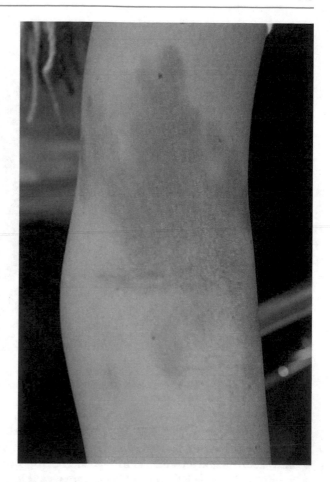

5.2.8   Zinc Deficiency

Despite the popularity of zinc as a supplement, zinc deficiency is fairly rare in the developed countries, specifically in otherwise healthy women complaining of hair loss. The daily requirement of zinc is 8 mg/day for women and 11 mg/day for men per day which is usually easily obtained with a normal omnivorous diet. The highest concentration of dietary zinc is found in oysters, meat, beans, and nuts. And yet, an estimated 25% of the world's population or up to 2 billion people worldwide may be at risk of zinc deficiency, while zinc is an essential trace mineral with wide clinical significance [165, 166].

Zinc deficiency can be caused by foods grown in zinc-deficient soil, a diet high in phytate-containing whole grains, or processed foods containing little or no zinc [167].

Soil zinc is an essential micronutrient for crops. Almost half of the world's cereal crops are deficient in zinc, leading to poor crop yields and to widespread human

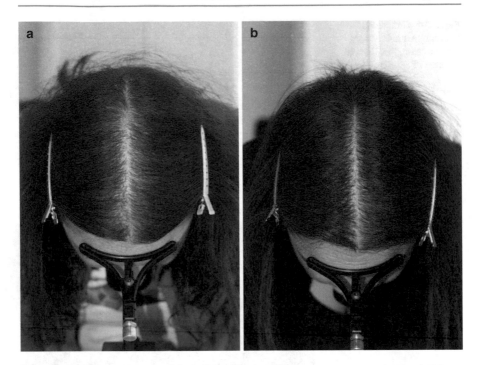

Fig. 5.15 (**a, b**) Successful treatment of alopecia in a female patient with anemic iron deficiency (serum ferritin: 4 μg/L, Hb: 81 g/L) due to ulcerative colitis: (**a**) before treatment, (**b**) regrowth of hair after treatment with iron infusion

zinc deficiency in areas with zinc-deficient soils. Adequate zinc uptake is imperative for good health during periods of rapid tissue growth, such as in childhood and adolescence. Stunted growth, and hypogonadism, especially in boys, has originally been observed in populations in which dietary zinc is low [168].

Despite some concerns [169], Western vegetarians and vegans do not suffer any more from overt zinc deficiency than meat eaters [170]. Major plant sources of zinc include cooked dried beans, sea vegetables, fortified cereals, soy foods, nuts, peas, and seeds. However, phytates in many whole grains and fibers may interfere with zinc absorption while the effects of marginal zinc intake are yet poorly understood.

Deficiency in zinc in the developed countries is predominantly seen with chronic alcoholism, anorexia nervosa, and drugs that chelate zinc (ACE inhibitors [171]), in association with pancreatitis, and following gastrointestinal bypass surgery. Vitamin and mineral supplements that contain iron-to-zinc ratios of greater than 3:1 may provide enough iron to inhibit zinc absorption. Ultimately, low levels of zinc may cause hypogeusia [172, 173] and reduce an individual's normal appetite for food [174]. In fact, the use of zinc in the treatment of anorexia has been advocated since 1979 by Bakan [175, 176].

Symptoms of zinc deficiency include diarrhea, diffuse alopecia [177], a peculiar acral and periorificial dermatitis (Fig. 5.16) with characteristic histopathologic

Fig. 5.16 Zinc deficiency (acquired acrodermatitis enteropathica): peculiar acral and periorificial dermatitis and alopecia with positive pull test

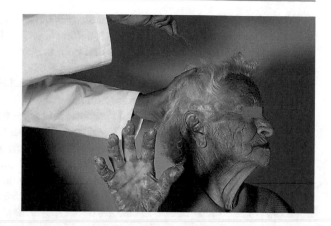

findings (necrobiosis of superficial layers of the epidermis), blepharoconjunctivitis, angular cheilitis and stomatitis, impaired wound healing, and overall compromised immune function, with a particular susceptibility to infections with *Candida* spp. and *Staph. aureus*. Finally, zinc is required to produce testosterone, and zinc deficiency can therefore lead to reduced circulating testosterone, which could lead to sexual immaturity, hypogonadism, and delayed puberty [178].

Differential diagnosis includes multiple other nutritional deficiencies including biotin, vitamin B2 (riboflavin), or essential fatty acid deficiency.

Zinc deficiency is defined either as insufficient zinc to meet the needs of the body or as a serum zinc level below the normal range. However, serum zinc is not a reliable biomarker for zinc status, and a decrease in the serum concentration is only detectable after long-term or severe depletion [179].

Prerequisite to the diagnosis is suspicion of inherited or acquired zinc deficiency based on clinical features, risk factors including geographical prevalence, age of presentation, dietary habits, and comorbidities. Ideal collection for serum studies includes using zinc-free vacuum tubes, stainless steel needles, avoiding contact with rubber stoppers, avoiding hemolysis, separating plasma or serum from cells within 45 min, use of anticoagulants low in zinc concentration, as well as morning fasting samples to optimize accuracy. Normal zinc levels are between 70 and 250 μg/dL in adults, and mild deficiency can manifest clinically when values decrease to 40–60 μg/dL. Ultimately, clinical improvement to zinc supplementation can be confirmatory.

Treatment begins with oral replacement. 2–3 mg/kg per day often cures all clinical manifestations within 1–2 weeks. Zinc supplements should only be ingested when there is zinc deficiency or increased zinc necessity, e.g., after surgery, trauma, or burn injury. Suggestions to help increase dietary zinc bioavailability are to include some form of animal food or vegetarian-acceptable fortified food in the diet each day, to avoid excessive consumption of alcohol and crash diets that are typically low in micronutrient content, and to take the dietary supplement of zinc separately from iron supplementations.

Arnaud et al. [180] evaluated the possible role of zinc deficiency in patients with idiopathic telogen effluvium ($n = 16$) and a control group. In addition to zinc determinations in blood plasma, blood cells, and hair, they measured serum albumin and alkaline phosphatase activity as functional indices. No significant differences between the two groups were noted, and the authors concluded that the involvement of zinc in telogen effluvium is therefore questionable.

Nevertheless, Karashima et al. [181] reported on the efficacy of oral zinc therapy for zinc deficiency-related telogen effluvium in five patients, and concluded that the administration of zinc for zinc deficiency-related alopecia may recover appropriate activities of metalloenzymes, hedgehog signaling, and immunomodulation, all of which are required for normal control of hair growth cycle.

Weisman et al. [182] reported on a 7-year-old girl with poor hair growth suffering from chronic diarrhea due to sucrase deficiency. Her scalp hair had a poor, colorless appearance with occipital alopecia. Microscopic hair examination, using polarized light, revealed well-defined abnormalities of the hair shafts, as originally reported by Dupré et al. in acrodermatitis enteropathica [183]: (1) a marked individual variation in diameter, (2) narrowing often associated with waving or sharp bending and broken ends, and (3) striation with a tendency to trichonodosis (Fig. 5.17a). Plasma zinc was low (7.9 μmol/L), whereas plasma albumin was normal. Oral zinc therapy, 40 mg daily, had a marked beneficial effect on her scalp hair, eyebrows, and eyelashes, which became thicker and pigmented. A rise in plasma zinc and serum alkaline phosphatase levels was observed during the zinc supplementation. The microscopic hair abnormalities were absent in the pigmented hair appearing after zinc therapy.

Traupe et al. [184] studied the hair of a 10-month-old girl who was suffering from acrodermatitis enteropathica, using light and polarizing microscopy before and after institution of zinc therapy. On light microscopy the shafts showed uneven diameter, atypical trichorrhexis nodosa with stretched fractures, and nodal swellings of the pseudomonilethrix type (Fig. 5.17b). Polarization microscopy disclosed

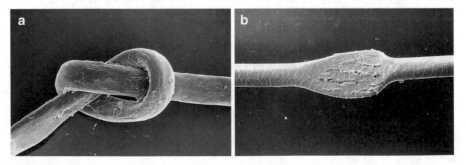

Fig. 5.17 (**a**, **b**) Hair shaft abnormalities reported in zinc deficiency (scanning electron microscopy). (**a**) Trichonodosis. (**b**) Pseudomonilethrix. The former is usually associated with a defective hair cuticle; the latter is with weakness of the hair shaft and is produced as an artifact when overlapped hairs are pressed together between glass slides while preparing hairs for microscopic examination

in 70% of all hair shafts an irregular pattern of alternating dark and bright bands. This anomaly but could no longer be detected after 2 years of zinc supplementation. Repeated determinations of hair probes before and after treatment gave a low cystine content, however, within the normal range. The authors assumed that the observed changes and the low hair cystine content could be attributed to the underlying zinc deficiency.

Slonim et al. [185] reported on two patients with dry brittle hair, alopecia, trichorrhexis nodosa, dry scaly skin, pigment dyschromia, short stature, and neurosecretory growth hormone deficiency. By means of the zinc tolerance test, one patient was shown to have zinc deficiency. In both patients, the hair and the skin abnormalities responded to oral zinc therapy.

Based on unconfirmed earlier reports [186, 187], oral zinc has traditionally been used for treating alopecia areata. Yet, Ead [188] had reported in 1981 that oral administration of zinc compounds had no therapeutic effect in a double-blind trial in alopecia areata. Since there are several reports stating that serum zinc levels may be low in alopecia areata patients [189–191], Park et al. [192] evaluated the therapeutic effects of oral zinc supplementation for 12 weeks in alopecia areata patients who had a low serum zinc level. Fifteen alopecia areata patients were enrolled in this study. After the therapy with oral zinc gluconate tablet (50 mg/day,) the serum zinc levels increased from 56.9 to 84.5 μg/dL. Positive therapeutic effects were observed for 9 out of 15 patients (66.7%). The patients with mild alopecia areata and who had a single alopecia areata patch displayed more positive results than the patients who had multiple alopecia areata patches. The serum zinc levels of the positive response group increased more than those of the negative response group.

Finally, considering the fact that zinc is essential in the regulation of a number of biological processes associated with normal growth and development, Baltaci et al. [193] reflected on the role of zinc on the endocrine system, since growth impairment, hypogonadism, and some endocrine diseases are associated with zinc deficiency. Zinc increases the synthesis of human growth hormone and its number of receptors and is therefore an important mediator in the binding of this hormone to its receptor. Found in a large quantity in the pancreas tissue, zinc has a part in the regulation of the effect of insulin. Zinc is involved in thyroid hormone metabolism, such as hormone synthesis, receptor activity, conversion of T4 to T3, and production of carrier proteins. Zinc is related to enzyme activity to melatonin synthesis. Zinc particularly affects the conversion of testosterone to dihydrotestosterone, as 5α-reductase is a zinc-dependent enzyme. In consideration of these relations, zinc may play critical roles in the endocrine system with possible implications for hormone-dependent hair growth and quality.

5.2.9   Copper Deficiency

Copper has frequently been described as the iron twin, because both iron and copper are metabolized in much the same manner, and both are components of cellular enzymes. Both are also involved in energy production and hemoglobin synthesis.

Because of its role in facilitating iron uptake, copper deficiency can produce anemia-like symptoms. The neurodegenerative syndrome of copper deficiency has been recognized for some time in ruminant animals, in which it is commonly known as swayback [194]. Copper (Cu) deficiency in a Norwegian red deer herd manifested as poor calf growth rate, low weights of adult hinds, dull and light-colored hair coats, and cases of diarrhea [195].

Copper is absorbed in the gut, and then transported to the liver bound to albumin. After processing in the liver, copper is distributed to other tissues in a second phase, which involves the protein ceruloplasmin, carrying the majority of copper in blood. Copper in the body normally undergoes enterohepatic circulation (about 5 mg a day, vs. about 1 mg per day absorbed in the diet and excreted from the body), and the body is able to excrete some excess copper, if needed, via bile, which carries some copper out of the liver that is not then reabsorbed by the intestine.

Bariatric surgery is a common cause of copper deficiency [196]. The disruption of the intestines and stomach from the surgery can cause absorption difficulties not only as regards copper, but also for iron and vitamin B12 and many other nutrients. The symptoms of copper deficiency myelopathy may take a long time to develop, sometimes decades before the myelopathy symptoms manifest.

Otherwise, copper deficiency in humans is rare and seen in premature babies, and severely malnourished children, with inadequately supplemented parenteral alimentation, and with prolonged oral zinc therapy without copper supplementation. Zinc is often used for the prevention or treatment of common colds, ulcers, sickle cell disease, celiac disease, memory impairment, and acne [197]. Zinc is found in many common vitamin supplements and is also found in denture creams. Recently, cases of copper-deficiency myeloneuropathy were found to be caused by use of denture creams containing high quantities of zinc [198].

Another rare cause of copper deficiency is celiac disease, probably due to malabsorption in the intestines. Still, a significant percentage, around 20%, of cases have unknown causes.

Clinical manifestations of acquired copper deficiency are fatigue and weakness, frequent sickness, weak and brittle bones, problems with memory and learning, difficulty walking, increased cold sensitivity, pale skin due to anemia, loss of vision, premature gray hair, and vision loss. Copper-deficiency myelopathy in humans was discovered and first described by Schleper and Stuerenburg in 2001 [199] who reported a patient with a history of gastrectomy and partial colonic resection. The patient presented with severe tetraparesis and painful paresthesia and was found on imaging to have dorsomedial cervical cord T2 hyperintensity. Upon further analysis, it was found that the patient had decreased levels of serum ceruloplasmin, serum copper, and cerebrospinal copper. The patient was successfully treated with parenteral copper. Since this discovery, there has been heightened and increasing awareness of copper-deficiency myelopathy and its treatment.

Copper deficiency is a very rare condition and therefore is often misdiagnosed several times by physicians. The diagnosis of copper deficiency may be supported by a person's report of compatible signs and symptoms, findings from a thorough physical examination, and supportive laboratory evidence. Low levels of copper and ceruloplasmin in the serum and low red blood cell superoxide dismutase levels are consistent with the diagnosis [200]. Additional supportive bloodwork findings also include anemia and neutropenia.

Copper deficiency can be treated with either oral copper supplementation or intravenous copper. If zinc intoxication is present, discontinuation of zinc may be sufficient to restore copper levels back to normal, but this usually takes long. People who suffer from zinc intoxication will usually have to take copper supplements in addition to ceasing intake of zinc.

The U.S. Institute of Medicine (IOM) updated the Estimated Average Requirements (EARs) and Recommended Dietary Allowances (RDAs) for copper in 2001. If there is no sufficient information to establish EARs and RDAs, an estimate designated adequate intake (AI) is used instead. The AIs for copper are 200 µg of copper for 0–6-month-old males and females, and 220 µg of copper for 7–12-month-old males and females. The RDAs for copper are 340 µg of copper for 1–3-year-old males, 440 µg of copper for 4–8-year-old males, 700 µg of copper for 9–13-year-old males, 890 µg of copper for 14–18-year-old males, and 900 µg of copper for males that are 19 years old and older. The RDAs for copper are 340 µg of copper for 1–3-year-old females, 440 µg of copper for 4–8-year-old females, 700 µg of copper for 9–13-year-old females, 890 µg of copper for 14–18-year-old females, and 900 µg of copper for females that are 19 years old and older. The RDAs for copper are 1000 µg of copper for 14–50-year-old pregnant females; furthermore, it is 1300 µg of copper for 14–50-year-old lactating females.

The European Food Safety Authority (EFSA) refers to the collective set of information as Dietary Reference Values, with Population Reference Intake (PRI) instead of RDA, and average requirement instead of EAR. AI and UL are defined the same as in the United States. For women and men aged 18 and older the AIs are set at 1.3 and 1.6 mg/day, respectively. AI for pregnancy and lactation is 1.5 mg/day. For children aged 1–17 years the AIs increase with age from 0.7 to 1.3 mg/day. These AIs are higher than the US RDAs.

5.2.10 Selenium Deficiency

Selenium intake varies greatly geographically depending on the soil selenium availability. Therefore, selenium deficiency is generally found in geographic area with a poor soil content of selenium, e.g., some areas in China (Jiangsu Province and Keshan County of Heilongjiang province), Yugoslavia [201], central Kenya Highlands [202], and Finland, where selenium salts are added to chemical fertilizers, as a way to increase selenium in soils [203].

Dietary deficiency of selenium due to poor soil content reported in Keshan, China, in combination with coxsackievirus infection can lead to Keshan disease [204]. The primary symptom of the disease is myocardial necrosis, leading to weakening of the heart. Clinical manifestations of disease are cardiomyopathy, muscle pain, and weakness with elevation of transaminase and creatine kinase levels. The condition is potentially fatal.

Along with iodine deficiency, selenium deficiency also contributes to Kashin-Beck disease [205], a chronic, endemic type of osteochondropathy that is mainly distributed from northeastern to southwestern China, Southeast Siberia, and North Korea. The condition usually involves children aged 5–15 with joint pain, morning stiffness, flexion and extension disturbances of the elbows, enlarged interphalangeal joints, and limited motion in many joints of the body due to death of cartilage cells of the growth plate and articular surface. This can result in growth retardation and secondary osteoarthrosis. This disease has been known for over 150 years but its cause has not yet been completely elucidated. Selenium and iodine have been considered as the major deficiencies. Currently, the accepted potential causes include mycotoxins present in grain, trace mineral deficiency in nutrition, and high levels of fulvic acid in drinking water. Mycotoxins produced by fungi that contaminate the grain cause the production of free radicals, while fulvic acid present in drinking water damages cartilage cells [206]. Selenium supplementation in selenium-deficient areas has been shown to prevent this disease.

Otherwise, selenium deficiency is relatively rare in healthy well-nourished individuals. It may occur in patients with severely compromised intestinal function, those undergoing total parenteral nutrition, those who have had gastrointestinal bypass surgery, and those of advanced age (over 90) [207].

Nevertheless, selenium has become a popular ingredient in many multivitamins and other dietary supplements, which typically contain 55 or 70 μg/serving. Selenium-specific supplements may contain up to 200 μg/serving, while the US Recommended Dietary Allowance (RDA) for teenagers and adults is 55 μg/day.

Cutaneous manifestations of selenium deficiency are white nails and hypopigmentation of skin and hair (pseudoalbinism) [208] with sparse, short, thin, light-colored hair in infants.

5.2.11 Vitamin D Deficiency

Vitamin D refers to a group of fat-soluble secosteroids responsible for multiple biological effects. The most important compounds within this group are vitamin D3 (cholecalciferol) and vitamin D2 (ergocalciferol). Both can be ingested from the diet, though only few foods contain vitamin D. The major natural source of vitamin D is the synthesis of cholecalciferol in the skin from cholesterol through a chemical reaction that is dependent on sun exposure, specifically to UVB radiation. Vitamin D from the diet or skin synthesis is biologically inactive. Enzymatic conversion (hydroxylation) in the liver and kidney is required for activation, with conversion in the liver of cholecalciferol to calcifediol (25-hydroxycholecalciferol) and of ergocalciferol to 25-hydroxyergocalciferol. Calcifediol is further hydroxylated by the kidneys to form calcitriol (1,25-dihydroxycholecalciferol), the biologically active form of vitamin D. Calcitriol circulates, by definition rather as a hormone than a vitamin, in the blood and produces effects via a nuclear receptor in multiple different target organs. It has a significant role in regulating the concentration of calcium and phosphate, and in promoting the healthy growth and remodeling of the bone.

Accordingly, its original discovery was due to the effort to find the dietary substance lacking in rickets (childhood osteomalacia). Nevertheless, calcitriol also has other effects, including some on cell growth, immune functions, and reduction of inflammation.

As vitamin D can be synthesized in adequate amounts by exposure to sufficient sunlight, it is not an essential dietary factor. Nevertheless, the dietary reference intake for vitamin D made by the National Academy Medicine assumes that all of a person's vitamin D is from oral intake, as recommendations about the amount of sun exposure required for optimal vitamin D levels are uncertain. Although vitamin D is not present naturally in most foods, it is commonly added as a fortification in various manufactured foods.

Vitamin D supplements are primarily given to treat or to prevent osteomalacia and rickets, but the evidence for other health effects of vitamin D supplementation in the general population remains inconsistent [209–212]; therefore as yet there exists no clear justification for recommending supplementation for preventing many diseases, before further research in these areas has supplied the respective data.

Vitamin D-dependent rickets is a rare genetic condition that may link hair growth to vitamin D. Vitamin D-dependent rickets type 2A (VDDR2A) is caused by a defect in the vitamin D receptor (VDR) gene. This defect leads to an increase in the circulating ligand, 1,25-dihydroxyvitamin D3. Most patients have total alopecia (Fig. 5.18) in addition to rickets [213].

The role of vitamin D in the proliferation and differentiation of keratinocytes is well appreciated within the field of dermatology, and lack of the VDR has been shown to be associated with reduced epidermal differentiation and hair follicle growth [214]. With this in mind, Amor et al. [215] sought to evaluate the role of vitamin D and its receptor in the hair cycle. Performing a MEDLINE search 1955–July 2009 to find relevant articles pertaining to vitamin D, VDR, and hair loss, they found that the VDR, independent of vitamin D, plays an important role in hair cycling, specifically anagen initiation, while the role of vitamin D in hair follicle cycling is not as well understood. They concluded that additional studies should be done to evaluate the role of vitamin D in the hair cycle, specifically on treatments that upregulate the VDR with the prospect of treating hair cycling disorders. Ultimately, Fawzi et al. [216] found serum and tissue VDR levels lower in alopecia areata, as well as androgenetic alopecia patients, when compared to healthy controls.

On another line of investigation, observations linking vitamin D deficiency to autoimmune diseases, such as multiple sclerosis, diabetes mellitus I, and inflammatory bowel disease in northern geographic regions with lower exposure to sunlight, led to the investigation of vitamin D levels in patients with alopecia areata: Yilmaz et al. [217] originally reported decreased vitamin D concentrations in patients with alopecia areata. The study, however, was performed in only 42 cases, and during summer. At this point, and after originally having reported on a statistical significant seasonality of alopecia areata in adult patients suffering from remitting-relapsing forms, independently from an atopic diathesis and seasonal telogen effluvium, d'Ovidio et al. [218] checked a larger group of 156 patients affected by chronic remitting-relapsing alopecia areata with involvement of more than 25% of scalp

Fig. 5.18 Universal
atrichia may be associated
with vitamin D-dependent
rickets type 2A caused by
a defect in the vitamin D
receptor gene

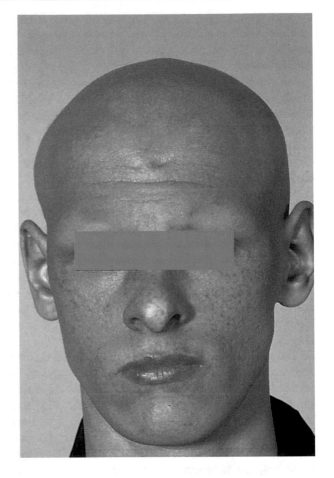

area. The authors confirmed presence of insufficiency/deficiency of
25-hydroxyvitamin D (25(OH)D) in the patients' group, although the results were
not significantly different compared with 148 controls. This was due to the universal
tendency to lower values of 25(OH)D also in the normal population of central
Europe. Subsequently, Aksu Cerman et al. [219] performed a cross-sectional study
on 86 patients with alopecia areata, 44 patients with vitiligo, and 58 healthy controls
to evaluate the status of vitamin D and the relationship between vitamin D levels
and disease severity in patients with alopecia areata. Serum 25(OH)D levels in
patients with alopecia areata were found to be significantly lower than those of the
patients with vitiligo and the healthy controls ($p = 0.001$ and $p < 0.001$, resp.). The
prevalence of 25(OH)D deficiency was significantly higher in the patients with alopecia areata (90.7%) compared with the patients with vitiligo (70.5%) and the
healthy controls (32.8%) ($p = 0.003$ and $p < 0.001$, resp.). Furthermore, a significant
inverse correlation was found between disease severity and serum 25(OH)D level in
the patients with alopecia areata ($r = -0.409$; $p < 0.001$). Subsequent authors

[220–223] came up with consistent results, including pediatric alopecia areata [224]. Accordingly, the general conclusion has been that screening alopecia areata patients for vitamin D deficiency is recommended for the possibility of respective supplementation, since patients with alopecia areata present deficient serum 25(OH) D levels that inversely correlate with disease severity.

However, Thompson et al. [225] have criticized that none of the studies reporting the increased prevalence of vitamin D deficiency in patients with alopecia areata have prospectively examined vitamin D status and incident alopecia areata. In 55,929 women in the Nurses' Health Study (NHS), they prospectively evaluated the association between estimated vitamin D status, derived from a prediction model incorporating lifestyle determinants of serum vitamin D, and self-reported incident alopecia areata, and evaluated dietary, supplemental, and total vitamin D intake as additional exposures. They found no significant association between dietary, supplemental, or total vitamin D intake and incident alopecia areata, disproving a preventive role for vitamin D in the risk of developing alopecia areata.

Finally, the number of studies on vitamin D levels in other hair loss conditions, such as female pattern hair loss and telogen effluvium, has been substantially lower than that for alopecia areata, though again lower levels of vitamin D in comparison to healthy controls have been identified both in female pattern hair loss [226, 227] and in telogen effluvium [226, 228, 229].

In a retrospective study of 444 female patients with either alopecia areata ($n = 95$), female pattern hair loss ($n = 294$), or telogen effluvium ($n = 93$) seen at the Center for Dermatology and Hair Disease Professor Trüeb in 2015, Speicher [230] found an inverse correlation between serum vitamin D levels and severity of female pattern hair loss (with levels of 70.01 nmol/L +/−33.9 SD in Ludwig I, 55.30 nmol/L +/−28.9 SD in Ludwig II, and 47.93 nmol/L +/−29.3 SD in Ludwig III) and of alopecia areata (with levels of 63.09 nmol/L +/−35.4 SD in alopecia areata <30% scalp surface, and 51.68 nmol/L +/−26.9 SD in alopecia areata >30% scalp surface but not alopecia totalis/universalis), possibly indicating a contributing role or threshold effect of vitamin D levels for hair growth and differentiation in female pattern hair loss, and for inflammation in alopecia areata. In analogy to the study of Kantor et al. on serum ferritin levels in women with alopecia [146], the mean vitamin D levels in women with telogen effluvium (66.0 nmol/L +/−33.9 SD) and alopecia areata totalis/universalis (68.05 nmol/L +/−33.4 SD) were not significantly lower than normal. In these cases, vitamin D levels do not seem to play a role, probably due to more important pathogenic factors overriding the effects of vitamin D.

The optimal level for 25-hydroxyvitamin D, the most stable and reliable parameter to evaluate vitamin D status, begins at 30 ng/mL even though the level required to maintain optimal immune system homeostasis has not been established yet, although several reports estimate that it would be superior to 40 ng/mL (or 100 nmol/ mL). The calculation formulas for saturation and maintenance therapy with vitamin D are the following (Box 5.1):

> **Box 5.1 Calculation formulas for saturation and maintenance therapy with vitamin D**
> Saturation dose in IU vitamin D
>
> $$= \left(40\,\text{ng}\,/\,\text{mL} - \text{patient's vitamin D level in ng}\,/\,\text{mL}\right)$$
> $$\times \frac{\text{patient's body weight in kg}}{70\,\text{kg}} \times \frac{10{,}000\,\text{IU}}{1\,\text{ng}\,/\,\text{mL}}$$
>
> Maintenance dose in IU vitamin D (per month)
>
> $$= 40\,\text{ng}\,/\,\text{mL} \times 0.2 \times \frac{\text{patient's body weight in kg}}{70\,\text{kg}} \times \frac{10{,}000\,\text{IU}}{1\,\text{ng}\,/\,\text{mL}}$$
>
> Vitamin D:
> 1 µg = 40 IU
> Vitamin D in blood levels:
> 1 ng/mL = 1 µg/L = 2.5 nml/L

Whether supplementation with vitamin D affects hair growth and shedding in alopecia areata (Fig. 5.19a,b), female pattern hair loss, or telogen effluvium remains to be elucidated. The optimal range for blood concentration is regarded to be 75.0–185.0 nmol/L. Based on risk assessment, a safe upper intake level of 250 µg (10,000 IU) per day in healthy adults has been suggested by nongovernment authors. However, no government has a suggested tolerable upper intake levels in excess of 4000 IU. Hypervitaminosis D is the state of vitamin D toxicity.

5.2.12 Multiple Nutritional Deficiencies

Finally, in real-time life, we are often confronted with multiple nutritional deficiencies rather than a single-deficiency disorder, depending on age, socioeconomic status, dietary habits, and comorbidities of the particular individual. Examples are morbid obesity [231], cancer patients [232], hospitalized patients [233], malnourished children [234], adolescents with eating disorders [235], inflammatory bowel disease [236], intestinal failure [237], dialysis [238], atopics with sensitization to multiple foodstuffs [239], neurologic disease [240], pregnancy and early childhood [241], geriatric population [242], dementia [243], chronic critical illness [244], homelessness [245], and chronic alcohol excess [246].

The multiple nutritional deficiencies may cause significant morbidity [247] and increased mortality, especially in the elderly, regardless of the cause of death [248]. Multiple nutritional deficiencies may affect the skin [87], whereby the condition of the skin and hair may be a presenting sign of the illness [249, 250]. Although some

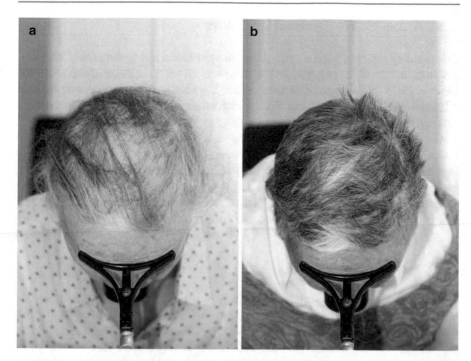

Fig. 5.19 (**a**, **b**) Successful treatment of diffuse alopecia areata in a 65-year-old female: (**a**) Before treatment the patient suffered from rapidly progressive diffuse hair loss associated with autoimmune thyroid disease, borrelia infection, and vitamin D deficiency. (**b**) Sustained regrowth of hair following topical clobetasol propionate 0.05% foam twice daily on 5 consecutive days per week for 6 months, thyroid supplementation therapy, intravenous ceftriaxone 2 g daily during 21 days, and oral vitamin D3 1500 IU per day

signs are characteristic of a specific single-nutrient deficiency, such as phrynoderma (vitamin A), pellagra (niacin), seborrheic-like dermatitis (biotin, zinc, essential fatty acids), glossitis (vitamin B12), and cheilosis (riboflavin), an overlap of skin manifestations is observed in multiple-deficiency states, while glossodynia [251] and hair loss are less specific markers for nutritional deficiencies. Therefore, specifically in these patient groups multiple nutrition screening should be performed as indicated to identify individuals who may require nutritional support for general health, hair growth, and quality.

Laboratory tests are useful when the probability of a disease being present is neither high nor low, since high degree of clinical certainty overrides the uncertainty of the laboratory data, e.g., in zinc deficiency. Clinical suspicion is the determinant, and knowledge of clinical dermatology is the prerequisite for combining medical sense with economic sense in requesting laboratory tests. The greater the number of different tests done, the greater the risk of getting irrelevant leads. The possibilities for laboratory errors increase in the automated multiple-screen procedures. Therefore, laboratory testing and interpretation must be kept focused on the medical history of the patient, clinical findings, and clinicopathological correlations.

5.3   Complex Nutritional Disorders

Accelerating economic development and modernization of agricultural, food processing, and food formulation techniques reduced single-nutrient-deficiency diseases globally. In response, nutrition science has shifted to the research on the role of nutrition in more complex conditions, such as gluten sensitivity, obesity, bariatric surgery, anorexia and bulimia, alcoholism, aging, and the oncological patient. Recognition of complexity is a key lesson of the past. Initial observations lead to reasonable, simplified theories that achieve certain practical benefits, which are then inevitably advanced by new knowledge and recognition of ever-increasing complexity.

Ultimately, additional complexity may arise in nutritional recommendations for general well-being versus the treatment of specific pathological conditions.

5.3.1   Gluten Sensitivity

Gluten is a composite of proteins stored together with starch in the endosperm of various grass-related grains with the function of nourishing the embryonic plant during germination. It is found in wheat, barley, rye, oat, related species and hybrids, and all products of these. In the food industry, it is appreciated for its viscoelastic properties giving elasticity to dough, helping it rise and keep its shape, and giving the final product, such as bread and imitation meats, a chewy texture. Finally, gluten may be present in beer and soy sauce, and is used as a stabilizing agent in more unexpected food products, such as ice cream and ketchup, where it may pose a hazard as hidden gluten for a small proportion of consumers suffering from gluten-sensitive enteropathy or celiac disease.

Gluten-related disorders is the umbrella term for all disease conditions triggered by gluten sensitivity, which include celiac disease, and non-celiac gluten sensitivity [252, 253].

Classical celiac disease is currently the least common of presentations, and affects predominantly children younger than 2 years of age with gastrointestinal manifestations, such as chronic diarrhea and abdominal distention, malabsorption, loss of appetite, and impaired growth [254].

Nonclassical celiac disease has evolved to be the more common clinical type occurring in all age groups with an estimated prevalence of 1–2% of the population. It is characterized by milder or even absent gastrointestinal symptoms and a variety of non-intestinal manifestations, including dermatitis herpetiformis Duhring (Fig. 5.20a–d) [255].

Untreated celiac disease may cause malabsorption, reduced quality of life, iron deficiency, osteoporosis, and an increased risk of intestinal lymphomas, with increased mortality [256].

Finally, celiac disease is associated with a number of other autoimmune diseases [257], including alopecia areata: Corazza et al. [258] originally reported on a possible association between celiac disease and alopecia areata. The authors initially

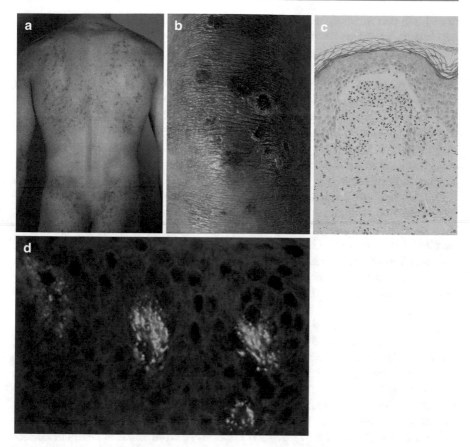

Fig. 5.20 (a–d) Dermatitis herpetiformis Duhring. (a) Typical clinical presentation. (b) Vesicular lesions on the elbow. (c) Histopathology: dermal papillary neutrophilic microabscess. (d) Direct immunofluorescence: granular IgA deposits in the dermal papillae

observed three patients with such an association. In one patient gluten-free diet resulted in complete regrowth of scalp and body hair. The authors subsequently set up a prospective screening program for celiac disease using antigliadin and antiendomysial antibodies in 256 consecutive outpatients with alopecia areata. Three patients that were completely asymptomatic for intestinal diseases were found to be positive and underwent biopsy. Histological analysis was consistent with the diagnosis of celiac disease. The authors concluded that alopecia areata may constitute the only clinical manifestation of celiac disease and that the association between these two conditions is a real one because the observed frequency of association was greater than that expected by chance. Naveh et al. [259] reported an association of celiac disease with alopecia in three children. In one, the alopecia developed after 4 years' nonadherence to a gluten-free diet, and the other two patients presented with alopecia. Administration of a gluten-free diet resulted in partial regrowth of hair in the first child and complete hair growth in the others. Ultimately, Ertekin et al. [260] performed a screening for celiac disease in children with alopecia areata, and found a prevalence of 41.7% celiac disease in 12 children with alopecia areata, while the prevalence of celiac disease in 1263 healthy children in the same city was 0.87%. The authors concluded that children with alopecia areata should be screened for celiac disease since the prevalence of silent celiac disease was very high among children with alopecia areata.

Making things more complicated is the concept of non-celiac gluten sensitivity that has evolved to describe a condition of multiple symptoms that improve when switching to a gluten-free diet, after exclusion of celiac disease. Acknowledged since 2010, with an alleged prevalence of 6–10% of the population, its pathogenesis remains as yet not understood. Symptoms include gastrointestinal symptoms, which resemble those of irritable bowel syndrome, and/or a wide variety of non-gastrointestinal symptoms, such as headaches, chronic fatigue, fibromyalgia, atopic disease, and others [261, 262]. People with non-celiac gluten sensitivity remain habitually in a no-man's-land, not being recognized by the respective specialists, and therefore lacking the medical care and treatment expected [263]. Most have a long history of health complaints and unsuccessful consultations with numerous physicians, and usually end up resorting to a self-diagnosis of gluten sensitivity, and a gluten-free diet.

The statement "Nothing is wrong with you" is dangerous on two accounts: first, it denies the fallibility of all physicians, and second, it splits the mind from the body [160]. Studies show that while it usually takes 20–30 min in a didactic exercise for the senior doctor and students to arrive at a working diagnosis, an expert clinician typically forms a notion of what is wrong with the patient within 20 s. However, physicians should caution themselves to be not so ready to match a patient's complaints against their mental templates or clinical prototypes [160]. In his publication *"How Doctors Think"* (2007), Jerome Groopman, from Harvard Medical School [160], focuses on the thinking errors in medicine: snap judgement, stereotypical thinking, premature conclusion, and herd instinct are only a few of the subtle traps that dangerously narrow the vision of the physician. Doctors, like everyone else, run the risk of being led astray by stereotypes that are based on an individual's appearance, emotional state, or circumstances. Most of us especially dislike patients whom we stereotype as neurotic and anxious. Ultimately, doctors who dislike their patients cut them short during the recitation of symptoms and complaints, and prefer to fix on a convenient diagnosis and treatment. This skewing of the physician's thinking potentially leads to poor care. Groopman describes this kind of attribution error in the case of a nervous young woman who kept losing weight even when prescribed a high-calorie diet. Her doctors, convinced that she was double-dealing about her food intake, attributed her symptoms to suspected anorexia or bulimia, while in fact her problem turned out to be celiac disease, diagnosed only after years of ill health [160].

Diagnosis of celiac disease may be difficult, with the risk of significant delay of diagnosis. Serological testing represents the first-line investigation. Its sensitivity correlates with the degree of histological lesions. Therefore, people who present minor damage of the small intestine may be seronegative. The level of symptoms will determine the order of tests, but all tests lose their usefulness if the person is already on a gluten-free diet. Intestinal damage begins to heal within weeks of gluten being removed from the diet, and antibody levels decline over months. In patients with villous atrophy, antiendomysial (EMA) antibodies of the immunoglobulin A (IgA) type can detect celiac disease with a sensitivity and specificity of 90% and 99%, respectively [264]. Serology for anti-transglutaminase antibodies (anti-tTG) was initially reported to have a higher sensitivity (99%) and specificity (>90%). However, it is now thought to have similar characteristics to antiendomysial antibody. Both anti-transglutaminase and antiendomysial antibodies have high sensitivity to diagnose people with classic symptoms and complete villous atrophy, but they are only found in 30–89% of the cases with partial villous atrophy and in less than 50% of the people who have minor mucosal lesions with normal villi, the so-called duodenal lymphocytosis [265]. Guidelines recommend that a total serum IgA level is checked in parallel, as people with IgA deficiency may be unable to produce the respective antibodies on which these tests depend resulting in false-negative rest results. In those people, IgG antibodies against transglutaminase (IgG-tTG) may be diagnostic. Because of the major implications of a diagnosis of celiac disease, professional guidelines recommend that a positive blood test is followed by an endoscopy and biopsy [266, 267].

For now, the only links between gluten sensitivity and hair loss are the association of celiac disease with alopecia areata, and nutritional hair loss resulting from malabsorption in celiac disease. Results of gluten-free diet on restoring hair growth in celiac disease-associated alopecia areata have so far been inconsistent [268–271]. Finally, there have so far been no reports on an association of hair loss with non-celiac gluten sensitivity.

At the time of diagnosis, further investigations are therefore recommended to identify complications, such as deficiency in iron, folic acid, and vitamin B12. Finally, thyroid function tests may also be required to identify hypothyroidism from associated autoimmune thyroid disease, which is more common in celiac disease [272], and may also affect the condition of the hair.

5.3.2   Junk Food and Obesity

Obesity is the clinical term for a medical condition in which excess body fat has accumulated to an extent that it may have a negative effect on health.

It is defined and classified by the body mass index (BMI), and further evaluated in terms of fat distribution via the waist–hip ratio. People are generally considered obese when their body mass index (BMI), a measurement obtained by dividing a person's weight by the square of the person's height, is over 30 kg/m^2; the range 25–30 kg/m^2 is defined as overweight, $\geq$35 kg/m^2 as severe obesity, and a BMI of $\geq$35 kg/m^2 in association with obesity-related health conditions or $\geq$40 kg/m^2 as morbid obesity. As Asian populations develop negative health consequences at a lower BMI than Caucasians, Japan has redefined obesity for its population as any BMI >25 kg/m^2 [273] and China a BMI >28 kg/m^2 [274].

The exclusive use of the BMI to define obesity has undergone criticism since it does not measure body fat but rather total body weight relative to height; specifically, for individuals with more muscle mass than the average person, the BMI may lose its reliability for assessing weight-associated risks. For increasing the accuracy of health risk assessment, the use of waist circumference has been introduced because it is understood that the greater the amount of adipose tissue stored within the abdominal region the higher the risk for comorbidities. Waist circumferences with increased risk are ≥100 cm (40 in.) for men, and ≥90 cm (35 in.) for women.

The waist–hip ratio (WHR) is the ratio of the circumference of the waist to that of the hips that is calculated as waist measurement divided by hip measurement ($W \div H$). Practically, the waist (W) is measured at the smallest circumference of the natural waist, usually just above the belly button, and the hip (H) circumference may likewise be measured at its widest part of the buttocks or hip. Abdominal obesity is defined as a waist–hip ratio >0.90 for males and >0.85 for females. WHRs of 0.9 for men and 0.7 for women correlate strongly with general health and fertility. Women within the 0.7 range have optimal levels of estrogen, and women with high WHR (0.80 or higher) have significantly lower pregnancy rates than women with lower WHRs (0.70–0.79), independent of their BMIs [275], while men with WHRs around 0.9, similarly, have been shown to be fertile with less prostate cancer and testicular cancer [276].

The hormonal changes associated with menopause, specifically the overall decrease in ovarian production of the hormones estradiol and progesterone, are also associated with an increase in WHR independent of increases in body mass [277]. Importantly, studies showed that large premenopausal WHRs are associated with lower estradiol levels and variation in age of menopause onset [278]. Circulating estrogen preferentially stores adipose tissue in the gluteofemoral region, including the buttocks and thighs, and there is evidence that menopause-associated estrogen deficiency results in an accumulation of adipose deposits around the abdomen [279].

Obesity is a leading preventable cause of death worldwide, with increasing rates in adults and children. Despite an apparent obsession with weight and a multibillion industry of weight-loss products, the trends in obesity continue to grow in an unfavorable direction. Currently 68.5% of adults in the United States are overweight, of which 35% are obese, and 6.4% extremely obese. 17% of children and adolescents between the ages of 2 and 19 years are also obese [280], and are significantly more likely to continue to suffer from obesity as they get older [281].

Obesity increases the risk of both physical and mental conditions. Important comorbidities are included in the metabolic syndrome, a combination of type 2 diabetes mellitus, arterial hypertension, and high blood cholesterol and triglyceride levels. Health consequences are either due to the effects of increased fat mass, such as osteoarthritis, obstructive sleep apnea, social stigmatization, and depression, or of those related to the increase in the number of adipose cells: diabetes, cancer, cardiovascular disease, nonalcoholic fatty liver disease, and insulin resistance. Increased fat also creates a pro-inflammatory [282] and a prothrombotic state [283].

Also, morbid obesity has been shown to be associated with a high prevalence of micronutrient deficiency, most commonly of vitamin D, iron, vitamin B12, and thiamine (vitamin B1), with the respective health sequelae. Inappropriate eating behavior; favoring foods with a high calorie density and poor micronutrient content; impaired expression of transporter proteins, e.g., for iron due to chronic inflammation; and small intestinal overgrowth syndrome, specifically following obesity surgery, may contribute. Small intestinal bacterial overgrowth results in malabsorption of thiamine due to bacterial thiaminases, of vitamin B12 due to bacterial cobamides, of biologically inactive vitamin B12 analogues, and of fat-soluble vitamins due to impaired micelle formation as a result of bacterial deconjugation of conjugated bile acids.

Associations of hair anomalies with obesity have been reported early on [284], and initially as ill-defined syndromes associated with hirsutism, such as the Achard-Thiers syndrome and the Morgagni-Stewart-Morel syndrome.

Achard-Thiers syndrome [285, 286] is a rare disorder that occurs primarily in postmenopausal women and is characterized by type 2 diabetes mellitus and signs of androgen excess, usually facial hirsutisms and receding hair line, and thus it is the synonymous term of the diabetic bearded woman syndrome (Fig. 5.21). The constellation of clinical androgen excess and hyperinsulinemia is now commonly identified earlier in a woman's life, typically during adolescence and young adulthood, as polycystic ovary syndrome (PCOS).

Morgagni-Stewart-Morel syndrome [287] is a disorder characterized by thickening of the frontal bone of the skull (internal frontal hyperostosis) causing headaches, in combination with obesity and excessive body hair growth. While individuals with Morgagni-Stewart-Morel syndrome nearly always have hyperostosis frontalis interna, the finding may be incidental on X-ray films, computed tomography, or magnetic resonance imaging of the head in 12–37% of women, and by itself is not indicative of any specific disease. The cause of Morgagni-Stewart-Morel is unknown, although some have suggested that a hormonal imbalance due to genetic and environmental factors may be causative.

More relevant are the obesity and hair anomalies (hirsutism and patterned hair loss) associated with the *Klein-Leventhal syndrome* or polycystic ovary syndrome (PCOS). Originally described by Irving Stein and Michael Leventhal in 1935 in a

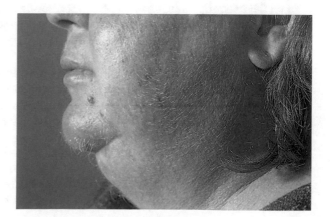

Fig. 5.21 Achard-Thiers syndrome

Table 5.3 2003 Rotterdam criteria for the diagnosis of polycystic ovary syndrome (PCOS)

1. Oligo- or anovulation:
• <9 menses a year or missed menses for ≥3 months
2. Clinical and/or biochemical signs of hyperandrogenism:
• Hirsutism, acne, alopecia
• Serum levels of androgens, including androstenedione and testosterone, may be elevated. The free testosterone level is thought to be the best measure, with ca. 60% of patients demonstrating elevated levels. Some other blood tests are suggestive but not diagnostic. The ratio of luteinizing hormone (LH) to follicle-stimulating hormone (FSH), when measured in international units, is elevated. Common cutoffs to designate abnormally high LH/FSH ratios are 2:1 or 3:1 as tested on day 3 of the menstrual cycle.
3. Echogenic evidence of polycystic ovaries and exclusion of other causes of hyperandrogenism and anovulation:
• Polycystic ovaries on ultrasound are defined by the presence of >12 follicles in each ovary (each follicle measuring 2–9 mm in diameter) and/or increased ovarian volume of >10 mL
• Differential diagnosis of PCOS (laboratory evaluation): pregnancy (elevated serum or urine HCG), premature ovarian failure (elevated FSH and LH, low-normal estradiol levels), hypothyroidism (elevated TSH, low thyroxine levels), hyperprolactinemia (elevated prolactin level), late-onset congenital adrenal hyperplasia (elevated day-5 morning level of 17-hydroxyprogesterone), virilizing ovarian/adrenal tumor (total testosterone >200 ng/dL, DHEAS >700 μg/L, and elevated androstenedione), Cushing's syndrome (elevated 24-h urine free cortisol level, unsuppressed morning serum cortisol during the low-dose dexamethasone suppression test, and elevated midnight salivary cortisol)
Requires 2 out of 3 for diagnosis of PCOS

case series of seven women with anovulation and polycystic ovaries discovered during surgery [288], the syndrome has more recently been defined by the Rotterdam criteria (Table 5.3) [289]. Given the broad definition described by the Rotterdam criteria, the prevalence of PCOS has been estimated to range from 15% to 18% [290].

PCOS represents a complex disorder with several aberrant hormonal and metabolic pathways. Hyperandrogenism is one of the most important clinical features of the syndrome and the most relevant to the role of the dermatologist in the diagnosis and management of the condition. The prevalence of hirsutism in PCOS ranges from 70 to 80%, vs. 4 to 11% in women in the general population [291], frequently seen on the upper lip, chin, areola, chest, back, lower abdomen, and thighs [292]. Acne is another common cutaneous manifestation of hyperandrogenism in PCOS, and originates or persists into adulthood while being refractory to conventional treatment (Fig. 5.22) [293].

Among women with PCOS, alopecia may be yet another manifestation of hyperandrogenism, though less frequent than hirsutism and acne are. Typically, it responds less well to topical minoxidil than in female androgenetic alopecia that is not associated with PCOS, and therefore should be treated with combined antiandrogen therapy [294].

Most importantly, PCOS presents with potentially serious systemic long-term implications, including risks of metabolic syndrome and of endometrial carcinoma [295]. PCOS is associated with several metabolic complications, including obesity, metabolic syndrome, and insulin resistance. Obesity is present in 75% of women

Fig. 5.22 Polycystic
ovary syndrome

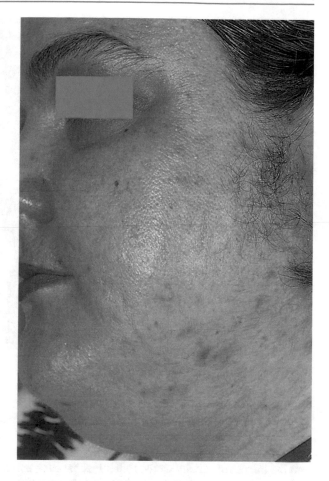

with PCOS, and up to 47% of women with PCOS have metabolic syndrome. Insulin resistance is common among patients with PCOS independent of obesity. The cutaneous signs of hyperinsulinemia include acanthosis nigricans and skin tags, basically the features of the *HAIR-AN (hyperandrogenism, insulin resistance, and acanthosis nigricans) syndrome* [296] (Fig. 5.23a,b). Insulin plays an important role in the development of anovulation and hyperandrogenism, which explains the ability of insulin-sensitizing agents, such as metformin, to lower androgen levels and induce ovulation.

Women with PCOS have an increased risk of cardiovascular disease; however it is not clear whether PCOS is an independent risk factor or whether cardiovascular disease results from the comorbidities associated with PCOS. In general, patients should be closely monitored and managed for obesity with weight loss and exercise, diabetes with insulin-sensitizing drugs such as metformin, hyperlipidemia, and hypertension. Although combined oral contraceptive pills are widely considered as first-line therapy in PCOS, a drawback may be the metabolic side effects, and risk of thromboembolism. The current recommendation suggests low-dose ethinyl

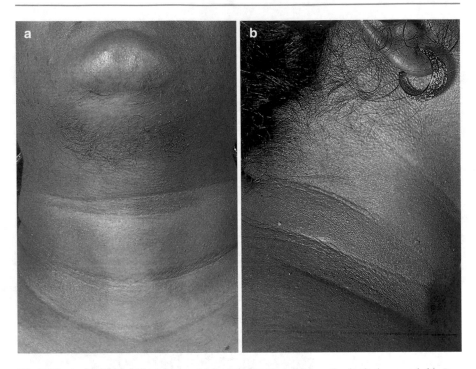

Fig. 5.23 (**a**, **b**) HAIR-AN syndrome. (**a**) Facial hirsutism. (**b**) Acanthosis nigricans and skin tags

estradiol (<50 microg), avoiding androgenic progestins, and addition of metformin to offset insulin resistance. There is as yet no evidence in the literature for the effect of weight loss or of metformin on alopecia associated with PCOS.

More recently, the association of obesity and alopecia has been scrutinized [297], and the impact of obesity on the folliculosebaceous unit has been discussed [298].

In a cross-sectional study conducted in Taiwan [299], the authors attempted to determine the association between BMI and alopecia severity in men with male-pattern androgenetic alopecia. The medical charts and photographs of 189 men with a clinical diagnosis of male-pattern androgenetic alopecia were reviewed. The men had a mean age of 30.8 years. In those with male-pattern androgenetic alopecia ($n = 142$), men with severe alopecia (grade V–VII) had higher BMI than those with mild-to-moderate alopecia (grade I–IV) (25.1 vs. 22.8 kg/m(2), $p = 0.01$). After multivariate adjustments, the risk for severe alopecia was higher in the overweight or obese (BMI ≥24 kg/m(2)) subjects with androgenetic alopecia (odds ratio 3.52, $p < 0.01$). In early-onset male-pattern androgenetic alopecia ($n = 46$), the risk for having severe alopecia was also higher in the overweight or obese subjects (odds ratio 4.97, $p = 0.03$). The authors concluded that higher BMI was significantly associated with greater severity of hair loss in men with male-pattern androgenetic alopecia, especially in those with early-onset androgenetic alopecia.

Since previous investigations had revealed an association of severe early-onset androgenetic alopecia with ischemic heart disease, Hirsso et al. [300] examined the possible association between early-onset alopecia and low-grade inflammation measured by high-sensitivity C-reactive protein (hs-CRP) that has been recommended for the assessment of the cardiovascular disease risk. The study population consisted of 727 young Finnish men, aged 25–34 years, participating in a national survey. The grade of alopecia was assessed by a trained nurse using the Hamilton-Norwood Classification Scale. Men with moderate-to-extensive alopecia (17%) had a BMI and larger waist, upper arm, hip, and waist circumference than those with little to no alopecia ($p < 0.05$), and statistically insignificant differences were seen in the waist-to-hip circumference ratio (WHR), diastolic blood pressure, and hs-CRP. With increasing hs-CRP, the mean WHR increased, but only among men with moderate-to-extensive alopecia ($p = 0.043$). The authors concluded that there is a relation between moderate-to-extensive alopecia and low-grade inflammation, a predictor of a future cardiovascular disease, especially combined with central obesity, among men younger than 35 years.

Ultimately, a study was performed to analyze the presence of cardiovascular risk factors included in the Adult Treatment Panel-III criteria for metabolic syndrome, prevalence of carotid atheromatosis, hormonal (aldosterone, insulin, testosterone, and sex hormone-binding globulin) factors, and acute-phase reactant (C-reactive protein, fibrinogen, D-dimers, erythrocyte sedimentation rate) variables in male and female patients with androgenetic alopecia and in a control group, and to analyze differences among the groups. The case-control study included 154 participants, 77 with early-onset androgenetic alopecia (40 male and 37 female) and 77 healthy control subjects (40 male and 37 female) from the Department of Dermatology at a University Hospital in Granada, Spain [301]. Metabolic syndrome was diagnosed in 60% of male patients with androgenetic alopecia (odds ratio [OR] = 10.5, 95% confidence interval [CI] 3.3–32.5), 48.6% of female patients with androgenetic alopecia (OR = 10.73, 95% CI 2.7–41.2), 12.5% of male control subjects, and 8.1% of female control subjects ($p < 0.0001$). Atheromatous plaques were observed in 32.5% of male patients with androgenetic alopecia (OR = 5.93, 95% CI 1.5–22.9) versus 7.5% of male control subjects ($p = 0.005$) and 27% of female patients with androgenetic alopecia (OR = 4.19, 95% CI 1.05–16.7) versus 8.1% of female control subjects ($p = 0.032$). Aldosterone and insulin levels were significantly higher in the male and female patients with androgenetic alopecia versus their respective control subjects. Mean values of fibrinogen were significantly higher in male patients with androgenetic alopecia, whereas values of fibrinogen, C-reactive protein, and D-dimers were significantly higher in female patients with androgenetic alopecia versus their respective control subjects. The authors concluded that the determination of metabolic syndrome and ultrasound study of carotid arteries may be useful screening methods to detect the risk of cardiovascular disease in male and female patients with early-onset androgenetic alopecia and signal a potential opportunity for early preventive treatment.

Finally, Starka et al. [302] suggested that premature androgenetic alopecia and insulin resistance may represent a clinical constellation that may be the male homologue or phenotype of PCOS.

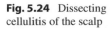

Fig. 5.24 Dissecting
cellulitis of the scalp

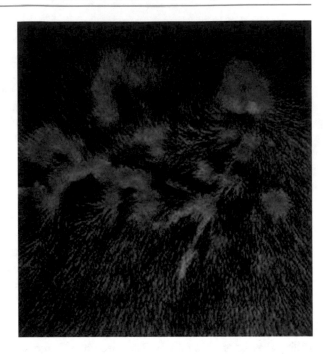

Lee et al. [303] suggested yet another scalp condition with a possible association with obesity. They conducted a hospital-based retrospective study of 66 patients (63 men/3 women) with a histopathological diagnosis or clinical features leading to diagnosis of dissecting cellulitis of the scalp (Fig. 5.24). Overweight and obesity were noted in 29 of 45 patients examined. There was comorbidity with acne conglobata in 15 of the 66 patients, 2 of whom had acne inversa. In contrast to acne inversa, they found no association with smoking in these patients.

The causes of obesity are multifactorial, and yet a major contributor to obesity in the Western world is physical inactivity. However genetic and environmental factors influence an individual's risk of obesity. Ultimately, family food and lifestyle patterns provide an environment that allows the genetic trait to manifest itself. Other environmental factors adding to the increasing problem of obesity are an increase in energy-dense food availability, low-cost fast and convenient foods, and increase in portion sizes, while the physical requirements of daily activities decrease, specifically domestic appliances, cars, delivery services, and elevators.

Junk food is the pejorative term used for food that is high in calories from sugar or fat, with little dietary fiber, protein, vitamins, and minerals of nutritional value (empty calories). Some high-protein foods, like meat prepared with saturated fat, may also be considered junk food. In general, most junk food is highly processed food, including the breakfast cereals that are mostly sugar or high-fructose corn syrup and white flour or milled corn. Junk food in its various forms is extremely popular, and an integral part of modern popular culture. As for junk food's appeal, there is no definitive scientific answer. The food industry invests multimillions of dollars on research and development to create flavor profiles that focus the human taste on sugar, salt, and fat. When junk food is consumed regularly, the excess fat, simple carbohydrates, and processed sugar in the junk food contribute to an increased risk of obesity and associated comorbidities. Therefore, concerns about the negative health effects resulting from a junk food-heavy diet have resulted in public health awareness campaigns.

Frantic attempts to lose weight may push people to extreme measures that may themselves pose health risks, specifically the fad diets.

A *fad diet* is a diet that is popular for a time, similar to fads in fashion, without being a standard or evidence-based dietary recommendation, and often promising unreasonably fast weight loss with little efforts. Therefore, there is a failure of educating consumers about whole-diet, whole-lifestyle changes necessary for sustainable results and health benefits.

Among the respective diets are the daily injections of human chorionic gonadotropin (hCG) to keep the body in an anabolic state and reduce appetite, combined with a very-low-calorie diet that promotes weight loss [304]. Telogen effluvium has been reported following hCG in combination with caloric restriction [305], and new-onset androgenic alopecia following hCG diet and testosterone pellet implantation in a male [306]. While the telogen effluvium may have been caused by caloric restriction, another proposed mechanism may be the induction of a pseudopregnancy state by hCG, thereby causing telogen effluvium after the cessation of hCG therapy similar to that experienced in postpartum effluvium. Administration of hCG is known to increase intratesticular testosterone levels, which correlates with serum testosterone levels after hCG administration, therefore providing an intuitive mechanism for how hCG may also precipitate androgenic alopecia in the genetically susceptible individual.

Others include Atkins, Dukan, Eat Right for Your Type, Paleo, The South Beach Diet, Whole30, and Zone 1-2-3 Program. Most have limited practicality in terms of limited food choices, and limited sustainability in terms of difficulties in maintenance, and fail on the accounts of scientific inaccuracies and misinformation, and failure to address the necessity of changing long-term habits and behavior.

Many fad dieters get caught in a vicious cycle of chronic dieting syndrome, defined as a cyclic pattern of weight loss by dieting followed by rapid weight gain and its harmful physical and psychological effects.

5.3.3   Deficiencies from Bariatric Surgery

Surgical procedures represent probably the only means of treating severe and morbid obesity effectively and in a sustained manner. They are usually reserved for the medical treatment of clinically severe obesity in patients who have not had success with other methods of long-term weight loss. There is ample evidence for the effectiveness of obesity surgery, both for weight reduction and more importantly in terms of decreasing the rates of morbidity and mortality in the severely obese patients [307]. And yet, a growing pool of data from long-term follow-up studies reveals evidence of potentially severe nutritional consequences, if not addressed specifically and professionally [308].

Since bariatric surgery patients sometimes present with hair loss following the procedure, it is of particular importance to consider the overall nutritional status of the patient.

Two primary types of surgical procedures are performed for weight loss: restrictive, i.e., making the stomach smaller (e.g., gastric banding), and combination of restrictive and malabsorptive procedures, i.e., making the stomach smaller and rearranging the small intestine to decrease the length and efficiency of the intestine for nutrient absorption (e.g., Roux-en-Y gastric bypass).

Macro- and micronutrient deficiencies are common following obesity surgery. The most important, depending on the surgical technique performed, are hypoalbuminemia in 3–18%, and deficiencies of vitamin B1 in up to 49%, of B12 in 19–35%, of vitamin D in 25–73%, of iron in 17–45%, and of zinc in 12–91% [308], with the respective effects on the general health and hair condition.

Protein malnutrition. Weight management strategies aim at reducing body fat mass while minimizing the loss of lean tissue mass. Yet obesity surgery is not infrequently associated with nutritional protein deficiency (<3.5 mg/dL), which occurs in 3–18% of bariatric surgery patients, and a substantial loss of lean tissue mass. In extreme cases, severe protein malnutrition may occur [309], usually 3–6 months following surgery, with an increase of morbidity and hospitalization rates [310]. While hair loss is an early clinical sign of protein malnutrition, presence of edema indicates severe protein malnutrition.

Both the frequency and the severity of protein malnutrition and lean tissue mass reduction are influenced by the type of surgical procedure, average of daily protein intake, and physical exercise. The highest rate of protein malnutrition is seen following distal Roux-en-Y gastric bypass (<150 cm small intestine remaining). Current recommendations aim at a daily protein intake of about 90 g to maximize postsurgical lean tissue mass. Since branched-chain amino acids, particularly leucine, have been demonstrated to stimulate muscle protein synthesis during catabolic periods [311], protein supplements should be rich in branched-chain amino acids, especially leucine. Finally, regular resistance training and aerobic exercise significantly improve the preservation of muscle mass during weight loss [312].

Vitamin B1 (thiamine) deficiency. Preoperative asymptomatic low thiamine concentrations have been observed in up to 29% of obese patients [313], and symptomatic thiamine deficiency occurs in up to 49% of patients following bariatric surgery [314]. Persistent postoperative vomiting represents one of the main risk factors, and occurs primarily with the restrictive procedures. Eating avoidance and noncompliance with oral supplementation have also been recognized as important factors causing thiamine deficiency. Further critical factors are the short half-life of the vitamin with body thiamine stores usually being sufficient only for 18–20 days, and small intestinal bacterial overgrowth resulting in malabsorption due to bacterial thiaminases. The clinical manifestations of thiamine deficiency (beriberi) are highly variable, involving the central and peripheral nervous system and the cardiovascular system. According to WHO, clinical diagnosis requires the presence of two of the following three categories of diagnostic findings: (1) bilateral lower limb edema, (2) labored respiration, and (3) paresthesia of hands or feet, motor deficiency, or loss of balance [315]. The most common early symptoms of thiamine deficiency are nausea, vomiting, and constipation [316]. The central nervous manifestations of thiamine deficiency are Wernicke's encephalopathy, a disorder affecting the eye movements due to oculomotor muscle paresis and double vision, and Korsakoff psychosis with antero- and retrograde amnesia and cerebellar ataxia. The two disorders commonly coexist, composing the Wernicke-Korsakoff syndrome.

Thiamine levels should be monitored postoperatively at 6-month intervals during the first 3 years after surgery. In subclinical cases, oral thiamine supplementation of 100 mg is usually sufficient; patients with suspected deficiency should receive daily thiamine supplementation of 100–200 mg i.m. or i.v. The Wernicke-Korsakoff syndrome necessitates inpatient therapy with i.v. administration of 200–300 mg of thiamine 3× daily for 3–5 days followed by 250 mg i.v. daily until clinical improvement is seen. Thereafter, an oral maintenance dose of 50–100 mg daily is recommended. Due to structural changes to the brain (damage to the mamillary bodies and cerebellum), anamnestic disorders and a chronic atactic gait disorder are irreversible in approximately 50% [317].

Vitamin B12 (cobalamin) deficiency. Preoperative vitamin B12 deficiency in obese patients undergoing bariatric surgery has been reported in up to 18% [318]. Risk factors include medication with proton pump inhibitors and metformin [319], frequently taken by obese patients, and small intestinal bacterial overgrowth. Besides iron deficiency, vitamin B12 deficiency is a common cause for anemia following Roux-en-Y stomach bypass and biliopancreatic diversion, with a prevalence of 4–62% after 2 years and of 19–35% after 5 years [320]. Early non-hematological, neurological, and psychiatric symptoms of vitamin B12 deficiency typically precede the anemia by months to years. These include acral paresthesia, disturbances affecting coordination and sense of position affecting the gait (funicular myelosis), concentration difficulties, memory disturbances, and lack of retentiveness, in some instances to the extent of overt dementia [321].

Daly and Daly [126] have found lower levels of vitamin B12 in patients with telogen effluvium and scalp dysesthesia that may respond to vitamin B12 supplementation, and vitamin B12 deficiency has been linked to premature graying [123, 322, 323], yet there is no evidence that treatment with vitamin B12 will reverse the graying.

It is recommended to screen baseline and postoperative vitamin B12 levels in all bariatric patients. Following malabsorptive procedures, oral supplementation at a dosage of 1000 μg is recommended to maintain normal levels of vitamin B12. In the case of existing vitamin B12 deficiency, parenteral (i.m. or s.c.) administration remains the preferred route, as is needed in autoimmune vitamin B12 deficiency to bypass the lack of intrinsic factor. To achieve a quick repletion of vitamin B12, 1000 μg of vitamin B12 is administered i.m. daily for 5–7 days, followed by 4–5 further weekly injections of 1000 μg.

Folate deficiency. Since folate is well absorbed throughout the intestine, including the colon [324], folate deficiency is thought to be due to a decreased intake rather than malabsorption, and therefore can be easily corrected by oral supplementation of the vitamin. The prevalence of folate deficiency after bariatric surgery has been estimated to be 9–39%, irrespective of the surgical procedure, and may indicate poor adherence to vitamin supplementation [325]. Since body stores of folate, likewise to thiamine and zinc, are marginal, folate deficiency occurs at an early postoperative stage. Folate deficiency may also arise as a consequence of vitamin B12 deficiency, since vitamin B12 is important for the conversion of inactive methyltetrahydrofolic acid to active tetrahydrofolic acid [326]. Ultimately, both vitamin B12 and folate deficiency result in a megaloblastic anemia. Women who become pregnant after bariatric surgery are at higher risk of folate deficiency [327].

Since folate is essential for prevention of neural tube defects in infants, counseling and prophylactic supplementation of women considering pregnancy after bariatric surgery with 1000 µg folic acid per day are of particular importance.

Vitamin C deficiency. While laboratory evidence of vitamin C deficiency is not uncommon with a prevalence of 10–50% of bariatric patients, only two cases of clinically manifest scurvy have been reported in the literature [328, 329]. Perifollicular petechiae and corkscrew hairs are important cutaneous clues to vitamin C deficiency. Early and unspecific symptoms of vitamin C deficiency occurring within 1–3 months of the deficiency are fatigue and myalgia. Later symptoms include gum disease, loosening of teeth, easy bruising, poor wound healing, easy breaking of bones with the respective radiological findings, personality changes, and ultimately death from infection or bleeding.

There are no data concerning the prevention or treatment of vitamin C deficiency in the bariatric population. The RDA for healthy subjects is 75 mg/day and in smokers 110 mg/day. Vitamin C deficiency in non-bariatric patients with scurvy is successfully treated with 500 mg of vitamin C daily, reaching complete remission with 14 days to 1 month.

Vitamin D deficiency. Vitamin D deficiency, secondary hyperparathyroidism (SHPT), and bone loss occur frequently following obesity surgery [330]. Increased postsurgical parathormone (PTH) levels have been reported in up to 53% of the bariatric population [331], depending on the surgical technique, being significantly higher following malabsorptive surgery. In addition, significant hypovitaminosis D from inadequate intake, reduced sun exposure, and decreased bioavailability of vitamin D due to its accumulation in adipose tissue is already present in a high proportion of patients before surgery.

To minimize the risk of bone loss following surgery, all patients should be screened for vitamin D deficiency prior to obesity surgery and treated accordingly. Since individual patients may require larger doses than others, 25-OH-vitamin D levels should be measured 2–4 weeks after initiation of supplementation and repeated every 3 months in the postoperative year. While most studies in nonobese patients have shown that serum levels of ≥50 nmol/L are adequate for prevention of osteoporosis [332], levels of around 100 nmol/L or higher seem to be more effective in the bariatric population for prevention of SHPT [333]. A number of other health conditions, including the condition of the hair in relation to vitamin D deficiency, have been the subject of recent debate. See respective chapter.

Vitamin A deficiency. As a fat-soluble vitamin, vitamin A needs micelle formation with conjugated bile acids, and is mainly absorbed in the proximal jejunum. Therefore, vitamin A deficiency is primarily observed after obesity surgery in the context of relative bile acid deficiency in patients with a short common channel after biliopancreatic diversion or extended Roux-en-Y bypass, and in association with bile acid deconjugation due to upper intestinal bacterial overgrowth. The clinical manifestations of vitamin A deficiency are night blindness (nyctalopia) followed by xerophthalmia, ulceration, and necrosis of the cornea. Vitamin A deficiency can also lead to impaired immune function, and birth defects. Cutaneous markers of hypovitaminosis A are a peculiar form of follicular hyperkeratosis characterized by excessive development of keratin in hair follicles, resulting in rough, cone-shaped, elevated papules called phrynoderma (Fig. 5.25), and dry hair. This condition has been shown to respond well to supplementation with vitamins and fats rich in essential fatty acids.

Measurements of serum retinol concentrations and/or assessment of the carrier protein retinol-binding protein (RBP) are the most used biomarkers for

Fig. 5.25 Vitamin A deficiency: phrynoderma.

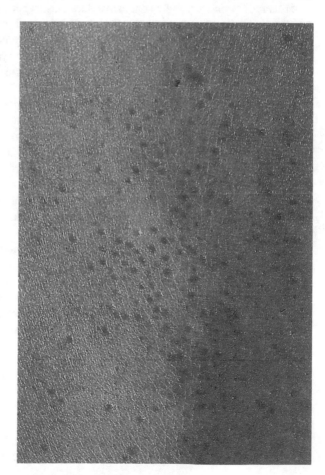

identification of patients at risk of vitamin A deficiency, with cutoff levels of serum retinol <0.35 μmol/L and/or RBP <4.8 μmol/L taken to define severe vitamin A deficiency. Since RBP is a negative acute-phase protein, retinol levels are decreased in the case of inflammation, which is why both markers should be evaluated only in the context of the CRP status. Rather, the detection of nyctalopia via standardized interview has been proven to be useful in the bariatric population before and after the surgery [334]. Currently, data are insufficient for general recommendations regarding the optimal daily supplementation of vitamin A in the bariatric population; however it has been shown that daily supplementation using over-the-counter multivitamins containing 5000 IU of retinol acetate fails to prevent vitamin A deficiency. Therefore, and in the light of the considerable impact of vitamin A deficiency on health and pregnancy, vitamin A status should be evaluated pre- and postoperatively and regularly monitored in individuals at risk. For the treatment of manifest hypovitaminosis A in the absence of corneal damage 10,000–25,000 IU/day vitamin A orally for 1–2 weeks is recommended, and in the presence of corneal lesions 50,000–1,000,000 IU i.m. followed by 50,000 IU i.m. daily for 2 weeks [335].

Vitamin E deficiency. Few conclusive data exist regarding vitamin E deficiency, and those existing are based on single case reports. And yet, reduced levels of vitamin E have been found in up to 22% of Roux-en-Y bypass patients post-surgery. Hemolytic anemia or neurological symptoms (ataxia, myopathy, absence of deep tendon reflexes, and loss of the ability to sense vibration) may indicate vitamin E deficiency.

Vitamin K deficiency. Since vitamin K acts as a key factor for the carboxylation of glutamic acid residues in proteins involved in blood clotting, as well as proteins involved in bone homoeostasis (osteocalcin), symptoms of vitamin K deficiency include bleeding and osteoporosis. Main sites of absorption of vitamin K are the distal jejunum and ileum. Like other fat-soluble vitamins requiring incorporation into micelles, vitamin K has a rapid turnover and minimal body reservoirs, resulting in a short half-life. And yet, apart from case reports, there is only one prospective trial demonstrating vitamin K deficiency after malabsorptive surgical procedures [336].

Vitamin K is largely supplied by dietary phylloquinones, while biosynthesis by colonic bacteria may contribute as a further important source of the vitamin. Vitamin K status is commonly assessed by functional assays, such as prothrombin time, which has been shown to underdetect vitamin K deficiency [337]. Better is the direct quantification of plasma vitamin K by means of high-performance liquid chromatography, with normal vitamin K plasma concentration ranging between 150 and 1150 ng/mL [338].

The role of vitamin K on hair growth is not understood, though traditional anticoagulant treatment with vitamin K antagonists is known to be able to cause reversible telogen effluvium [339].

Vitamin K deficiency is initially replenished with 10 mg i.m. or s.c., followed by 1–2 mg/week orally.

Deficiencies in essential minerals and trace elements. Besides the deficiencies in protein and vitamins, bariatric surgery may lead to deficiencies in essential minerals and trace elements, specifically of calcium (in approx. 10%), magnesium (in 32%), iron (in 17% following sleeve gastrectomy, and in 30% and 45%, respectively, after 2 years following Roux-en-Y bypass and biliopancreatic diversion), zinc (in 12% following sleeve gastrectomy, 21–33% following Roux-en-Y bypass, and 74–91% following biliopancreatic diversion with duodenal switch), and copper (in 2% following Roux-en-Y bypass, and in 10–24% following biliopancreatic diversion with duodenal switch), of which deficiencies of iron and of zinc are particularly relevant to hair health.

Calcium. The four basic functions of calcium in the body are bone and tooth formation, blood clotting, muscle and nerve action, and metabolic reactions. The intestinal absorption of dietary calcium depends on the food and hormonal control. The daily dietary calcium intake is approximately 1000 mg, of which 400 mg is absorbed in the ileum and jejunum via a passive paracellular route, and in the duodenum via an active transcellular calcium transport that is regulated by 1,25-OH-vitamin D. Calcium deficiency after obesity surgery may be due to malabsorption of calcium and vitamin D following malabsorptive procedures, steatorrhea due to the interaction of dietary calcium with fatty acids, and low-lactose diets rigorously excluding milk products. In 50% of bypass patients secondary lactose intolerance may develop, or an existing minor lactase deficiency may manifest postoperatively [340]. Consequent avoidance of milk and milk products results in an average calcium intake of approximately 250–300 mg, whereas 1000–1200 mg is actually required. Long-term calcium deficiency results in decreased bone mineral density with an increased risk of fractures due to osteoporosis. Since serum calcium levels are of limited diagnostic value in determining calcium status, serum parathyroid hormone (PTH) determination [333] and measurement of bone density by axial DEXA (spine and hip) [341] are recommended. Decreases in calcium levels are compensated by a PTH-vitamin D-controlled increase in intestinal absorption, reduction in renal elimination, and intensified osteolysis. Therefore, serum PTH levels may indicate increased bone turnover and decreased bone mineral density. Finally, since more than 90% of body calcium is stored in the bone, measurement of bone density represents yet another reliable marker.

Daily calcium supplementation of 1200–1500 mg or up to 2000 mg calcium, preferably calcium citrate for its bioavailability, is recommended for prevention and effective treatment of calcium deficiency following bariatric surgery. It must be kept in mind though that oral calcium may hamper intestinal absorption of iron, zinc, and copper.

Magnesium. Magnesium represents one of the major minerals composing approximately 0.1% of the adult body weight, and 60% of that magnesium being found again in the bones. Magnesium has widespread metabolic functions, and is a necessary cofactor for more than 300 enzymatic reactions involved in protein synthesis, muscle action, and basal energy expenditure. Magnesium deficiency not only directly influences bone crystal formation, but also impacts the secretion and activity of PTH, thus also contributing to osteoporosis [342]. Severe deficiency symptoms include muscle weakness, tetany, and potentially fatal ventricular arrhythmia. In a significant proportion of bariatric patients, magnesium deficiency may have already been manifest preoperatively [343]. Long-term intake of proton pump inhibitors (PPIs) has been shown to induce magnesium depletion [344].

Clinical awareness of hypomagnesemia in bariatric patients, especially those on PPIs, is essential. Serum magnesium levels <0.75 mmol/L are regarded as a useful marker for severe deficiency. As for calcium, the bioavailability of magnesium citrate has been found to be superior to that of other preparations [345].

Iron. Along with vitamin B12 deficiency, iron deficiency represents a leading cause of anemia in the bariatric population, and is one of the most prevalent long-term complications of obesity surgery. Causative factors include reduced iron absorption due to malabsorptive surgery, hindrance of iron resorption due to a chronic inflammatory status and release of stored iron, diminished gastric acid secretion, and frequent intolerance of red meat. For the effects of iron deficiency and iron-deficiency anemia on the general health status and the condition of hair (telogen effluvium), see the respective chapter.

Due to the causative factors, it is not surprising that oral iron substitution is ineffective in bariatric patients. In addition, oral iron is associated with significant gastrointestinal side effects, such as nausea, abdominal pain, and diarrhea. Rather i.v. substitution should be preferred in the bariatric population, using the traditional Ganzoni equation (Box 5.2) [346].

Box 5.2 Ganzoni equation for intravenous iron substitution

$$\text{Body weight in kg} \times (\text{target Hb} - \text{actual Hb in g / dL})$$
$$\times 0.24 + 500\,\text{mg iron stores} = \text{total iron deficit in mg.}$$

Zinc. Analogous to iron, zinc is absorbed in the duodenum. Due to decreased intestinal absorption, specially following malabsorptive procedures, and lack of functional body reserves, zinc deficiency may develop early after obesity surgery. Clinical symptoms of zinc deficiency are alopecia, glossitis, nail dystrophy, and a peculiar acral dermatitis.

There are no standardized recommendations for zinc supplementation; however standard multivitamin formulations usually only contain small amounts of zinc, so that it seems questionable whether these would be sufficient to prevent zinc deficiency if recommended. Zinc deficiency is treated with 50 mg oral zinc gluconate or 30 mg zinc histidine daily to be taken approximately 45 min before breakfast. It must be borne in mind that oral zinc substitution may, if carried out over a longer period of time, lead to a reduced intestinal absorption of copper and iron that share the cation transporter DMT-1 resulting in respective deficiencies. Therefore, patients receiving zinc supplements on a long-term basis should receive 1–2 mg of copper for each 15 mg of zinc [347].

Copper. Only few instances of copper deficiency following obesity surgery have been reported. It is important to consider though that hematological (iron-resistant microcytic anemia, neutropenia) and/or neurologic disorders (myeloneuropathy) related to copper deficiency may occur only many years (mean onset 11.4 years) after obesity surgery [348]. Copper levels should be monitored in patients taking zinc supplementation over a longer period of time, as this may cause impairment of intestinal copper absorption. It has been hypothesized that because copper plays an important role in melanin formation, a lack of copper can affect a person's hair color, potentially leading to premature graying hair.

Recent guidelines recommend that copper supplementation (2 mg/day) should be included as part of routine multivitamin and mineral supplementation in bariatric surgery patients [347].

Selenium. There is insufficient evidence to support routine selenium screening or supplementation after obesity surgery.

In summary, all of the procedures currently performed in obesity surgery involve radical changes of the gastrointestinal anatomy and physiology, and have the potential to cause nutritional deficiencies. Therefore, individuals who have undergone any form of obesity surgery require professional guidance and close monitoring with respect to nutrient levels, and rigorous lifelong adherence to nutritional supplementation regimens.

Since hair loss may be a symptom of a specific, i.e., of protein, iron, zinc, or a combined, nutritional deficiency, it has to be systematically investigated and treated, respectively. In addition, seborrheic-like dermatitis may point to deficiencies of biotin, zinc, or essential fatty acids; follicular hyperkeratosis and dry hair due to vitamin A deficiency; and perifollicular petechiae and corkscrew hairs due to vitamin C deficiency.

Prevention, recognition, and treatment of nutritional deficiencies in bariatric patients are of utmost importance considering the potential serious health issues connected to them, such as the Wernicke-Korsakoff syndrome (vitamin B1), funicular myelosis (vitamin B12), dementia (vitamin B1, vitamin B12), birth defects (folate), scurvy (vitamin C), osteoporosis (vitamin D, calcium, magnesium), keratomalacia (vitamin A), anemia (vitamin B12, folate, iron, copper), and cardiomyopathy (selenium).

5.3.4   Anorexia and Bulimia

By definition, eating disorders are mental disorders characterized by abnormal eating habits that negatively affect an individual's physical or mental health. They include anorexia nervosa, where people eat very little due to a fear of gaining weight and thus have a low body weight; bulimia nervosa, where people eat a lot and then try to rid themselves of the food; binge eating disorder, where people eat a large amount in a short period of time; and pica, where people eat nonfood items. The eating disorders do not include obesity.

Mortality from eating disorders is significant compared with other psychological disorders: 4.37% for anorexia nervosa and 2.33% for bulimia nervosa [349]. There have been no published studies on mortality in binge eating disorder, although its comorbidities may increase mortality risks.

Pica is most commonly seen in pregnant women, small children, and persons with developmental disabilities such as autism. Children eating painted plaster containing lead may suffer from lead poisoning. In addition to poisoning, there is a risk of serious gastrointestinal complications, for instance *Toxocara* infection from ingestion of soil (geophagia), or gastrointestinal obstruction from eating hair (trichophagia) resulting in a hair ball (trichobezoar: Fig. 5.26), the so-called Rapunzel syndrome [350].

Pica has been linked to mental and emotional disorders. Stressors such as emotional trauma, maternal deprivation, family issues, parental neglect, and pregnancy are strongly linked to pica as a form of comfort. More recently, cases of pica have been tied to the obsessive–compulsive spectrum [351]. People practicing certain forms of pica, such as geophagy, pagophagy (appetite for ice), and amylophagy (appetite for starch), are more likely to be anemic with low hemoglobin and hematocrit levels, or have lower plasma zinc concentrations [352]. Additionally, being a

Fig. 5.26 Trichobezoar (private collection)

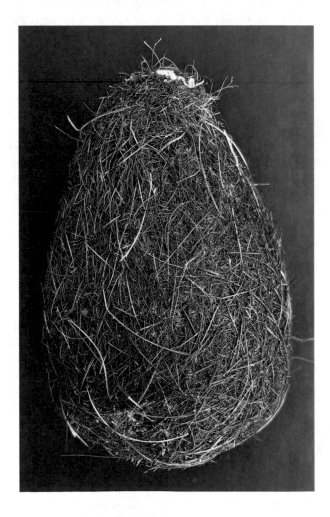

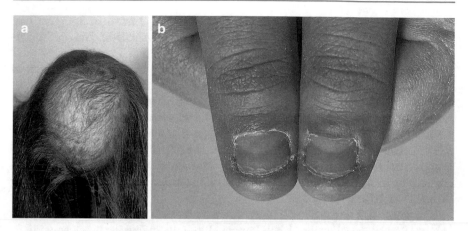

Fig. 5.27 (**a**, **b**) Trichotillomania. (**a**) Tonsure trichotillomania. (**b**) Associated onychophagia

child or pregnant woman practicing pica was associated with a higher chance of being anemic or having low hemoglobin relative to the general population.

Trichotillomania involves the repetitive, uncontrollable pulling of one's hair, resulting in noticeable hair loss (Fig. 5.27a). Like pica, it represents a disorder of impulse control. Associated features of trichotillomania may include excoriations of the scalp, nail biting (onychophagy: Fig. 5.27b), and eating hairs (trichophagy).

In trichophagy, it is not clear whether iron deficiency may be a cause of the eating disorder [353] or rather an effect of the trichobezoar [354]. In the first case it has been hypothesized whether in cases of such psychic anomalies the iron content of the iron-rich cerebral ganglia is lower than normal and the disturbance could be ceased by the administration of iron [355, 356].

The primary treatment approach for trichotillomania is habit reversal combined with stress management and behavioral contracting. Early work focused on the serotonin reuptake inhibitors, yet the majority of the trials have been negative. Newer therapies have been based on the glutamate modulator N-acetylcysteine [357, 358] and on the cannabinoid agonist dronabinol [359]. It is hypothesized that N-acetylcysteine, an amino acid, restores the extracellular glutamate concentration in the nucleus accumbens of the brain and, therefore, offers promise in the reduction of compulsive behavior, while dronabinol reduces the excitotoxic damage caused by glutamate release in the striatum.

With the exception of pica, the eating disorders have similar risk factors, including negative self-evaluation in view of media exposure for idealization of thinness, perfectionism, and negative impulsivity [360]. Eating disorders occur more frequently among females than males, and homosexual males are at higher risk than heterosexuals [361]. Anorexia nervosa is more likely to occur in a person's pubertal years.

The nutrition-related clinical signs commonly associated with anorexia nervosa are protein-energy malnutrition, various micronutrient deficiencies, hypokalemia, hypomagnesemia, hypophosphatemia, hypotension, orthostasis, sinus bradycardia, constipation, vomiting, cold sensitivity, hypoglycemia, menstrual irregularities, osteopenia or osteoporosis, muscular wasting and weakness, and an under-weight state.

The skin and hair signs associated with anorexia nervosa are the expression of the medical consequences of starvation, vomiting, abuse of laxatives and diuretics, and psychiatric morbidity [362]. In a study of dermatological changes in 21 young female anorectics aged 19–24, the most common dermatological findings were xerosis in 71%, cheilitis in 76%, diffuse lanugo-like hypertrichosis (Fig. 5.28) in 62%, telogen effluvium in 24%, dry scalp hair in 48%, acral coldness in 38%, acro-cyanosis in 33%, periungual erythema in 48%, gingival changes in 37%, nail changes in 29%, and calluses on dorsum of hand due to self-induced vomiting (Russell's sign) in 67% [363].

Symptoms due to psychiatric morbidity may include the consequences of self-induced trauma, specifically trichotillomania [364], including the pubic area [365].

In the so far largest study available on micronutrient status in anorexia nervosa patients evaluated before initiation of treatment [366], roughly one-half of patients

Fig. 5.28 Anorexia nervosa: Lanugo-like hypertrichosis

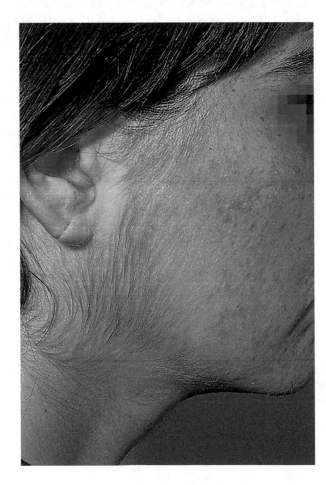

presented with at least one deficit in trace elements and/or vitamins, the most frequent being selenium deficit (40% of patients), and vitamin A and folic acid, respectively. Surprisingly, the other half of patients presented with normal micronutrient concentrations despite severe malnutrition witnessed by a mean 20% of weight loss. Zinc deficiency was not observed in the study, while authors have suggested that zinc deficiency could be a causative or perpetuation factor in anorexia nervosa [175]. Indeed, zinc deficiency may cause taste alterations and contribute to a variety of neuropsychiatric symptoms [367, 368]. Some early reports supported the benefit of zinc supplementation on clinical outcome of anorexia [369, 370], including a randomized, double-blind, placebo-controlled trial: use of zinc supplements (15 mg b.i.d.) improved the rate of weight gain by an unknown mechanism [176]. Zinc has been reported to be an appetite stimulator and to play also a role to limit the progression of cachexia and sarcopenia in other disease conditions [174]. It has also been proposed that low zinc intake may adversely affect neurotransmitters such as gamma-aminobutyric acid (GABA) in different parts of the human brain and affect amygdala functions [371], an important structure for the central regulation of the autonomic nervous system, which is often affected in anorexia nervosa [372, 373].

Recommendations on energy requirements vary from 5 to 10 kcal/kg/day in the critically ill with the risk of electrolyte imbalances during refeeding (hypokalemia, hypomagnesemia, hypophosphatemia) to 1900 kcal/day [374]. Monitoring of micronutrients and correction of deficits should be included in the routine care of anorexia nervosa patients. Finally, despite an incomplete understanding of the mechanisms underlying the actions of zinc, oral supplementation (15 mg daily) during refeeding should be considered as an integrative part of the treatment plan. Patients with eating disorders often have neurobiological aberrations. These chemical disturbances were initially suspected to be the cause of the disordered eating behavior. However, researchers have found that when a normal weight and eating pattern are re-established, the neurologic chemistry returns to normal [375].

5.3.5   Deficiencies of Alcoholism

Alcoholism, also known as alcohol-use disorder, is by definition any drinking of alcohol that results in mental or physical health problems. The *Dietary Guidelines for Americans* defines moderate use as no more than two alcoholic beverages a day for men and no more than one alcoholic beverage a day for women [376]. According to the *National Institute on Alcohol Abuse and Alcoholism*, men may be at risk for alcohol-related problems if their alcohol consumption exceeds 14 standard drinks per week or 4 drinks per day, and women may be at risk if they have more than 7 standard drinks per week or 3 drinks per day. It defines a standard drink as one 12-ounce (350 mL) bottle of beer, one 5-ounce (150 mL) glass of wine, or 1.5 ounces (40 mL) of distilled spirits [377].

Alcohol contributes to the overall energy intake in the form of calories, and yields 7 kcal/g. This is more than both carbohydrates and protein, which yield 4 kcal/g each. And yet, alcohol is not a nutrient, but represents empty calories.

Unlike carbohydrates, fats, proteins, vitamins, minerals, and water, alcohol performs no essential function in the body. Alcohol is not stored in the body; in fact, the by-products of alcohol metabolism can accumulate to toxic amounts when alcohol is consumed in large quantities, the primary by-product being acetaldehyde. Acetaldehyde is the culprit for the destruction of healthy tissue that is associated with alcoholism. Alcohol metabolism is a priority for the liver. After detoxifying the alcohol the liver uses remaining by-products to produce fatty acids. Fatty acids are combined with glycerol through lipogenesis to form triglycerides that are stored in the liver. Repeated episodes of drinking binge over time can therefore lead to fatty liver disease.

Long-term alcohol abuse can cause a number of physical and mental effects, including cirrhosis of the liver, pancreatitis, epilepsy, polyneuropathy, alcoholic dementia, heart disease, nutritional deficiencies, peptic ulcers, and several cancers. The most prevalent psychiatric symptoms are anxiety and depression disorders. Social skills are significantly impaired with dysfunction or other problems at work, marital and economic problems, loss of interest in personal appearance or hygiene including the condition of the hair, and loss of appetite.

Nutrition disorders in the patient with alcoholism can include malnutrition, micronutrient deficiencies, overweight, and obesity. Chronic alcoholics frequently have evidence of nutritional deficiency due to decreased intake, reduced uptake, and impaired utilization of nutrients. The alcoholic has increased nutrient requirements due to greater metabolic demands and need for tissue repair. Serious health conditions, such as the Wernicke-Korsakoff syndrome, dementia, pellagra, and scurvy, can be a direct result of either specific nutrient deficiencies of vitamin B1, vitamin B6, vitamin B12 [378], folic acid [379], niacinamide [380], vitamin C [381], vitamin A [382], magnesium [383], vitamin D [384], zinc [385], vitamin E and selenium [386], vitamin K [387], and copper [388] or multiple vitamin deficiencies [246].

Bahmer and Bader [389] reported on 52 dermatologic patients suffering from chronic alcoholism. The skin changes observed consisted of interfollicular erythrosis of the neck, scleral icterus, telangiectatic erythema of the face, and diminished secondary body hair. In 29 out of 44 sera investigated, they found elevation of the gamma-glutamyl transferase as evidence of alcoholic liver disease. In 17 patients, serum samples were analyzed for zinc. In 16 cases, the zinc levels were slightly decreased but still within the normal range, i.e., below 100 micrograms/dL. The biotin levels in the 48 serum samples varied; however 6 patients showed definitely decreased values. Bader et al. [390] reported on seven patients with chronic alcohol abuse and ichthyosiform erythroderma. In another study of 200 alcoholics examined for cutaneous changes, 182 (91%) had cutaneous, nail, hair, or oral cavity changes. Nail changes were found in 51 (25.5%) with koilonychia being the commonest (16%). Oral changes were present in 107 (53.5%), and changes due to nutritional deficiency in 20 (10%). Diseases due to poor hygiene were seen in 55 (27.5%) alcoholics. Pityriasis versicolor (14%) and seborrheic dermatitis (11.5%) were the commonest cutaneous changes noted. The authors concluded that even though alcohol abuse has a variety of cutaneous manifestations, there are no specific cutaneous signs of alcoholism [391]. Cutaneous signs of specific nutritional deficiencies that may be observed in alcoholics are xerosis and follicular keratosis (vitamin A), cheilosis (vitamin B2 and vitamin B6), pellagra (niacin), seborrheic-like dermatitis (vitamin B6, biotin, zinc), atrophic glossitis (vitamin B12), follicular petechiae and corkscrew hairs (vitamin C), alopecia, glossitis, and acral dermatitis (zinc). Other common skin changes in alcoholism not related to nutrition are urticaria, porphyria cutanea tarda, flushing, cutaneous stigmata of cirrhosis (spider telangiectasias, caput medusae, palmar erythema, gynecomastia, abdominal alopecia, white nails, disappearance of lunulae), treatment-resistant psoriasis, pruritus, rosacea, Madelung's disease, and benign symmetric lipomatosis (Launois–Bensaude) [392]. The clinical features of benign symmetric lipomatosis are reminiscent of the Egyptian graphic representation of gluteal femoral obesity, hyperlordosis, and symmetrical deposits of fat on the trunk, limbs, and thighs in the Queen Ati of the Land of Punt, as depicted on Pharaoh Hatshepsut's (1507–1458 BC) temple at Deir el-Bahri [393].

Physicians who see patients with these particular skin and hair conditions should be aware that there is a greater probability that the individual at hand is an alcoholic. This additional risk factor needs to be considered when physicians design a treatment plan to include the nutritional status of the patient.

Quantification of ethyl glucuronide (EtG) in hair (hEtG) samples has established itself as one of the most reliable biomarkers of long-term alcohol consumption habits for assessment of both abstinence and heavy drinking [394]. Ethyl glucuronide is a minor, non-oxidative ethanol metabolite that can be reliably detected in several matrices, including the blood, urine, hair, and meconium, for variable periods of time. However, prolonged exposition of hair to alcohol-based perfumes may increase hEtG levels, resulting in false-positive results [395], while detox shampoos sold online may have the potential to alter EtG concentrations in hair [396].

5.3.6   Aging and Diet

Aging is the process of becoming older. It results from the accumulation of changes in a person over time. Aging in humans represents a multidimensional process of physical, psychological, and social changes. Ultimately, aging is among the largest known health risk factors for most human diseases, ultimately leading to death.

Life expectancy has dramatically increased during the past century. One of the primary goals is to reach high-quality, longer lives that are free of preventable disease, disability, injury, and premature death. Achieving this objective requires proper nutrition, among other healthy lifestyle habits. The overall process of human aging has the unique potential for growth and fulfilment at every stage of life. At each life stage, four basic areas of adult life shape general growth and development: physical, psychosocial, socioeconomic, and nutritional.

In biology, senescence denotes the state or process of aging. Cellular senescence is a phenomenon where isolated cells demonstrate a limited capacity to divide in culture (the Hayflick limit, discovered by Leonard Hayflick in 1961 [397]), while organismal senescence is the aging of organisms. After a period of near-perfect renewal between 20 and 35 years of age in humans, organismal senescence is characterized by the declining ability to respond to stress, increasing homeostatic imbalance, and increasing risk of disease.

Physical growth is no longer a process of increasing numbers of cells, but rather involves the vital growth of new cells to replace old ones. Adjustment to the gradually declining metabolic rate requires fewer kilocalories. Approximately 45–65% of total kilocalories should come from carbohydrates, with an emphasis on complex carbohydrates, e.g., whole grains and vegetables. High-quality dietary fat provides a backup energy source, important fat-soluble vitamins, and essential fatty acids. With 1.5 g/kg body weight/day the protein needs of older adults ($\geq$65 years) [398] are higher per kilogram of body weight than the DRIs recommend of protein intake of 0.8 g per kilogram of body weight in adults, because of a decreased metabolic performance and sarcopenia. Finally, some essential nutrients may require special attention because of their relationship with possible health problems in the aging adult and morbidity or medication interactions. Specifically, physiologic changes associated with aging are known to alter the bioavailability of vitamin B12 [399], and the endogenous synthesis of vitamin D [400].

While with age the needs for types and quantities of nutrients change, it has been found that as many as 50% of older adults have a vitamin and mineral intake less than the recommended dietary allowance, and as many as 30% of the elderly population have subnormal levels of vitamins and minerals [401]. A physiologic decline in food intake is seen in people as they age, regardless of illness, and is often referred to as anorexia of aging. It probably involves alterations in neurotransmitters and hormones that affect the central feeding drive and the peripheral satiation system. Moreover, sensory decline in both olfaction and taste decreases the enjoyment of food and dietary variety. Problems with dentition and disorders of the gastrointestinal system are related to poor intake and malabsorption of nutrients. Many diseases (i.e., thyroid, cardiovascular, and pulmonary disease) lead to an increased metabolic demand, and at the same time decreased appetite and caloric intake [402]. Finally, drugs may affect nutritional status through side effects (i.e., anorexia, nausea, and altered taste perception) and through alteration of nutrient absorption, metabolism, and excretion.

In addition, socioeconomic status and functional ability have an important influence on nutritional status. When financial concerns are present, meals are skipped and food that is purchased may not provide a nutritionally adequate diet. Declines in both physical and cognitive functional status affect an individual's ability to shop for food and to prepare meals. Nutritional problems are further compromised by social isolation, which commonly leads to apathy about food and decreased intake. The older person has experienced change and loss through retirement, disability and death of friends and family, as well as change in financial, social, and physical health status. These changes may lead to depression. Depression is often unrecognized in older persons. Malnutrition may be a presenting symptom of depression in the elderly.

Ultimately, dementia is the progressive decline in cognitive function due to damage or disease of the brain beyond what might be expected from normal aging. It represents a nonspecific set of symptoms in which affected areas of cognition may be memory, attention, language, and problem-solving. Higher mental functions are affected first in the process; in the later stages of the condition, affected persons may be disoriented in time, place, and person. Steady decline in cognitive processes is seen across the life span, accelerating from the 20s or even 30s. Research has focused in particular on memory and has found decline of memory with aging, but not of general knowledge, such as vocabulary definitions, which typically increases or remains steady until the late adulthood. In fact, some dimensions of aging naturally grow and expand over time, while the others decline. Reaction time, for example, slows with age, while knowledge of world events and wisdom may expand. Research shows that even late in life, potential exists for mental and social growth and development, and some cases of apparent dementia may be due to specific disease processes that may be amenable to treatment. Therefore, routine blood tests are recommended to rule out treatable causes. These include vitamin B12, folic acid, thyroid-stimulating hormone (TSH), C-reactive protein (CRP), full blood count, electrolytes, calcium, renal function, liver enzymes, and syphilis serology. Also, mental illnesses that include depression and psychosis may produce symptoms of pseudodementia, which must be differentiated from dementia. Chronic abuse of substances, such as alcohol, can also predispose to cognitive changes suggestive of dementia.

In addition to age-, disease-, and nutritional deficiency-related changes of hair growth and quality, neglect of hair and hair care in the elderly may be manifestations of dementia or of pseudodementia from depression, psychosis, or chronic alcoholism.

The Mini Nutritional Assessment (MNA®) is one of the standard assessment tools to evaluate nutritional risk in the elderly residing in nursing homes that is highly sensitive in detecting the risk of malnutrition early. It represents a 7-point questionnaire including (A) decline of food intake due to loss of appetite, digestive problems, and chewing or swallowing difficulties; (B) weight loss; (C) mobility; (D) psychological stress or acute disease; (E) neuropsychological problems (dementia or depression); (F1) body mass index (BMI); and (F2) calf circumference [403].

With technologic advances and improvements in medical care, an increasing number of patients survive medical conditions that used to be fatal. This fact combined with the aging of the population means that a growing proportion of patients have multiple concurrent medical conditions [404]. The term multimorbidity means several concurrent medical conditions within one person. According to a survey done in Canada in 1998, 30% of the population reported suffering from more than one chronic health problem, and the percentage increased with age. In the United States, the prevalence of multimorbidity among those 65 and older has been estimated at 65% [402]. The increasing number of chronic conditions per patient and the increasing amount of multimorbidity in the elderly population lead to a more complex approach to successful treatment of hair problems in the elderly. In addition, multiple medications (polypharmacy) may affect the overall nutritional status when drug–nutrient interactions occur. In the United States as many as 39% of adults ≥65 years old take five or more prescription drugs on a regular basis [405]. Many of the medications can affect the fluid balance, appetite, and absorption and utilization of nutrients, thereby contributing to dehydration and malnutrition.

In summary, older patients may suffer from a variety of conditions that affect the hair. Sometimes, symptoms of overt pathologic conditions may be misinterpreted as signs of normal aging, ignored, and left untreated. In taking care of the elderly with hair problems, it is therefore important to be suspicious of the possibility of a more general problem underlying the patient's complaint, including the nutritional status.

Aging hair is characterized by loss of follicle rigor, consistent with age-dependent slowing of other body activities, failure to pigment the hair shaft, decrease in hair growth, and reduction in the diameter of the hair shaft. The condition of the hair depends on hereditary and ethnic factors with great interindividual variability, condition of the scalp, hair care and styling habits, external factors and hair damage, nutritional status, and overall health status.

The original studies into hair aging were performed in the 1980s by Pinkus [406], Ebling [407], and Kligman [408]. Ebling's estimation of the diameters of plucked scalp hairs is the first credible attempt to measurement in the literature. He found that, regardless of age, hairs from the same individual showed a wide diversity of diameters, with a shift towards smaller diameters with old age. While Pinkus originally coined the term senile alopecia, Kligman performed the first comparative histopathology of male pattern baldness and senescent alopecia with the conclusion that male pattern baldness and senescent alopecia are clearly different processes: while he found that hair follicle miniaturization, inflammation, and fibrosis are the hallmarks of male pattern baldness, senescent alopecia was characterized by a modest reduction in the size of follicles that were otherwise normal. Therefore, he considered what Pinkus had described as a "fibrosing alopecia, the result of a prominent increase in collagen which choked the epithelium of the follicle till it disappeared, leaving only a collapsed fibrous sheath" rather to be a late stage of male pattern baldness in the elderly than senescent alopecia. Since streamer fibrosis was not a feature of senescent alopecia, he considered that "theoretically at least, hair growth in senescent alopecia could be stimulated by pharmacological means, because scarring does not stand in the way."

In contrast to the skin, aging of the hair has seemingly only recently found the attention of major dermatological meetings, mainly promoted by the cosmetic industry for global marketing purposes. Since the appearance of hair plays an important role in people's overall physical appearance and self-perception, and aging of the hair is particularly visible, the hair care industry has a substantial interest in delivering products that are directed towards meeting this consumer demand.

Meanwhile, basic scientists interested in the biology of hair growth and pigmentation have exposed the hair follicle as a highly accessible model with unique opportunities for the study of the age-related effects [409]: the hair follicle's complex multicell-type interaction system involving epithelium, mesenchyme, and neuroectoderm and its unique cyclical activity of growth, regression, rest, and regrowth provide the investigator with a range of stem, differentiating, mitotic, and postmitotic terminally differentiated cells, including cells with variable susceptibility to apoptosis, for study. In fact, Tobin and Paus ultimately established the study of the aging hair follicle as a science they called gerontobiology of the hair follicle on the basis of their investigations into hair graying [410]. As opposed to the continuous cutaneous melanogenesis, the coupling of hair follicle melanogenesis to the hair growth cycle is a distinguishing feature of follicular melanogenesis. This cycle involves periods of melanocyte proliferation and maturation during anagen, and melanocyte death via apoptosis during catagen. Each hair cycle is associated with the reconstruction of an intact hair follicle pigmentary unit at least for the first ten cycles; thereafter white hairs appear suggesting an age-related exhaustion of the pigmentary potential in the individual hair follicle.

Hair graying is closely related to chronological age, and the age of its onset is largely controlled by genetics. The normal incidence of hair graying is 34 ± 9.6 years in Caucasians and 43.9 ± 10.3 years in Africans [411]. As a rule of thumb, by 50 years of age, 50% of people have 50% gray hair. This graying incidence appears irrespective of sex and hair color. Hair is said to gray prematurely if it occurs before the age of 20 in Caucasians, 25 in Asians, and 30 in Africans. While premature graying most commonly appears without underlying pathology, presumably inherited in an autosomal dominant manner (familial premature greying: Fig. 5.29), it has also been linked to a similar cluster of autoimmune disorders observed in association

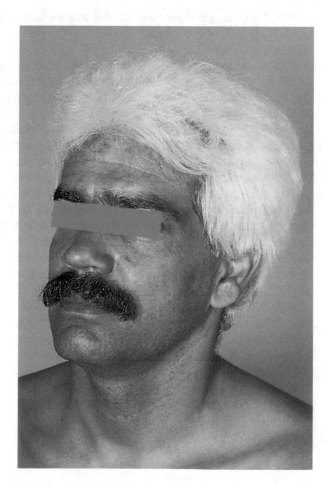

Fig. 5.29 Familial premature graying

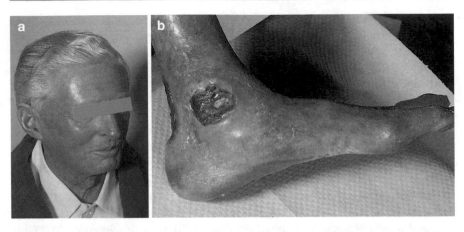

Fig. 5.30 (**a**, **b**) Progeria adultorum (Werner's syndrome). (**a**) Premature graying and syndromic facial features. (**b**) Pseudoscleroderma with skin ulceration

with vitiligo, i.e., pernicious anemia and autoimmune thyroid disease, as well as with the rare premature aging syndromes (progeria), Hutchinson-Gilford and Werner's syndrome (Fig. 5.30).

Reports linking cigarette smoking with premature hair graying [412] have drawn on the one hand the attention to gray hair as a marker for the general health status, and on the other to the role of oxidative stress on hair growth and pigmentation. A possible explanation of the observation may be that smoking-related diseases increase aging in general, including pigmentation. Whether gray hair, premature or otherwise, is a predictor or risk marker for disease remains controversial, mainly due to poor epidemiologic study design. However, more direct effects, e.g., via smoke genotoxin-induced apoptosis and oxidative stress, may also be involved.

So far, the process of hair graying has been attributed to the loss of the pigment-forming melanocytes from the aging hair follicle [413]. The net effect of this reduction is that fewer melanosomes are incorporated into cortical keratinocytes of the hair shaft. In addition, there appears also to be a defect of melanosome transfer, as keratinocytes may not contain melanin despite their proximity to melanocytes with remaining melanosomes. This defect is further corroborated by the observation of melanin debris in and sometimes around the graying hair bulb. This anomaly is due to either defective melanosomal transfer to the cortical keratinocytes or melanin incontinence due to melanocyte degeneration. Eventually, no melanogenic melanocytes remain in the hair bulb. This decrease of melanin synthesis is associated with a decrease in tyrosinase activity. Ultrastructural studies have eventually shown that remaining melanocytes not only contain fewer melanosomes, but the residual melanosomes may be packaged within autophagolysosomes. This removal of melanosomes into autophagolysosomes suggests that they are defective, possibly with reactive melanin metabolites. This interpretation is supported by the observation that melanocytes in graying hair bulbs are frequently highly vacuolated, a common cellular response to increased oxidative stress [414].

By analogy to Harman's original free radical theory of aging [415], Arck et al. proposed a free radical theory of graying [416]: the extraordinary melanogenic activity of pigmented bulbar melanocytes, continuing for up to 10 years in some hair follicles, is likely to generate large amounts of reactive oxygen species via the hydroxylation of tyrosine and the oxidation of DOPA to melanin. If not adequately removed by an efficient antioxidant system, an accumulation of these reactive oxidative species will generate significant oxidative stress. It is possible that the antioxidant system becomes impaired with age leading to damage to the melanocyte itself from its own melanogenesis-related oxidative stress. Since mutations occur at a higher rate in tissue exposed to high levels of oxidative stress, and these accumulate with age, the induction of replicative senescence with apoptosis is likely to be an important protective mechanism against cell transformation.

Wood et al. [417] originally demonstrated for the first time that human white scalp hair shafts accumulate hydrogen peroxide (H_2O_2) in millimolar concentrations, and almost absent catalase and methionine sulfoxide reductase (MSR) protein expression in association with functional loss of methionine sulfoxide repair in the entire gray hair follicle. Accordingly, methionine sulfoxide formation of methionine residues (Met), including Met 374 in the active site of tyrosinase, the key enzyme in melanogenesis, limits enzyme functionality, which eventually leads to loss of hair color. While the entire hair follicle is subject to H_2O_2-mediated stress, it is tempting to assume that, besides tyrosinase and MSR, other proteins and peptides, including anti-apoptotic Bcl-2 protein, are targets for oxidation, which in turn could explain melanocyte apoptosis in the gray hair follicle. Moreover, H_2O_2-mediated oxidation has been documented for many other important regulators of pigmentation, including the proopiomelanocortins alpha-melanocyte-stimulating hormone (MSH) and beta-endorphin, the prohormone convertases, and the synthesis and recycling of the ubiquitous cofactor 6-tetrahydrobiopterin.

Since the discovery of unpigmented melanocyte stem cells located within the hair follicle by Nishimura et al. [418], the question arose whether the process underlying hair graying arises specifically from changes in differentiated, pigmented melanocytes or unpigmented progenitors which provide them. Utilizing melanocyte-tagged transgenic mice and aging human hair follicles, Nishimura et al. [419] demonstrated that hair graying is caused by defective self-maintenance of melanocyte stem cells, and not of differentiated melanocytes. This process was accelerated dramatically with Bcl-2 deficiency, which causes selective apoptosis of melanocyte stem cells, but not of differentiated melanocytes, within the niche at their entry into the dormant state.

Gray hair has been found to have increased sensitivity to weathering, increased cysteic acid residues and decreased cystine, and increased fiber reactivity to reducing and oxidizing agents [420]. Moreover, gray hair is more sensitive to UVR. Photochemical impairment of the hair includes degradation and loss of hair proteins as well as degradation of hair pigment. UVB radiation is responsible for hair protein loss and UVA radiation is responsible for hair color changes. Absorption of radiation in photosensitive amino acids of the hair and their photochemical degradation produce free radicals. They have adverse impact on hair proteins, especially keratin, while melanin can partially immobilize free radicals and block their entrance in keratin matrix [421].

Hair thinning is one of the most typical signs of aging in both humans and many long-lived mammals. Hair diameter changes with age are likely to impart the largest impact on overall perception of hair aging. The largest study on female hair diameter in relation to age was performed in 1988 by Otsuka and Nemoto [422] on >18,000 Japanese females aged 10 through 60 years. The study showed that hair diameter versus age does not represent a linear relationship, but rather a curvature that increases to a maximum near the age of 40 and thereafter decreases. The second largest study performed more recently by Robbins et al. [423] on 1099 Caucasian females aged 18 through 66 years with perceived hair loss revealed the age for maximum diameter to be 43–46 years. Several smaller studies on age versus diameter were in reasonable agreement with the conclusions of these two large studies, indicating that the age of maximum diameter for females is near the 40s. One exception is the study of Birch et al. [424] on >300 Caucasian females concluding that the age for maximum hair diameter was near the 30s. Postmenopausal women were shown to have significantly lower hair fiber diameters (lower frontal scalp hair density, and lower growth rates) than premenopausal women for the frontal but not the occipital scalp region. This effect was independent of age, together with the co-localization with androgenetic alopecia, suggesting an impact of the hormonal effects of menopause on hair diameter. In males, Otsuko and Nemoto found scalp hair fiber diameter in Japanese men to increase to a maximum in the late teenage years and then to decrease relatively rapidly with increasing age [425]. Courtois et al. [426] studied ten French male subjects aged 25–49 over a period of 14 years, and demonstrated that the diameter of hair shafts decreased with increasing age beginning at age 25.

At the turn of the last millennium, some controversy arose with regard to the concept of senescent alopecia, specifically whether pattern hair loss and senescent alopecia represented two distinct entities: in a study performed in 2001, Price et al. [427] compared men aged 60 years or older with presumed senescent alopecia with younger men with typical male pattern hair loss, and found in scalp biopsies from patients with senescent alopecia follicular miniaturization that was indistinguishable from male pattern baldness. The histopathology of aging hair was further scrutinized in 2003 by Sperling [428], in 2005 by Sinclair et al. [429], and in 2011 by Whiting [430], who all found modest changes in total hair counts, anagen-to-telogen ratios, and terminal-to-vellus hair ratios in senescent alopecia and a significant overlap with pattern hair loss. Furthermore, inflammation was not a feature. Ultimately, Whiting concluded that old age was not a significant cause of hair loss.

And yet, data comparing senescent alopecia with pattern hair loss using microarray analysis have eventually demonstrated significant differences in the gene expression profiles suggesting that they do represent different entities [431]: in senescent alopecia, genes involved in epithelial signal to dermal papilla (FGF5), actin cytoskeleton (DST, ACTN2, TNNI3, PARVB), and mitochondrial function (JAK2, PRKD3, AK2, TRAP1, TRIO, ATP12A, MLL4, STK22B) were downregulated, while oxidative stress and inflammatory response genes were upregulated. In pattern hair loss, genes required for anagen onset (Wnt-beta-catenin, TGF-alpha, TGF-beta, Stat-3, Stat-1), epithelial signal to dermal papilla (PPARd, IGF-1), hair shaft differentiation (Notch, Msx2, KRTs, KAPs), and anagen maintenance (Msx2, activin, IGF-1) were downregulated, while genes for catagen (BDNF, BMP2, BMP7, VDR, IL-1, ER) and telogen induction and maintenance (VDR, RAR) were upregulated.

Additional changes in hair fiber curvature with age have an important effect on hair cosmetic properties. Nagase et al. [432] studied hair curvature of hair from 132 Japanese females aged 10 through 70 years, and found an increase in curvature with age. In a different publication by the same authors, frizziness was explained as a lack of synchronization in the curvature of neighboring hair fibers in an assembly of hair. Changes in hair fiber diameter and curvature with age also affect structural properties of hairs increasing combing forces and therefore breakage. Combing forces have been shown to increase with decreasing fiber curvature and increasing fiber curvature. Therefore, combing forces can be expected to increase with age, leading to increase in breakage of hair.

Age-related lipid changes affect hair greasiness, shine, softness, and smoothness. The two major sources of hair lipids are the hair matrix cells (cholesterol, cholesterol sulfate, ceramides, covalent fatty acids, 18-methyl eicosanoic acid) and the hair follicle-associated sebaceous glands (squalene, wax esters, triglycerides, total fatty acids). The amount of sebum produced varies with the size of sebaceous glands, being low before puberty, rapidly increasing at puberty, and remaining at a high level until 45–50 where it declines. The decline is greater in females than in males [433].

Miniaturization of hair follicles has long been considered the hallmark of androgenetic alopecia. The studies of Nishimura et al. [434] reveal that mammalian hair follicles do miniaturize and often disappear from the skin in the course of aging. Nishimura found mouse hair follicles to age through defective renewal of hair follicle stem cells much in the manner as maintenance of melanocyte stem cells becomes incomplete with aging. Hair production is fueled by stem cells, which transition between cyclical bouts of rest and activity. Aged hair follicle stem cells exhibit enhanced resting and abbreviated growth phases and are delayed in response to tissue-regenerating cues. Ultimately, aged hair follicle stem cells are poor at initiating proliferation and show diminished self-renewing capacity upon extensive use. Aging-related loss of hair follicle stem cell marker expression starts well before hair follicles have shortened. Using genomic instability syndromes and exposure to ionizing radiation as models, Nishimura proposed an accumulation of DNA damage to be involved in the aging process [435]. Further, Nishimura et al. [434] found that hair follicle stem cell aging resulted from proteolysis of type XVII collagen (COL17A1/BP180) by protease expression in response to DNA damage in stem cells and their commitment to epidermal differentiation. This enables the transepidermal elimination of damaged stem cells as shed corneocytes from the skin surface. Ultimately, hair follicle aging can be recapitulated by COL17A deficiency, and conversely can be prevented by forced maintenance of COL17A1 in hair follicle stem cells, thereby indicating a potential for antiaging therapeutic intervention [436].

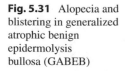

Fig. 5.31 Alopecia and blistering in generalized atrophic benign epidermolysis bullosa (GABEB)

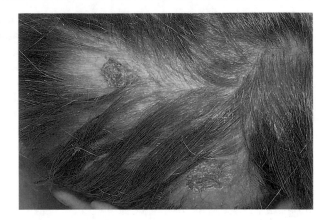

The earlier discovery of a mutation of the collagen COL17A1 gene in generalized atrophic benign epidermolysis bullosa (GABEB) [437], a benign form of hereditary junctional epidermolysis bullosa [438], led to the anticipation of a critical role of collagen XVII in epidermal physiology and hair growth, since affected patients suffer from blistering skin disease and alopecia (Fig. 5.31) [439].

Finally, though being exceedingly rare, the progeroid syndromes (Hutchinson-Gilford and Werner), together with other rare conditions associated with premature hair loss, such as the Laron syndrome and myotonic dystrophy (Curschmann-Steinert, Fig. 5.32), give insights into the roles of telomeres [440, 441], mitochondrial function [442], human growth hormone (HGH) [443, 444], and insulin-like growth factor 1 (IGF-1) [445] for the growth and aging of hair (Fig. 5.33).

Replications errors, reactive oxygen species, eroded telomeres, and chromosome breaks represent sources of accumulated DNA damage. The aging phenotypes, including graying and hair loss, are accelerated by intrinsic genomic instability in the progeroid syndromes (and their mouse models), as well as by extrinsic genomic instability, such as by ionizing radiation, and others. Accumulation of DNA damage is implicated in tissue damage. Physiological hair cycling itself is sufficient to induce DNA damage foci formation in renewing hair follicle stem cells. Accumulation of unrepaired DNA damage in the hair follicle stem cells over anagen phases causes the hair follicle stem cell-aging state that is characterized by COL17A1 depletion with sustained DNA damage response, loss of stem cell signature, and epidermal commitment. Nishimura et al. did not detect any significant increase in markers of apoptosis or cellular senescence, indicating that cell death and cellular senescence are not likely to be the major fate of hair follicle stem cells during hair follicle aging. Aged hair follicle stem cell-derived progeny migrate up towards the skin surface through the junction zone and epidermis without renewing themselves in the stem cell niche upon induction of a hair cycle. This elimination of stressed and damaged hair follicle stem cells through terminal epidermal differentiation as shed corneocytes at the skin surface may be understood to maintain the high quality of hair follicle stem cells and as a cancer barrier [434].

Fig. 5.32 Myotonic
dystrophy type 1
(Curschmann-Steinert
syndrome): premature
alopecia and
myopathic face

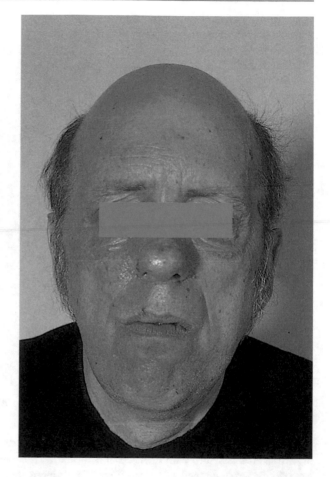

In summary, the elderly often suffer from a variety of conditions that may affect the hair beyond physiological aging: nutritional deficiency, endocrine disorders, psychological problems, and drug-related adverse effects. Therefore, one must remain suspicious of the possibility of a more general problem underlying the patient's complaint in taking care of the elderly with hair problems.

Topical minoxidil has not been studied in the specific perspective of aging and senescent alopecia. In an analysis of clinical trial data in 636 males and 630 females a therapeutic benefit of topical 2% and 5% minoxidil solution was compared to age, duration of balding, and diameter of balding vertex area in males, and age and duration of hair loss in females [446]: age was found to be the denominator for predicting treatment success for both males and females. The younger subjects experienced better efficacy than the older subjects. Nevertheless, clear treatment benefits of topical minoxidil solution are also noted in the older age group that has retained some hair. Males showed an inverse relationship between effect and duration of balding. Males with duration of balding <5 years showed a significantly better effect than those with duration of balding >21 years. Females, in contrast, showed no

Fig. 5.33 Hypotrichosis
in male child with primary
growth hormone resistance
and low IGF-1 levels

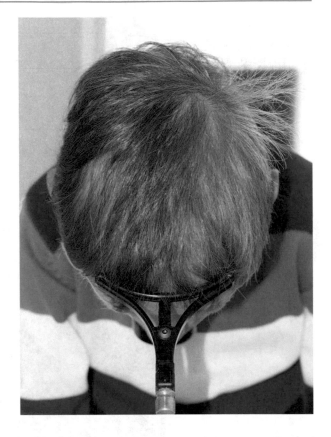

correlation with duration of balding. The diameter of vertex balding in men showed
an inverse relationship with efficacy of minoxidil. Males with <5 cm diameter vertex balding area showed a better effect of treatment than subjects with diameters
>15 cm. Finally, duration of hair loss less than 1 year compared to more than
10 years at the onset of treatment resulted in a significantly more effective treatment
with respect to stabilization of alopecia and new hair growth.

CG 210® represents a novel hair growth-promoting formulation differing from
the mechanism of action of existing treatment options for androgenetic alopecia.
The lotion is a botanical based on *Allium cepa* (onion), *Citrus medica Limonium*
(lemon), *Theobroma cacao* (cocoa), and *Paullinia cupana* (guarana) with a proposed three-level mechanism of action including (1) regulation of the intracellular
anti-apoptotic Bcl-2 protein, (2) reduction of micro-inflammation, and (3) increase
of collagen content and collagen remodeling [447], designed from an extended
understanding of the pathogenic mechanisms underlying androgenetic alopecia, to
include apoptosis, inflammation, and fibrosis (Fig. 5.34) for multitargeted treatment
as formerly proposed by Trüeb [448].

The mechanisms of action, efficacy, and safety of the product were evaluated in
both females and males with androgenetic alopecia, either as monotherapy [449] or
as combination therapy with either topical minoxidil [450, 451] or oral finasteride

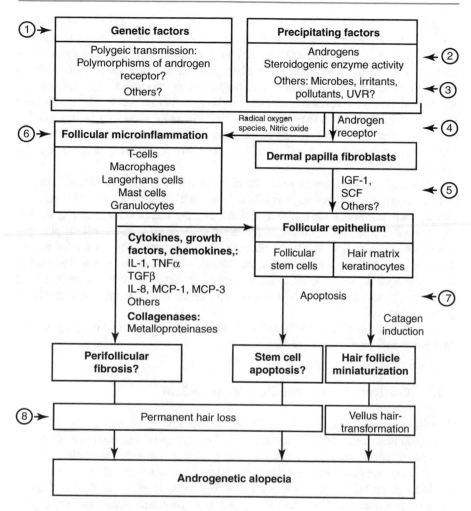

Fig. 5.34 Androgenetic alopecia: pathogenic mechanisms and therapeutic strategies (from Trüeb RM. Molecular mechanisms of androgenetic alopecia. Exp Gerontol. 37:981–990 (2002)): 1. Targeted gene therapy? 2. Modifiers of androgen metabolism, 3. Antimicrobials, detox shampoos, UVR-protection, 4. Antiandrogens, 5. Hair growth promoting agents, 6. Antiinflammatory agents, 7. Apoptosis modulating agents, 8. Autologous hair transplantation, implantation of dermal papilla cells or cells of follicular dermal-sheath

[452]. In an open prospective study of 20 males with androgenetic alopecia, immunohistochemical analyses of scalp biopsies showed an increase in CD1A+ Langerhans cells, in the cellular proliferation marker Ki-67+, and in BCL-2+ anti-apoptotic protein in accordance with the proposed multidimensional mode of action [453].

 Coenzyme Q10 (CoQ10) has previously been used for its antiaging effects on aging skin, where it has been theorized that there is an increase in anaerobic metabolism due to a decrease in mitochondrial function as a result of oxidative damage [454]. Expanding the cutaneous application to the hair, it has been shown with quantitative polymerase chain reaction techniques that CoQ10 administration results in an increase in particular keratins in the hair root compared to placebo [455]. Specific keratin and keratin-associated protein levels have been found to be decreased in aged hair compared to fibers from a younger individual [456]. A decrease in keratin levels correlates with a decrease in interactions between the filaments and keratin-associated proteins resulting in a decline in the mechanical strength of the hair fiber. However, as with all cosmetic antiaging treatments, the question arises as to whether and to what extent a quantifiable improvement in a particular parameter measured translates into improvement perceived by the consumer.

The use of *oral collagen* as a nutraceutical for skincare has been rising, but regulations on quality, absorption, and efficacy are lacking. Choi et al. [457] recently performed a literature search with PubMed using the search criteria collagen AND supplement OR food OR nutrition. Inclusion criteria were randomized, placebo-controlled trials using collagen supplementation in human subjects related to dermatology and written in English. Eleven studies with a total of 805 patients using either collagen hydrolysate or collagen tripeptide were included for review. Oral collagen supplements were found to increase skin elasticity, hydration, and dermal collagen density.

Oral collagen has as yet to be studied in the specific perspective of aging-related changes in hair growth and quality.

5.3.7   Controversies in the Oncologic Patient

Oncologic patients are at risk of losing vital body resources, especially with advanced disease. Cancer cachexia is a multifactorial condition that is characterized by systemic inflammation, weight loss, and profound metabolic alterations, which may or may not affect hair growth and quality. The metabolic alterations include myofibrillar protein breakdown, increased lipolysis, insulin resistance, elevated energy expenditure, and reduced food intake. The symptoms of cachexia are dependent on the type of tumor, its stage, and the individual patient's response to cancer therapy. Individual nutrition problems throughout the continuum of care for cancer patients will therefore vary greatly. By definition, an involuntary weight loss >5% of the premorbid weight within a 1-month period or >10% in the previous 6 months is indicative of cachexia. Cancer cachexia greatly increases morbidity and mortality, and contributes to poor quality of life [458]. The 1-year mortality rate is estimated to be between 20% and 80% [459]. The best way to treat cancer-related cachexia is of course to alleviate the underlying cancer and the metabolic derangements associated with it. However, since this is not always possible, professional medical nutrition therapy is indicated with the objective of preventing weight loss, maintaining lean body mass, and identifying and managing treatment-related side effects, including hair loss. The particular medical nutrition therapy will vary depending on the cancer site, stage of disease, treatment modality, and nutritional state of the patient.

In general, more kilocalories may be needed depending on the degree of metabolic stress, the amount of tissue buildup that is taking place, and the physical activity level of the patient. Patients receiving chemotherapy or radiation therapy, hypermetabolic patients, and severely stressed patients may have energy requirements up to 35 kcal/kg [460]. Essential amino acids and nitrogen are essential for tissue building and healing. Finally, key vitamins and minerals help to control protein and energy metabolism through their coenzyme roles in the specific cell enzyme pathways, and also may play a role in building and maintaining strong tissue.

On the other hand, as the link between obesity and metabolic syndrome and cancer unravels, an increasing interest is arising in how to incorporate dietary manipulations in the treatment of cancer patients. Caloric restriction and intermittent fasting [461] have the ability to decrease the incidence of spontaneous tumors and slow the growth of primary tumors, and may have an effect on distant metastases in animal models [462]. Cancer cells usually have a higher metabolic rate than the surrounding normal tissue, and as glucose is their main source of fuel, intermittent fasting aims to reduce circulating glucose levels. It has been shown that fasting causes a reduction in insulin-like growth factor 1 (IGF-1) which results in cell death [463]. Despite the abundance of preclinical data demonstrating the benefit of dietary modification for cancer, to date there are few clinical trials targeting diet as an intervention for cancer patients [464].

The risk of hair loss during fasting is of theoretical consideration. Blackburn et al. commented on diffuse hair loss following rapid weight loss making the statement that telogen effluvium is observed in patients in whom weight loss is associated with loss of body cell mass, i.e., significant negative nitrogen balance. With an increase in protein intake during fasting to preserve nitrogen balance, hair loss may be almost completely eliminated [465].

As many as 48% of cancer patients follow popular diets, including the alkaline, Paleolithic, ketogenic, vegan, and macrobiotic diets, with the hope of preventing recurrence and improving survival [466]. Drawbacks of these diets are pseudoscientific rationales for their anticancer properties, limited evidence that they improve cancer outcomes, and risk of nutrient deficiencies.

Specifically, the vegan diet entails total dietary abstinence from all animal products. Adhering to a vegan diet is believed to increase the consumption of cancer-fighting foods, such as berries, greens, whole grains, nuts, and seeds, while excluding foods such as dairy products and red and processed meats that may increase cancer risk. A meta-analysis of 24 cross-sectional studies and 4 prospective cohort studies found that vegan diets were associated with a 15% risk reduction in total cancer incidence, although no difference was observed for mortality [467]. Vegan diets can be low in calcium (from dairy products) and vitamin B12 (from meats), although this can be checked by appropriate dietary advice and supplementation.

There is up to date no evidence that a vegan diet has a negative effect on hair growth.

Also, nutritional supplements are widely used among patients with cancer who perceive them to have anticancer and/or antitoxic properties [468]. A significant proportion of people with cancer have been found to supplement their diets with antioxidants and immune system-stabilizing micronutrients, depending on the type of malignancy and the gender of the patient [469] often without consulting their attending physician. However, from the oncological viewpoint, there have been concerns that dietary supplements may decrease the effectiveness of chemotherapy and radiotherapy, specifically the antioxidants may reduce toxicity of chemotherapy and radiotherapy at the cost of reduced treatment efficacy since radiotherapy and many chemotherapy agents exert their anticancer effects by production of reactive oxygen species and apoptosis [470]. Recent studies, however, have provided evidence of improved patient compliance, fewer adverse effects, and, subsequently, a lower rate of treatment discontinuations, when selected micronutrients, such as selenium and vitamin D, were added to an adequate supply of energy substrates (proteins, fats, and carbohydrate) [471]. Moreover, a majority of cytostatics used in treatment today, specifically the antimetabolites (methotrexate), nitrogen mustard derivatives (cyclophosphamide), platinum complexes (cisplatin), vinca alkaloids (vinorelbine), taxanes (paclitaxel), and anthracyclines (epirubicin), do not primarily act through oxidative stress. Therefore, the often uncritical blanket renunciation of dietary supplements with antioxidant and immunomodulating micronutrients during chemotherapy does not seem justified [472]. In fact, the success of treatment and the healing process in cancer patients are significantly influenced by the nutritional status of patients [473]. Depending on the nature, site, and stage of the malignancy, 30–90% of patients have a cancer-associated nutritional deficiency [474] that in its most severe form is seen physically as cachexia, especially with bronchial, gastric, pancreatic, and prostate cancer [475].

Therefore, there is a need of an open dialogue between oncologists and cancer patients, addressing the needs of the patient while dealing with issues related to the efficacy and safety of nutritional supplements. Simply administering supplements to unselected patients, often with an adequate vitamin status, has not been successful. Rather, identifying and replenishing individuals with specific nutritional deficiencies may be appropriate and beneficial; that is, future research should develop targeted therapies tailored to background diet, patient's genetic makeup, tumor histology, and treatments. A targeted approach may yield benefits in subsets of patients in the same way that the pharmaceutical industry has developed more effective cancer therapies targeted to variations in the individual and tumor type [476]. Precision medicine refers to the customization of medical care to the patient's individual characteristics based on the patient's genetic background and other molecular or cellular analysis while classifying patients into subpopulations that differ in their susceptibility to a particular medical condition, in the biology or prognosis of those medical conditions, or in their response to a specific treatment. The concept has evolved from cancer medicine, where it is also referred to as precision oncology and has paved the way to targeted cancer therapies with success. With the advances in hair research, powerful tools of molecular biology and genetics, and innovative technologies, we have the robust scientific data and tools to adapt the concept for the management of specific hair derangements. Finally, databases pertaining to the development and efficacy of precision medicine must be analyzed and be used to form the basis of evidence-based personalized treatments [477].

Chemotherapy-induced hair loss is considered as one of the most traumatic factors in cancer patient care, since hair loss negatively affects a patient's perception of appearance, body image, sexuality, and self-esteem, and patients feel deprived of their privacy because hair loss is readily interpreted by the lay public as associated with having cancer. 47% of female cancer patients consider hair loss as the most traumatic aspect of chemotherapy, and 8% would even decline chemotherapy because of this fear of hair loss [478].

Chemotherapy-induced hair loss is a consequence of direct toxic insult to the rapidly dividing cells of the hair follicle. While chemotherapy-induced hair loss has traditionally been categorized as acute diffuse hair loss caused by dystrophic anagen effluvium, more recently it has been pointed out that, in fact, chemotherapy-induced hair loss may present with different pathomechanisms and clinical patterns. Evidence exists that the hair follicle may respond to the same insult capable of stopping mitosis with shedding patterns, dystrophic anagen effluvium, and telogen effluvium. Accordingly, the hair may fall out very quickly in clumps or gradually. When mitotic activity is arrested, numerous and interacting factors may influence the shedding pattern. One of these factors is the mitotic activity of the hair follicle at the moment of the insult.

It is a major characteristic of the anagen hair follicle that the epithelial compartment undergoes proliferation, with the bulb matrix cells showing the greatest proliferative activity in building up the hair shaft. The abrupt cessation of mitotic activity leads to the weakening of the partially keratinized proximal portion of the hair shaft, a narrowing, and a subsequent breakage within the hair canal. The consequence is hair shedding that usually begins at 1–3 weeks after initiation of chemotherapy. Due to its long anagen phase, the scalp is the most common location for hair loss, while other terminal hairs are variably affected depending on the percentage of hairs in anagen. Since normally up to 90% of scalp hair is in the anagen phase, hair loss is usually copious and the resulting alopecia is quite obvious. Nevertheless, chemotherapy given at high doses for a sufficiently long time and with multiple exposures may also affect the beard, eyebrows, eyelashes, axillary, and pubic hairs.

Finally, when the hair is in its late anagen phase, in which the mitotic rate is slowing down spontaneously, it simply accelerates its normal path to telogen, while mitotically inactive phases (catagen and telogen) are not affected. Since anagen duration is diminished in androgenetic alopecia, the probability is increased that the antimitotic insult strikes the hair close to the resting phase resulting in telogen effluvium. While synchronization of hair cycles also plays a role, and again in androgenetic alopecia, the hair cycles tend to synchronize due to the diminished duration of anagen; even a minor antimitotic insult may produce marked hair loss [479].

Chemotherapy-induced hair loss occurs with an estimated overall incidence of 65%. The incidence and severity of the hair loss are variable and related to the particular chemotherapeutic agent and protocol: multiple classes of anticancer drugs induce alopecia, with frequencies of chemotherapy-induced hair loss differing for the four major drug classes: more than 80% for antimicrotubule agents (for example, paclitaxel), 60–100% for topoisomerase inhibitors (for example, doxorubicin), more than 60% for alkylators (for example, cyclophosphamide), and 10–50% for antimetabolites (for example, 5-fluorouracil plus leucovorin). Combination therapy consisting of two or more agents usually produces greater incidences of more severe hair loss compared with single-agent therapy [480].

The hair loss has traditionally been regarded as usually being reversible, with hair regrowth typically occurring after a delay of 3–6 months. In some patients, the regrown hair shows changes in color and/or texture. It might be curlier than it was before, or it could be gray until the follicular melanocytes begin functioning again. But the difference is usually temporary. And yet, permanent alopecia has been reported after chemotherapy, originally reported from busulfan and cyclophosphamide after bone marrow transplantation [481], and has been associated with particular risk factors, including age of patients, previous exposure to X-ray, and chronic graft-versus-host reaction [482]. More recently, permanent chemotherapy-induced alopecia has also been reported in women treated for breast cancer [483]. Miteva et al. [484] studied scalp biopsies from the affected scalp areas of permanent alopecia after systemic chemotherapy. The histology was characterized by a non-scarring pattern with a preserved number of follicular units and lack of fibrosis. The hair count revealed a decreased number of terminal hairs, an increased number of telogen, and miniaturized vellus-like hairs. There was an increased number of fibrous streamers (stelae) in both the reticular dermis and the subcutis, with Arao-Perkins bodies found in the subcutaneous portions of the streamers. The histological findings of permanent alopecia after chemotherapy are similar to those in androgenetic alopecia. It may be speculated that exposure to chemotherapy may lead to an accumulation of DNA damage with defective renewal of hair follicle stem cells.

A number of preventive measures have been proposed and tried to reduce chemotherapy-induced hair loss. Nevertheless, no treatment exists that can guarantee to prevent chemotherapy-induced hair loss. Of the treatments so far investigated, scalp cooling (hypothermia) has been the most widely used and studied. Of 53 multiple patient studies published between 1973 and 2003 on the results of scalp cooling for the prevention of chemotherapy-induced hair loss seven trials were randomized. In six of the seven randomized studies, a significant advantage was observed with scalp cooling. The positive results were most evident when anthracyclines or taxanes were the chemotherapeutic agents. In the most recent open-label, prospective, non-randomized clinical trial, patients with solid tumors receiving docetaxel in a palliative setting were allocated according to patients' preference to short-term cooling (over 45 min postinfusion) with a Paxman® PSC-2 machine (PAX), with cold cap (CC), or with no cooling. The combined endpoint was alopecia World Health Organization (WHO) III or IV, or the necessity to wear a wig. Two hundred thirty-eight patients were included in the trial (128 patients PAX, 71 CC, and 39 no cooling). The number of cycles (median 4) and median docetaxel doses were similar across the three groups (55–60 mg/day on weekly therapy, 135–140 mg/day on 3-weekly therapy). Alopecia occurred with PAX, CC, and no cooling under 3-weekly docetaxel in 23, 27, and 74%, and under weekly docetaxel in 7, 8, and 17%, respectively. Overall, cooling (PAX and CC combined) reduced the risk of alopecia by 78% (hazard ratio 0.22; 95% confidence interval 0.12–0.41). CC and PAX prophylaxis led to the same degree of prevention of alopecia. In this first comparison study published to date, both PAX and CC offered efficacious protection against hair loss, in particular when docetaxel was administered in a 3-weekly interval [485].

So far, no approved pharmacologic treatment or nutrient exists for chemotherapy-induced hair loss, despite some experimental trials in animal models. In one study, the in vivo effects of oral zinc using the C57BL/6 mouse model for hair research were explored; specifically, the researchers investigated whether continuous administration of high-dose $ZnSO(4) \times 7H(2)O$ (20 mg/mL) in drinking water affects hair follicle cycling, whether it retards or inhibits chemotherapy-induced alopecia, and whether it modulates the subsequent hair regrowth pattern. They showed that high doses of oral zinc significantly inhibited hair growth by retardation of anagen development in mice. However, oral zinc also significantly retarded and prolonged spontaneous, apoptosis-driven hair follicle regression (catagen). Oral zinc could also retard, but not prevent, the onset of chemotherapy-induced alopecia in mice. Interestingly, $Zn(2+)$ treatment of cyclophosphamide-damaged HFs also significantly accelerated the regrowth of normally pigmented hair shafts, which reflected a promotion of hair follicle recovery. However, if given for a more extended time period, zinc actually retarded hair regrowth. Thus, high-dose oral zinc proved to be a powerful, yet ambivalent, hair growth modulator in mice, whose ultimate effects on the hair follicle greatly depended on the timing and duration of zinc administration. The authors suggested that this study would encourage one to explore whether oral zinc can mitigate chemotherapy-induced hair loss in humans and/or can stimulate hair regrowth [486].

In another animal study, soymetide-4, an immunostimulating peptide from soy protein, inhibited chemotherapy-induced alopecia from etoposide in neonatal rats [487]. As yet, no respective clinical study has followed up on these findings.

Sieja et al. [488] gave selenium to accompany chemotherapy with cisplatin and cyclophosphamide in patients with ovarian cancer, and found a significant reduction both in hematotoxicity and alopecia.

Among the agents that so far have been evaluated in cancer patients, the topical hair growth-promoting agent minoxidil was able to shorten the duration, though it did not prevent chemotherapy-induced hair loss [489]. Minoxidil also fails to induce significant regrowth of hair in busulfan- and cyclophosphamide-induced permanent alopecia [490].

Nevertheless, topical minoxidil has proven to be effective in the management of endocrine therapy-induced alopecia in patients with breast cancer (Fig. 5.35a,b). Freites-Martinez et al. [491] reported on patients with endocrine therapy-induced alopecia ($n = 112$) with information on the drug-related frequencies, clinical features, impact on quality of life, and response to dermatologic therapy. Alopecia was attributed to aromatase inhibitors in 67% and tamoxifen in 33% of patients; the presentation was androgenetic alopecia-like, both clinically and on trichoscopic examination; negative impact on quality of life was significant; and topical minoxidil improved alopecia in 80% of treated patients. Patients who had previously received cytotoxic therapy were excluded from the study. However, patients with breast cancer often receive a combination of chemotherapy and endocrine therapy.

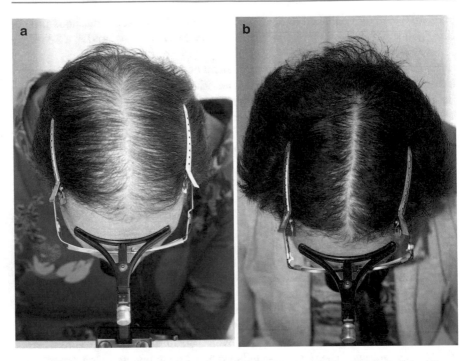

Fig. 5.35 (**a**, **b**) Successful treatment of endocrine therapy-induced alopecia in a female on letro-
zole with 5% topical minoxidil b.i.d. associated with a L-cystine, nutritional yeast, pantothenic
acid, and thiamine-based nutritional supplement (**a**) before and (**b**) after 12 months of treatment

While in many instances chemotherapy-induced alopecia is reversible, permanent
chemotherapy-induced alopecia has been reported in women treated for breast cancer [492]. While permanent chemotherapy-induced alopecia is irreversible, endocrine therapy-induced alopecia is amenable to treatment with minoxidil in the same
way androgenetic alopecia is, if treated timely. At the time point of the clinical
consultation, the pattern of hair loss is not always reliable to distinguish the two
conditions, since chemotherapy-induced alopecia is not always diffuse, but can also
be patterned [479]. Rather, the chronology of events will help prognostication, since
a history of recovery from chemotherapy-induced alopecia with worsening following initiation of endocrine therapy will point to endocrine therapy-induced alopecia
and potential improvement with topical minoxidil. The mean time to development
of alopecia from endocrine therapy initiation has been 16.8 months (range
1–91 months) with 58% reporting alopecia within the first 12 months of endocrine
therapy. Minoxidil should be used for the whole duration of endocrine therapy to
preserve the hairs that are at risk of gradually being permanently lost in the course
of endocrine therapy-induced alopecia, just as in androgenetic alopecia. Furthermore,
after cessation of endocrine therapy, there is the potential for further and sustained
recovery of hair, irrespective of duration (usually from 5 to 10 years) of endocrine
therapy.

   In summary, the incidence and severity of hair loss in patients treated for breast cancer with either chemotherapy, endocrine therapy, or both are variable and related to the particular treatment protocol. Even if the hair loss cannot be totally prevented, it can be managed, and patients can be given hope and confidence. Anticipating hair loss, coming to terms with it, and taking control are the key steps in coping with the condition [493]. Nutritional supplement advice needs to be individualized to the particular patient at hand, needs to come from a credible source, and needs to be communicated by the patient's oncologist.

References

1. Androutsos G, Karamanou M, Stefanadis C. William Harvey (1578-1657): discoverer of blood circulation. Hellenic J Cardiol. 2012;53:6–9.
2. Dronamraju K. Profiles in genetics: Archibald E. Garrod (1857-1936). Am J Hum Genet. 1992;1992(5):216–9.
3. Menkes JH, Alter M, Steigleder GK, Weakley DR, Sung JH. A sex-linked recessive disorder with retardation of growth, peculiar hair, and focal cerebral and cerebellar degeneration. Pediatrics. 1962;29:764–79.
4. de Bie P, Muller P, Wijmenga C, Klomp LW. Molecular pathogenesis of Wilson and Menkes disease: correlation of mutations with molecular defects and disease phenotypes. J Med Genet. 2007;44:673–88.
5. Ivo S, Ralf D, Mercer Julian FB. Chapter 11. Copper: effects of deficiency and overload. In: Sigel A, Sigel H, Sigel RKO, editors. Interrelations between essential metal ions and human diseases. Metal ions in life sciences, vol. 13. Dordrecht: Springer; 2013. p. 359–87.
6. Kaler SG, Gallo LK, Proud VK, Percy AK, Mark Y, Segal NA, Goldstein DS, Holmes CS, Gahl WA. Occipital horn syndrome and a mild Menkes phenotype associated with splice site mutations at the MNK locus. Nat Genet. 1994;8:195–202.
7. Tønnesen T, Kleijer WJ, Horn N. Incidence of Menkes disease. Hum Genet. 1991;86:408–10.
8. Kaler SG, Holmes CS, Goldstein DS. Neonatal diagnosis and treatment of Menkes disease. N Engl J Med. 2008;358:605–14.
9. Moore CM, Howell RR. Ectodermal manifestations in Menkes disease. Clin Genet. 1985;28:532–40.
10. Kumar V, Abbas AK, Fausto N. Robbins & Cotran. Pathologic basis of disease. 7th ed. Philadelphia: Elsevier; 2008. p. 16.
11. Lapointe M. Iron supplementation in the intensive care unit: when, how much, and by what route? Crit Care. 2004;8:S37–41.
12. Merle U, Schaefer M, Ferenci P, Stremmel W. Clinical presentation, diagnosis and long-term outcome of Wilson's disease: a cohort study. Gut. 2007;56:115–20.
13. Ala A, Walker AP, Ashkan K, Dooley JS, Schilsky ML. Wilson's disease. Lancet. 2007;369:397–408.
14. Roberts EA, Schilsky ML. A practice guideline on Wilson disease. Hepatology. 2003;37:1475–92.
15. Kuruvilla A, Joseph S. Face of the giant panda sign in Wilson's disease: revisited. Neurol India. 2000;48:395–6.
16. Talhout R, Schulz T, Florek E, Van Benthem J, Wester P, Opperhuizen A. Hazardous compounds in tobacco smoke. Int J Environ Res Public Health. 2011;8:613–28.
17. Bernhard D, Rossmann A, Wick G. Metals in cigarette smoke. IUBMB Life. 2005;57:805–9.
18. Sehgal VN, Jain S. Acrodermatitis enteropathica. Clin Dermatol. 2000;18:745–8.

19. Kasana S, Din J, Maret W. Genetic causes and gene–nutrient interactions in mammalian zinc deficiencies: acrodermatitis enteropathica and transient neonatal zinc deficiency as examples. J Trace Elem Med Biol. 2015;29:47–62.

20. Ciampo IRLD, Sawamura R, Ciampo LAD, Fernandes MIM. Acrodermatitis enteropathica: clinical manifestations and pediatric diagnosis. Rev Paul Pediatr. 2018;36:238–41.

21. Ranugha P, Sethi P, Shastry V. Acrodermatitis enteropathica: the need for sustained high dose zinc supplementation. Dermatol Online J. 2018;24:12.

22. Secor McVoy JRS, Levy HL, Lawler M, Schmidt MA, Ebers DD, Hart S, Pettit DD, Blitzer MG, Wolf B. Partial biotinidase deficiency: clinical and biochemical features. J Pediatr. 1990;116:78–83.

23. Wolf B, Norrgard K, Pomponio RJ, Mock DM, Secor Mcvoy JR, Fleischhauer K, Shapiro S, Blitzer MG, Hymes J. Profound biotinidase deficiency in two asymptomatic adults. Am J Med Genet. 1997;73:5–9.

24. Forman DT, Bankson DD, Highsmith WE Jr. Neonatal screening for biotinidase deficiency. Ann Clin Lab Sci. 1992;22:144–54.

25. Porta F, Pagliardini V, Celestino I, Pavanello E, Pagliardini S, Guardamagna O, Ponzone A, Spada M. Neonatal screening for biotinidase deficiency: a 30-year single center experience. Mol Genet Metab Rep. 2017;13:80–2.

26. Wolf B. Worldwide survey of neonatal screening for biotinidase deficiency. J Inherit Metab Dis. 1991;14:923–7.

27. Michalski AJ, Berry GT, Segal S. Holocarboxylase synthetase deficiency: 9-year follow-up of a patient on chronic biotin therapy and a review of the literature. J Inherit Metab Dis. 1989;12:312–6.

28. McCoy RH, Meyer CE, Rose WC. Feeding experiments with mixtures of highly purified amino acids. VIII. Isolation and identification of a new essential amino acid. J Biol Chem. 1935;112:283–302.

29. Holtcamp W. The emerging science of BMAA: do cyanobacteria contribute to neurodegenerative disease? Environ Health Perspect. 2012;120:A110–6.

30. Cox PA, Davis DA, Mash DC, Metcalf JS, Banack SA. Dietary exposure to an environmental toxin triggers neurofibrillary tangles and amyloid deposits in the brain. Proc Biol Sci. 2016;283(1823):20152397.

31. Holtcamp W. Shark fin consumption may expose people to neurotoxic BMAA. Environ Health Perspect. 2012;120:A191.

32. Wiest LG, Lutz P, Jung EG, Paweletz N. Morphological and biochemical investigations of hairs in inborn errors of amino acid metabolism (author's transl). Arch Dermatol Res. 1976;256:53–65.

33. Morris AA, Kožich V, Santra S, Andria G, Ben-Omran TI, Chakrapani AB, Crushell E, Henderson MJ, Hochuli M, Huemer M, Janssen MC, Maillot F, Mayne PD, McNulty J, Morrison TM, Ogier H, O'Sullivan S, Pavlíková M, de Almeida IT, Terry A, Yap S, Blom HJ, Chapman KA. Guidelines for the diagnosis and management of cystathionine beta-synthase deficiency. J Inherit Metab Dis. 2017;40:49–74.

34. Cavka M, Kelava T. Homocystinuria, a possible solution of the Akhenaten's mystery. Coll Antropol. 2010;34:255–8.

35. Freud S. The standard edition of the complete psychological works of sigmund Freud, volume XXIII (1937–1939), "Moses and monotheism". London: Hogarth Press; 1964.

36. Dever WG. What remains of the house that Albright built? In: Wright GE, Cross FM, Campbell EF, Filson FV, editors. The biblical archaeologist, American Schools of Oriental Research, vol. 56: Scholars Press; 1993. p. 25–35, No. 1, p. 33.

37. Dever WG. What did the biblical writers know and when did they know it? What archeology can tell us about the reality of ancient Israel. Michigan: WM. B. Eerdmans Publishing; 2001. p. 99. ISBN: 978-0-8028-2126-3.

38. Barber GW, Spaeth GL. The successful treatment of homocystinuria with pyridoxine. J Pediatr. 1969;75:463–78.

39. Valayannopoulos V, Schiff M, Guffon N, Nadjar Y, García-Cazorla A, Martinez-Pardo Casanova M, Cano A, Couce ML, Dalmau J, Peña-Quintana L, Rigalleau V, Touati G, Aldamiz-Echevarria L, Cathebras P, Eyer D, Brunet D, Damaj L, Dobbelaere D, Gay C, Hiéronimus S, Levrat V, Maillot F. Betaine anhydrous in homocystinuria: results from the RoCH registry. Orphanet J Rare Dis. 2019;4:66.
40. Milne MD, Crawford MA, Girao CB, Loughridge L. The metabolic disorder of the Hartnup disease. Q J Med. 1961;29:407–21.
41. Gounelle H, Mitrovic M, Demarne M. On the vitamin B complex content of the hair of normal and pellagrous subjects. Am J Clin Nutr. 1961;9:746–51.
42. Snyderman SE. The dietary therapy of inherited metabolic disease. Prog Food Nutr Sci. 1975;1:507–30.
43. Gonzalez J, Willis MS. Ivar Asbjörn Følling. Lab Med. 2010;41:118–9.
44. Macleod EL, Ney DM. Nutritional management of phenylketonuria. Ann Nestle Eng. 2010;68:58–69.
45. Michals-Matalon K. Sapropterin dihydrochloride, 6-R-L-erythro-5,6,7,8-tetrahydrobiopterin, in the treatment of phenylketonuria. Expert Opin Investig Drugs. 2008;17:245–51.
46. Mitchell JJ, Trakadis YJ, Scriver CR. Phenylalanine hydroxylase deficiency. Genet Med. 2011;13:697–707.
47. Buck PS. The child who never grew. New York: John Day; 1950.
48. Smith AJ, Strang LB. An inborn error of metabolism with the urinary excretion of alpha-hydroxy-butyric acid and phenylpyruvic acid. Arch Dis Child. 1958;33:109–13.
49. Chayet NL. Absorption of amino acids. N Engl J Med. 1965;273:560–1.
50. Bonafe JL, Pieraggi MT, Abravanel M, Benque A, Abravanel G. Skin, hair and nail changes in a case of citrullinemia with late manifestation. Dermatologica. 1984;168:213–8.
51. Patel HP, Unis ME. Pili torti in association with citrullinemia and arginine succinic aciduria. J Am Acad Dermatol. 1985;12(1 Pt 2):203–6.
52. Phillips ME, Barrie H, Cream JJ. Argininosuccinic aciduria with pili torti. J R Soc Med. 1981;74:221–2.
53. Yazaki M, Hineno A, Matsushima A, Ozawa K, Kishida D, Tazawa K, Fukushima K, Urata K, Ikegami T, Miyagawa S, Ikeda S. First two cases of adult-onset type II citrullinemia successfully treated by deceased-donor liver transplantation in Japan. Hepatol Res. 2012;42:934–9.
54. Shelley WB, Rawnsley HM. Aminogenic alopecia. Loss of hair associated with argininosuccinic aciduria. Lancet. 1965;2:1327–8.
55. Bachmann C. Long-term outcome of patients with urea cycle disorders and the question of neonatal screening. Eur J Pediatr. 2003;162:S29–33.
56. Liu T, Howard RM, Mancini AJ, Weston WL, Paller AS, Drolet BA, Esterly NB, Levy ML, et al. Kwashiorkor in the United States: fad diets, perceived and true milk allergy, and nutritional ignorance. Arch Dermatol. 2001;137:630–6.
57. Badaloo AV, Forrester T, Reid M, Jahoor F. Lipid kinetic differences between children with kwashiorkor and those with marasmus. Am J Clin Nutr. 2006;83:1283–8.
58. Williams CD, Oxon BM, Lond H. Kwashiorkor: a nutritional disease of children associated with a maize diet. Bull World Health Organ. 1935;81:912–3.
59. Stanton J. Listening to the Ga: Cicely Williams' discovery of kwashiorkor on the Gold Coast. Clio Med. 2001;61:149–71.
60. McLaren DS. Skin in protein energy malnutrition. Arch Dermatol. 1987;123:1674–1676a.
61. Sims RT. Hair growth in kwashiorkor. Arch Dis Child. 1967;42:397–400.
62. Wyness LA, McNeill G, Prescott GJ. Trichotillometry: the reliability and practicality of hair pluckability as a method of nutritional assessment. Nutr J. 2007;6:9.
63. Johnson AA, Latham MC, Roe DA. An evaluation of the use of changes in hair root morphology in the assessment of protein-calorie malnutrition. Am J Clin Nutr. 1976;29:502–11.
64. Bradfield RB. Hair tissue as a medium for the differential diagnosis of protein-calorie malnutrition: a commentary. J Pediatr. 1974;84:294–6.
65. Williams CD. Fifty years ago. Archives of diseases in childhood 1933. A nutritional disease of childhood associated with a maize diet. Arch Dis Child. 1983;58:550–60.

66. No authors listed. Kwashiorkor. A nutritional disease of children associated with a maize diet by Cicely D. Williams from the Lancet, Nov. 16, 1935, p. 1151. Nutr Rev 1973;31:350–1.
67. Konotey-Ahulu, Felix. There is nothing mysterious about kwashiorkor. Br Med J 2005. Accessed 28 July 2012
68. Müller O, Krawinkel M. Malnutrition and health in developing countries. Can Med Assoc J. 2005;173:279–86.
69. Bradfield RB. Hair tissue in the diagnosis of marasmus and kwashiorkor. J Am Med Womens Assoc. 1973;28:393–4.
70. Steinbart JW. Intermediary forms of malnutrition between kwashiorkor and marasmus [article in German]. Monatsschr Kinderheilkd. 1975;123:285–7.
71. Bergstrom S, Danielson H, Klenberg D, Samuelsson B. The enzymatic conversion of essential fatty acids into prostaglandins. J Biol Chem. 1964;239:PC4006–8.
72. Lands WE. Biochemistry and physiology of n-3 fatty acids. FASEB J. 1992;6:2530–6.
73. Kuda O. Bioactive metabolites of docosahexaenoic acid (Review). Biochimie. 2017;136:12–20.
74. Truchetet E, Brändle I, Grosshans E. Skin changes, pathophysiology and therapy in deficiency of essential fatty acids. Z Hautkr. 1988;63:290–301.
75. Schroeter AL, Tucker SB. Essential fatty acid deficiency. Arch Dermatol. 1978;114:800–1.
76. Burns-Whitmore B, Froyen E, Heskey C, Parker T, San PG. Alpha-linolenic and linoleic fatty acids in the vegan diet: do they require dietary reference intake/adequate intake special consideration? Nutrients. 2019;11:2365.
77. Le Floc'h C, Cheniti A, Connétable C, Piccardi N, Vincenzi C, Tosti A. Effect of a nutritional supplement on hair loss in women. J Cosmet Dermatol. 2015;14:76–82.
78. Floersheim GL. Treatment of brittle fingernails with biotin. Z Hautkr. 1989;64:41–8.
79. Colombo VE, Gerber F, Bronhofer M, Floersheim GL. Treatment of brittle fingernails and onychoschizia with biotin: scanning electron microscopy. J Am Acad Dermatol. 1990;23:1127–32.
80. Hochman LG, Scher RK, Meyerson MS. Brittle nails: response to daily biotin supplementation. Cutis. 1993;51:303–5.
81. Iorizzo M, Pazzaglia M, Piraccini B, Tullo S, Tosti A. Brittle nails. J Cosmet Dermatol. 2004;3:138–4.
82. Floersheim GL. Prüfung der Wirkung von Biotin auf Haarausfall und Haarqualität. Z Hautkr. 1991;67:246–55.
83. Patel DP, Swink SM, Castelo-Soccio L. A review of the use of biotin for hair loss. Skin Appendage Disord. 2017;3:166–9.
84. Piraccini BM, Berardesca E, Fabbrocini G, Micali G, Tosti A. Biotin: overview of the treatment of diseases of cutaneous appendages and of hyperseborrhea. G Ital Dermatol Venereol. 2019;154:557–66.
85. Shelley WB, Shelley ED. Uncombable hair syndrome: observations on response to biotin and occurrence in siblings with ectodermal dysplasia. J Am Acad Dermatol. 1985;13:97–102.
86. Limat A, Suormala T, Hunziker T, Waelti ER, Braathen LR, Baumgartner R. Proliferation and differentiation of cultured human follicular keratinocytes are not influenced by biotin. Arch Dermatol Res. 1996;288:31–8.
87. Prendiville JS, Manfredi LN. Skin signs of nutritional disorders. Semin Dermatol. 1992;11:88–97.
88. György P, Rose CS, Eakin RE, Snell EE, Williams RJ. Egg-white injury as the result of non-absorption or inactivation of biotin. Science. 1941;93:477–8.
89. Subramanya SB, Subramanian VS, Kumar JS, Hoiness R, Said HM. Inhibition of intestinal biotin absorption by chronic alcohol feeding: cellular and molecular mechanisms. Am J Physiol Gastrointest Liver Physiol. 2011;300:G494–501.
90. Sealey WM, Teague AM, Stratton SL, Mock DM. Smoking accelerates biotin catabolism in women. Am J Clin Nutr. 2004;80:932–5.

91. Mock DM, Baswell DL, Baker H, Holman RT, Sweetman L. Biotin deficiency complicating parenteral alimentation: diagnosis, metabolic repercussions, and treatment. J Pediatr. 1985;106:762–9.
92. Greenway FL, Ingram DK, Ravussin E, Hausmann M, Smith SR, Cox L, Tomayko K, Treadwell BV. Loss of taste responds to high-dose biotin treatment. J Am Coll Nutr. 2011;30:178–81.
93. Mock DM, Dyken ME. Biotin catabolism is accelerated in adults receiving long-term therapy with anticonvulsants. Neurology. 1997;49:1444–7.
94. Schulpis KH, Karikas GA, Tjamouranis J, Regoutas S, Tsakiris S. Low serum biotinidase activity in children with valproic acid monotherapy. Epilepsia. 2001;42:1359–62.
95. Schulpis KH, Georgala S, Papakonstantinou ED, Michas T, Karikas GA. The effect of isotretinoin on biotinidase activity. Skin Pharmacol Appl Skin Physiol. 1999;12:28–33.
96. Mock DM, Quirk JG, Mock NI. Marginal biotin deficiency during normal pregnancy. Am J Clin Nutr. 2002;75:295–9.
97. Mock DM. Skin manifestations of biotin deficiency. Semin Dermatol. 1991;10:296–302.
98. Coulter DL, Beals TF, Allen RJ. Neurotrichosis: hair-shaft abnormalities associated with neurological diseases. Dev Med Child Neurol. 1982;24:634–44.
99. Seymons K, De Moor A, De Raeve H, Lambert J. Dermatologic signs of biotin deficiency leading to the diagnosis of multiple carboxylase deficiency. Pediatr Dermatol. 2004;21:231–5.
100. Trüeb RM. Serum biotin levels in women complaining of hair loss. Int J Trichology. 2016;8:73–7.
101. Said HM. Biotin: biochemical, physiological and clinical aspects. Subcell Biochem. 2012;56:1–19.
102. Clevidence BA, Marshall MW, Canary JJ. Biotin levels in plasma and urine of heathy adults consuming physiological doses of biotin. Nutr Res. 1988;8:1109–18.
103. Bitsch RSI, Hötzel D. Studies on bioavailability of oral biotin doses for humans. Int J Vit Nutr Res. 1989;59:65–71.
104. Zempleni JM, Mock DM. Bioavailability of biotin given orally to humans in pharmacologic doses. Am J Clin Nutr. 1999;69:504–8.
105. Stone I. On the genetic etiology of scurvy. Acta Genet Med Gemellol (Roma). 1966;15:345–50.
106. Lind J. A treatise on the scurvy. 3rd ed. G. Pearch and W. Woodfall: London, England; 1772.
107. Ashhurst J, editor. The international encyclopedia of surgery, vol. 1. New York, NY: William Wood and Co.; 1881. p. 278.
108. Toler PD. Mankind: the story of all of us. Philadelphia: Running Press; 2012. p. 296. ISBN: 978-0762447176
109. Milne I. Who was James Lind, and what exactly did he achieve. J R Soc Med. 2012;105:503–8.
110. Renzaho AMN. Globalisation, migration and health: challenges and opportunities: World Scientific; 2016. p. 94. ISBN: 978-1-78326-889-4
111. Hürlimann R, Salomon F. Scurvy—a mistakenly forgotten disease [article in German]. Schweiz Med Wochenschr. 1994;124:1373–80.
112. Agarwal A, Shaharya A, Kumar A, Bhat MS, Mishra M. Scurvy in pediatric age group—a disease often forgotten? J Clin Orthop Trauma. 2015;6:101–7.
113. Fuchs J. Vitamins and skin [article in German]. Ther Umsch. 1994;51:489–95.
114. Lessing JN, LaMotte ED, Moshiri AS, Mark NM. Perifollicular haemorrhage with corkscrew hair due to scurvy. Postgrad Med J. 2015;91:719–20.
115. Hunt A, Harrington D, Robinson S. Vitamin B12 deficiency. BMJ. 2014;349:g5226.
116. Pawlak R, Parrott SJ, Raj S, Cullum-Dugan D, Lucus D. How prevalent is vitamin B(12) deficiency among vegetarians? Nutr Rev. 2013;71:110–7.
117. Miller JW. Proton pump inhibitors, H2-receptor antagonists, metformin, and vitamin B-12 deficiency: clinical implications. Adv Nutr (Bethesda, MD). 2018;9:511S–8S.
118. Wang H, Li LL, Qin LL, Song Y, Vidal-Alaball V, Liu TH. Oral vitamin B12 versus intramuscular vitamin B12 for vitamin B12 deficiency. Cochrane Database Syst Rev. 2018;3:CD004655.
119. Hunt A, Harrington D, Robinson S. Vitamin B12 deficiency. BMJ. 2014;349:g5226.

120. Herrmann W, Obeid R. Causes and early diagnosis of vitamin B12 deficiency. Deutsches Arzteblatt international. 2008;105:680–5.
121. Jarquin Campos A, Risch L, Nydegger U, Wiesner J, Vazquez Van Dyck M, Renz H, Stanga Z, Risch M. Diagnostic accuracy of holotranscobalamin, vitamin B12, methylmalonic acid, and homocysteine in detecting B12 deficiency in a large, mixed patient population. Dis Markers. 2020;2020:7468506.
122. Dietary Supplement Fact Sheet: Vitamin B12—Health Professional Fact Sheet. National Institutes of Health: Office of Dietary Supplements. 2016-02-11. Archived from the original on 2016-07-27. Accessed 15 July 2016.
123. Sonthalia S, Priya A, Tobin DJ. Demographic characteristics and association of serum vitamin B12, ferritin and thyroid function with premature canities in indian patients from an urban skin clinic of North India: a retrospective analysis of 71 cases. Indian J Dermatol. 2017;62:304–8.
124. Capo A, Amerio P. Polyglandular autoimmune syndrome type III with a prevalence of cutaneous features. Clin Exp Dermatol. 2017;42:61–3.
125. Kumar B, Sharma VK, Sehgal S. Antismooth muscle and antiparietal cell antibodies in Indians with alopecia areata. Int J Dermatol. 1995;34:542–5.
126. Daly T, Daly K. Telogen effluvium with dysesthesia (TED) has lower B12 levels and may respond to B12 supplementation. J Drugs Dermatol. 2018;17:1236–40.
127. Devalia V, Hamilton MS, Molloy AM. Guidelines for the diagnosis and treatment of cobalamin and folate disorders. Br J Haematol. 2014;166:496–513.
128. Holm RP. The corn-skin connection. S D Med. 2009;62:449.
129. Portale S, Sculati M, Stanford FC, Cena H. Pellagra and anorexia nervosa: a case report. Eat Weight Disord. 2019; https://doi.org/10.1007/s40519-019-00781-x. [Epub ahead of print]
130. Zaki I, Millard L. Pellagra complicating Crohn's disease. Postgrad Med J. 1995;71:496–7.
131. Bilgili SG, Karadag AS, Calka O, Altun F. Isoniazid-induced pellagra. Cutan Ocul Toxicol. 2011;30:317–9.
132. Bell HK, Poston GJ, Vora J, Wilson NJ. Cutaneous manifestations of the malignant carcinoid syndrome. Br J Dermatol. 2005;152:71–5.
133. Creamer D. Malnutrition and skin disease in Far East prisoners-of-war in World War II. Clin Exp Dermatol. 2018;43:766–9.
134. Chaidemenos GC, Mourellou O, Karakatsanis G, Koussidou T, Xenidis E, Charalampidou H, Avgoloupis D. Acute hemorrhagic pellagra in an Albanian refugee. Cutis. 2002;69:96–8.
135. Licata M, Iorio S. What disease did Goethe witness during his journey through the Italian Alps? Was it pellagra or another disease of malnutrition? Nutr Diet. 2018;75:541.
136. Williams AC, Hill LJ. The 4 D's of pellagra and progress. Int J Tryptophan Res. 2020;13:1178646920910159.
137. Hegyi J, Schwartz RA, Hegyi V. Pellagra: dermatitis, dementia, and diarrhea. Int J Dermatol. 2004;43:1–5.
138. Spivak JL, Jackson DL. Pellagra: an analysis of 18 patients and a review of the literature. Johns Hopkins Med J. 1977;140:295–309.
139. World Health Organization (2009). In: Stuart MC, Kouimtzi M, Hill SR (editors). WHO Model Formulary 2008. World Health Organization, pp. 496, 500
140. Centers for Disease Control (CDC). Iron deficiency–United States, 1999–2000. Morb Mortal Wkly Rep. 2002;51:897–9.
141. Hard S. Non-anemic iron deficiency as an etiologic factor in diffuse loss of hair of the scalp in women. Acta Derm Venereol. 1963;43:562–9.
142. Aguilera MC. Diffuse alopecia in women and hyposideremia [article in Spanish]. Actas Dermosifiliogr. 1966;57:169–80.
143. Rushton DH, Ramsay ID, James KC, Norris MJ, Gilkes JJ. Biochemical and trichological characterization of diffuse alopecia in women. Br J Dermatol. 1990;123:187–97.
144. Aydingoz I, Ferhanoglu B, Guney O. Does tissue iron status have a role in female alopecia? J Eur Acad Dermatol Venereol. 1999;13:65–7.

145. Sinclair R. There is no clear association between low serum ferritin and chronic diffuse telogen hair loss. Br J Dermatol. 2002;147:982–4.
146. Kantor J, Kessler LJ, Brooks DG, Cotsarelis G. Decreased serum ferritin is associated with alopecia in women. J Invest Dermatol. 2003;121:985–8.
147. Chamberlain AJ, Dawber RP. Significance of iron status in hair loss in women. Br J Dermatol. 2003;149:428.
148. Rushton DH. Decreased serum ferritin and alopecia in women. J Invest Dermatol. 2003;121:xvii–xviii.
149. Trost LB, Bergfeld WF, Calogeras E. The diagnosis and treatment of iron deficiency and its potential relationship to hair loss. J Am Acad Dermatol. 2006;54:824–44.
150. Deloche C, Bastien P, Chadoutaud S, Galan P, Bertrais S, Hercberg S, de Lacharrière O. Low iron stores: a risk factor for excessive hair loss in non-menopausal women. Eur J Dermatol. 2007;17:507–12.
151. Moeinvaziri M, Mansoori P, Holakooee K, Safaee Naraghi Z, Abbasi A. Iron status in diffuse telogen hair loss among women. Acta Dermatovenerol Croat. 2009;17:279–84.
152. Olsen EA, Reed KB, Cacchio PB, Caudill L. Iron deficiency in female pattern hair loss, chronic telogen effluvium, and control groups. J Am Acad Dermatol. 2010;63:991–9.
153. St Pierre SA, Vercellotti GM, Donovan JC, Hordinsky MK. Iron deficiency and diffuse nonscarring scalp alopecia in women: more pieces to the puzzle. J Am Acad Dermatol. 2010;63:1070–6.
154. Wang W, Knovich MA, Coffman LG, Torti FM, Torti SV. Serum ferritin: past, present and future. Biochim Biophys Acta. 2010;1800:760–9.
155. Firkin F, Rush B. Interpretation of biochemical tests for iron deficiency: diagnostic difficulties related to limitations of individual tests. Aust Prescr. 1997;20:74–6.
156. Waalen J, Felitti V, Beutler E. Haemoglobin and ferritin concentrations in men and women: cross sectional study. BMJ. 2002;325:137.
157. Schrier SL. Causes and diagnosis of anaemia due to iron deficiency. www.UpToDate.com, last updated 6 Nov 2003.
158. Centers for Disease Control (CDC). Recommendations to prevent and control iron deficiency in the Unites States. Morb Mortal Wkly Rep. 1998;47:1–36.
159. Bregy A, Trüeb RM. No association between serum ferritin levels >10 microg/l and hair loss activity in women. Dermatology. 2008;217:1–6.
160. Groopman J. How doctors think. Boston, NY: Houghton Mifflin Company; 2007.
161. DeLoughery TG. Safety of oral and intravenous iron. Acta Haematol. 2019;142:8–12.
162. Rampton D, Folkersen J, Fishbane S, Hedenus M, Howaldt S, Locatelli F, Patni S, Szebeni J, Weiss G. Hypersensitivity reactions to intravenous iron: guidance for risk minimization and management. Haematologica. 2014;99:1671–6.
163. Wong M, Bryson M. Extensive skin hyperpigmentation following intravenous iron infusion. Br J Haematol. 2019;184:709.
164. Moltz L. Hormonal diagnosis in so-called androgenetic alopecia in the female [Article in German]. Geburtshilfe Frauenheilkd. 1988;48:203–14.
165. Maret W, Sandstead HH. Zinc requirements and the risks and benefits of zinc supplementation. J Trace Elem Med Biol. 2006;20:3–18.
166. Prasad AS. Discovery of human zinc deficiency: 50 years later. J Trace Elem Med Biol. 2012;26:66–9.
167. Solomons NW. Dietary sources of zinc and factors affecting its bioavailability. Food Nutr Bull. 2001;22:138–54.
168. Prasad AS, Miale A, Farid Z, Sandstead HH, Schulert AR. Zinc metabolism in patients with the syndrome of iron deficiency anemia, hepatosplenomegaly, dwarfism, and hypogonadism. J Lab Clin Med. 1963;61:537–49.
169. American Dietetic Association. Position of the American Dietetic Association and Dietitians of Canada: vegetarian diets. J Am Diet Assoc. 2003;103:748–65.
170. Freeland-Graves JH, Bodzy PW, Epright MA. Zinc status of vegetarians. J Am Diet Assoc. 1980;77:655–61.

171. Smit AJ, Hoorntje SJ, Donker AJ. Zinc deficiency during captopril treatment. Nephron. 1983;34:196–7.
172. Ikeda M, Ikui A, Komiyama A, Kobayashi D, Tanaka M. Causative factors of taste disorders in the elderly, and therapeutic effects of zinc. J Laryngol Otol. 2008;122:155–60.
173. Stewart-Knox BJ, Simpson EE, Parr H, Rae G, Polito A, Intorre F, Andriollo Sanchez M, Meunier N, O'Connor JM, Maiani G, Coudray C, Strain JJ. Taste acuity in response to zinc supplementation in older Europeans. Br J Nutr. 2008;99:129–36.
174. Suzuki H, Asakawa A, Li JB, Tsai M, Amitani H, Ohinata K, Komai M, Inui A. Zinc as an appetite stimulator - the possible role of zinc in the progression of diseases such as cachexia and sarcopenia. Recent Pat Food Nutr Agric. 2011;3:226–31.
175. Bakan R. The role of zinc in anorexia nervosa: etiology and treatment. Med Hypotheses. 1979;5:731–6.
176. Birmingham CL, Goldner EM, Bakan R. Controlled trial of zinc supplementation in anorexia nervosa. Int J Eat Disord. 1994;15:251–5.
177. Alhaj E, Alhaj N, Alhaj NE. Diffuse alopecia in a child due to dietary zinc deficiency. Skinmed. 2007;6:199–200.
178. Prasad AS. Discovery of human zinc deficiency: its impact on human health and disease. Adv Nutr. 2013;4:176–90.
179. Hess SY, Peerson JM, King JC, Brown KH. Use of serum zinc concentration as an indicator of population zinc status. Food Nutr Bull. 2007;28(3 Suppl):S403–29.
180. Arnaud J, Beani JC, Favier AE, Amblard P. Zinc status in patients with telogen defluvium. Acta Derm Venereol. 1995;75:248–9.
181. Karashima T, Tsuruta D, Hamada T, Ono F, Ishii N, Abe T, Ohyama B, Nakama T, Dainichi T, Hashimoto T. Oral zinc therapy for zinc deficiency-related telogen effluvium. Dermatol Ther. 2012;25:210–3.
182. Weismann K, Hagdrup HK. Hair changes due to zinc deficiency in a case of sucrose malabsorption. Acta Derm Venereol. 1981;61:444–7.
183. Dupré A, Bonafé JL, Carriere JP. The hair in acrodermatitis enteropathica—a disease indicator? Acta Derm Venereol. 1979;59:177–8.
184. Traupe H, Happle R, Gröbe H, Bertram HP. Polarization microscopy of hair in acrodermatitis enteropathica. Pediatr Dermatol. 1986;3:300–3.
185. Slonim AE, Sadick N, Pugliese M, Meyers-Seifer CH. Clinical response of alopecia, trichorrhexis nodosa, and dry, scaly skin to zinc supplementation. J Pediatr. 1992;121:890–5.
186. Wolowa F, Jablonska S. Zinc in the treatment of alopecia areata. In: Kobori T, Montagna W, Toda K, editors. Biology and disease of the hair. 2nd ed. Tokyo: University of Tokyo Press; 1976. p. 305–8.
187. Camacho FM, Garcia-Hernandez MJ. Zinc aspartate, biotin, and clobetasol propionate in the treatment of alopecia areata in childhood. Pediatr Dermatol. 1999;16:336–8.
188. Ead RD. Oral zinc sulphate in alopecia areata-a double blind trial. Br J Dermatol. 1981;104:483–4.
189. Lee SY, Nam KS, Seo YW, Lee JS, Chung H. Analysis of serum zinc and copper levels in alopecia areata. Ann Dermatol. 1997;9:239–41.
190. Malanin K, Telegdy E, Qazaq H. Hair loss and serum zinc values among Arab females in Al Ain region, United Arab Emirates. Eur J Dermatol. 2007;17:446–7.
191. Mussalo-Rauhamaa H, Lakomaa EL, Kianto U, Lehto J. Element concentrations in serum, erythrocytes, hair and urine of alopecia patients. Acta Derm Venereol. 1986;66:103–9.
192. Park H, Kim CW, Kim SS, Park CW. The therapeutic effect and the changed serum zinc level after zinc supplementation in alopecia areata patients who had a low serum zinc level. Ann Dermatol. 2009;21:142–6.
193. Baltaci AK, Mogulkoc R, Baltaci SB. Review: the role of zinc in the endocrine system. Pak J Pharm Sci. 2019;32:231–9.
194. Jaiser SR, Winston GP. Copper deficiency myelopathy. [Review]. J Neurol. 2010;257:869–81.
195. Handeland K, Bernhoft A, Aartun MS. A copper deficiency and effects of copper supplementation in a herd of Red Deer (Cervus Elaphus). Acta Vet Scand. 2008;50:8.

196. Jaiser SR, Winston GP. Copper deficiency myelopathy [Review]. J Neurol. 2010;257:869–81.
197. Kumar N. Copper deficiency myelopathy (human swayback). Mayo Clin Proc. 2006;81:1371–84.
198. Hedera P, Peltier A, Fink JK, Wilcock S, London Z, Brewer GJ. Myelopolyneuropathy and pancytopenia due to copper deficiency and high zinc levels of unknown origin II. The denture cream is a primary source of excessive zinc. Neurotoxicology (Amsterdam). 2009;30:996–9.
199. Schleper B, Stuerenburg HJ. Copper deficiency-associated myelopathy in a 46-year-old woman. J Neurol. 2001;248:705–6.
200. Goodman JC. Neurological complications of bariatric surgery. Curr Neurol Neurosci Rep. 2015;15:79.
201. Maksimović J, Djujić I, Jović V, Rsumović M. A selenium deficiency in Yugoslavia. Biol Trace Elem Res. 1992;33:187–96.
202. Ngigi PB, Du Laing G, Masinde PW, Lachat C. Selenium deficiency risk in central Kenya highlands: an assessment from the soil to the body. Environ Geochem Health. 2019; https://doi.org/10.1007/s10653-019-00494-1. Online ahead of print.
203. Var P, Alfihan G, Ekholm P, Aro A, Koivistoinen P. Selenium intake and serum selenium in Finland: effects of soil fertilization with selenium. Am J Clin Nutr. 1988;48:324–9.
204. Beck MA, Levander OA, Handy J. Selenium deficiency and viral infection. J Nutr. 2003;133:1463S–7S.
205. Moreno-Reyes R, Carl S, Mathieu F, Begaux F, Zhu D, Rivera MT, Boelaer M, Nève J, et al. Kashin–Beck osteoarthropathy in rural tibet in relation to selenium and iodine status. N Engl J Med. 1998;339:1112–20.
206. Yao PF, Kang P. Selenium, iodine, and the relation with Kashin–Beck disease. Nutrition. 2011;27:1095–100.
207. Ravaglia G, Forti P, Maioli F, Bastagli L, Facchini A, Mariani E, Savarino L, Sassi S, et al. Effect of micronutrient status on natural killer cell immune function in healthy free-living subjects aged ≥90 y. Am J Clin Nutr. 2000;71:590–8.
208. Kanekura T, Yotsumoto S, Maeno N, Kamenosono A, Saruwatari H, Uchino Y, Mera Y, Kanzaki T. Selenium deficiency: report of a case. Clin Exp Dermatol. 2005;30:346–8.
209. Pittas AG, Chung M, Trikalinos T, Mitri J, Brendel M, Patel K, Lichtenstein AH, Lau J, Balk EM. Systematic review: vitamin D and cardiometabolic outcomes. Ann Intern Med. 2010;152:307–14.
210. Chung M, Balk EM, Brendel M, Ip S, Lau J, Lee J, Lichtenstein A, Patel K, Raman G, Tatsioni A, Terasawa T, Trikalinos TA. Vitamin D and calcium: a systematic review of health outcomes. Evid Rep Technol Assess. 2009;183:1–420.
211. Bjelakovic G, Gluud LL, Nikolova D, Whitfield K, Wetterslev J, Simonetti RG, Bjelakovic M, Gluud C. Vitamin D supplementation for prevention of mortality in adults. Cochrane Database Syst Rev. 2014;1:CD007470.
212. Bolland MJ, Grey A, Gamble GD, Reid IR. The effect of vitamin D supplementation on skeletal, vascular, or cancer outcomes: a trial sequential meta-analysis. Lancet Diabet& Endocrinol. 2014;2:307–20.
213. Tamura M, Ishizawa M, Isojima T, Özen S, Oka A, Makishima M, Kitanaka S. Functional analyses of a novel missense and other mutations of the vitamin D receptor in association with alopecia. Sci Rep. 2017;7:5102.
214. Xie Z, Komuves L, Yu Q-C, Elalieh H, Ng DC, Leary C, et al. Lack of the vitamin D receptor is associated with reduced epidermal differentiation and hair follicle growth. J Invest Dermatol. 2002;118:11–6.
215. Amor KT, Rashid RM, Mirmirani P. Does D matter? The role of vitamin D in hair disorders and hair follicle cycling. Dermatol Online J. 2010;16:3.
216. Fawzi MM, Mahmoud SB, Ahmed SF, Shaker OG. Assessment of vitamin D receptors in alopecia areata and androgenetic alopecia. J Cosmet Dermatol. 2016;15:318–23.
217. Yilmaz N, Serarslan G, Gokce C. Vitamin D concentration are decreased in patients with alopecia areata. Vitam Trace Elem. 2019;1:105–9.

218. d'Ovidio R, Vessio M, d'Ovidio FD. Reduced level of 25-hydroxyvitamin D in chronic/relapsing alopecia areata. Dermatoendocrinol. 2013;5:271–3.
219. Aksu Cerman A, Sarikaya Solak S, Kivanc Altunay I. Vitamin D deficiency in alopecia areata. Br J Dermatol. 2014;170:1299–304.
220. Mahamid M, Abu-Elhija O, Samamra M, Mahamid A, Nseir W. Association between vitamin D levels and alopecia areata. Isr Med Assoc J. 2014;16:367–70.
221. Bakry OA, El Farargy SM, El Shafiee MK, Soliman A. Serum Vitamin D in patients with alopecia areata. Indian Dermatol Online J. 2016;7:371–7.
222. Ghafoor R, Anwar MI. Vitamin D deficiency in alopecia areata. J Coll Physicians Surg Pak. 2017;27:200–2.
223. Erpolat S, Sarifakioglu E, Ayyildiz A. 25-Hydroxyvitamin D status in patients with alopecia areata. Postepy Dermatol Alergol. 2017;34:248–52.
224. Unal M, Gonulalan G. Serum vitamin D level is related to disease severity in pediatric alopecia areata. J Cosmet Dermatol. 2018;17:101–4.
225. Thompson JM, Li T, Park MK, Qureshi AA, Cho E. Estimated serum vitamin D status, vitamin D intake, and risk of incident alopecia areata among US women. Arch Dermatol Res. 2016;308:671–6.
226. Rasheed H, Mahgoub D, Hegazy R, El-Komy M, Abdel Hay R, Hamid MA, et al. Serum ferritin and vitamin D in female hair loss: do they play a role? Skin Pharmacol Physiol. 2013;26:101–7.
227. Banihashemi M, Nahidi Y, Meibodi NT, Jarahi L, Dolatkhah M. Serum vitamin D3 level in patients with female pattern hair loss. Int J Trichology. 2016;8:116–20.
228. Cheung E, Sink J, English Lii J. Vitamin and mineral deficiencies in patients with telogen effluvium: a retrospective cross-sectional study. J Drugs Dermatol. 2016;15(10):1235–7.
229. Nayak K, Garg A, Mithra P, Manjrekar P. Serum vitamin D3 levels and diffuse hair fall among the student population in south India: a case-control study. Int J Trichology. 2016;8:160–4.
230. Speicher P. Serum vitamin D levels in women with hair loss. Inaugural Dissertation, University of Zurich, in preparation.
231. O'Brien KF, Maiman RE, DeWitt CA. Multiple nutritional deficiencies in a morbidly obese patient. Am J Gastroenterol. 2019;114:11.
232. Argilés JM. Cancer-associated malnutrition. Eur J Oncol Nurs. 2005;9(Suppl 2):S39–50.
233. Leandro-Merhi VA, Costa CL, Saragiotto L, Aquino JLB. Nutritional indicators of malnutrition in hospitalized patients. Arq Gastroenterol. 2019;56:447–50.
234. Khor GL. Update on the prevalence of malnutrition among children in Asia. Nepal Med Coll J. 2003;5:113–22.
235. Aparicio E, Canals J, Pérez S, Arija V. Dietary intake and nutritional risk in Mediterranean adolescents in relation to the severity of the eating disorder. Public Health Nutr. 2015;18:1461–73.
236. Li S, Ney M, Eslamparast T, Vandermeer B, Ismond KP, Kroeker K, Halloran B, Raman M, Tandon P. Systematic review of nutrition screening and assessment in inflammatory bowel disease. World J Gastroenterol. 2019;25:3823–37.
237. Mziray-Andrew CH, Sentongo TA. Nutritional deficiencies in intestinal failure. Pediatr Clin North Am. 2009;56:1185–200.
238. Cano NJ, Heng AE, Pison C. Multimodal approach to malnutrition in malnourished maintenance hemodialysis patients. J Ren Nutr. 2011;21:23–6.
239. Shaker M, Venter C. The ins and outs of managing avoidance diets for food allergies. Curr Opin Pediatr. 2016;28:567–72.
240. Redondo Robles L, Pintor de la Maza B, Tejada García J, García Vieitez JJ, Fernández Gómez MJ, Barrera Mellado I, Ballesteros Pomar MD. Nutritional profile of multiple sclerosis. Nutr Hosp. 2019;36:340–9.
241. Imdad A, Bhutta ZA. Intervention strategies to address multiple micronutrient deficiencies in pregnancy and early childhood. Nestle Nutr Inst Workshop Ser. 2012;70:61–73.
242. Beck AM. Nutritional interventions among old people receiving support at home. Proc Nutr Soc. 2018;77:265–9.

243. Park M, Song JA, Lee M, Jeong H, Lim S, Lee H, Kim CG, Kim JS, Kim KS, Lee YW, Lim YM, Park YS, Yoon JC, Kim KW, Hong GS. National study of the nutritional status of Korean older adults with dementia who are living in long-term care settings. Jpn J Nurs Sci. 2018;15:318–29.

244. Pingleton SK. Nutrition in chronic critical illness. Clin Chest Med. 2001;22:149–63.

245. Darmon N. A fortified street food to prevent nutritional deficiencies in homeless men in France. J Am Coll Nutr. 2009;28:196–202.

246. Dickson JM, Naylor G, Colver G, Powers HJ, Masters P. Multiple vitamin deficiencies in a patient with a history of chronic alcohol excess and self-neglect in the UK. BMJ Case Rep. 2014;2014:bcr2014204523.

247. Kuroda T, Uenishi K, Ohta H, Shiraki M. Multiple vitamin deficiencies additively increase the risk of incident fractures in Japanese postmenopausal women. Osteoporos Int. 2019;30:593–9.

248. Söderström L, Rosenblad A, Thors Adolfsson E, Bergkvist L. Malnutrition is associated with increased mortality in older adults regardless of the cause of death. Br J Nutr. 2017;117:532–40.

249. Heath ML, Sidbury R. Cutaneous manifestations of nutritional deficiency. Curr Opin Pediatr. 2006;18:417–22.

250. Goskowicz M, Eichenfield LF. Cutaneous findings of nutritional deficiencies in children. Curr Opin Pediatr. 1993;5:441–5.

251. Huber MA, Hall EH. Glossodynia in patients with nutritional deficiencies. Ear Nose Throat J. 1989;68:771–5.

252. Sapone A, Bai JC, Ciacci C, Dolinsek J, Green PH, Hadjivassiliou M, Kaukinen K, Rostami K, Sanders DS, Schumann M, Ullrich R, Villalta D, Volta U, Catassi C, Fasano A. Spectrum of gluten-related disorders: consensus on new nomenclature and classification. BMC Med. 2012;10:13.

253. Lebwohl B, Ludvigsson JF, Green PH. Celiac disease and non-celiac gluten sensitivity. BMJ. 2015;351:h4347.

254. Fasano A. Clinical presentation of celiac disease in the pediatric population. Gastroenterology. 2005;128(4 Suppl 1):S68–73.

255. Lionetti E, Gatti S, Pulvirenti A, Catassi C. Celiac disease from a global perspective. Best Pract Res Clin Gastroenterol. 2015;29:365–79.

256. Ludvigsson JF, Card T, Ciclitira PJ, Swift GL, Nasr I, Sanders DS, Ciacci C. Support for patients with celiac disease: a literature review. United Eur Gastroenterol J. 2015;3:146–59.

257. Lundin KE, Wijmenga C. Coeliac disease and autoimmune disease-genetic overlap and screening. Nat Rev Gastroenterol Hepatol. 2015;12:507–15.

258. Corazza GR, Andreani ML, Venturo N, et al. Celiac disease and alopecia areata: report of a new association. Gastroenterology. 1995;109(4):1333–7.

259. Naveh Y, Rosenthal E, Ben-Arieh Y, Etzioni A. Celiac disease-associated alopecia in childhood. J Pediatr. 1999;134:362–4.

260. Ertekin V, Tosun MS, Erdem T. Screening of celiac disease in children with alopecia areata. Indian J Dermatol. 2014;59(3):317.

261. Catassi C, Bai JC, Bonaz B, Bouma G, Calabrò A, Carroccio A, Castillejo G, Ciacci C, Cristofori F, Dolinsek J, Francavilla R, Elli L, Green P, Holtmeier W, Koehler P, Koletzko S, Meinhold C, Sanders D, Schumann M, Schuppan D, Ullrich R, Vécsei A, Volta U, Zevallos V, Sapone A, Fasano A. Non-celiac gluten sensitivity: the new frontier of gluten related disorders. Nutrients. 2013;5:3839–53.

262. Mansueto P, Seidita A, D'Alcamo A, Carroccio A. Non-celiac gluten sensitivity: literature review. J Am Coll Nutr. 2014;33:39–54.

263. Verdu EF, Armstrong D, Murray JA. Between celiac disease and irritable bowel syndrome: the "no man's land" of gluten sensitivity. Am J Gastroenterol. 2009;104:1587–94.

264. van der Windt DA, Jellema P, Mulder CJ, Kneepkens CM, van der Horst HE. Diagnostic testing for celiac disease among patients with abdominal symptoms: a systematic review. JAMA. 2010;303:1738–46.

265. Lewis NR, Scott BB. Systematic review: the use of serology to exclude or diagnose coeliac disease (a comparison of the endomysial and tissue transglutaminase antibody tests). Aliment Pharmacol Ther. 2006;24:47–54.
266. Rostom A, Murray JA, Kagnoff MF. American Gastroenterological Association (AGA) Institute technical review on the diagnosis and management of celiac disease. Gastroenterology. 2006;131:1981–2002.
267. Hill ID, Dirks MH, Liptak GS, Colletti RB, Fasano A, Guandalini S, Hoffenberg EJ, Horvath K, Murray JA, Pivor M, Seidman EG. Guideline for the diagnosis and treatment of celiac disease in children: recommendations of the North American Society for Pediatric Gastroenterology, Hepatology and Nutrition. J Pediatr Gastroenterol Nutr. 2005;40:1–19.
268. Bondavalli P, Quadri G, Parodi A, Rebora A. Failure of gluten-free diet in celiac disease-associated alopecia areata. Acta Derm Venereol. 1998;78:319.
269. Viola F, Barbato M, Formisano M, et al. Reappearance of alopecia areata in a coeliac patient during an unintentional challenge with gluten. Minerva Gastroenterol Dietol. 1999;45:283–5.
270. Bardella MT, Marino R, Barbareschi M, et al. Alopecia areata and coeliac disease: no effect of a gluten-free diet on hair growth. Dermatology. 2000;200:108–10.
271. Zampetti M, Filippetti R. Alopecia areata and celiac disease. G Ital Dermatol Venereol. 2008;143(2):168.
272. Sun X, Lu L, Yang R, Li Y, Shan L, Wang Y. Increased incidence of thyroid disease in patients with celiac disease: a systematic review and meta-analysis. PLoS One. 2016;11:e0168708.
273. Kanazawa M, Yoshiike N, Osaka T, Numba Y, Zimmet P, Inoue S. Criteria and classification of obesity in Japan and Asia-Oceania. Nutrition and fitness: obesity, the metabolic syndrome, cardiovascular disease, and cancer. World Rev Nutr Diet. 2005;94:1–12.
274. Zhou BF. Predictive values of body mass index and waist circumference for risk factors of certain related diseases in Chinese adults—study on optimal cut-off points of body mass index and waist circumference in Chinese adults. Biomed Environ Sci. 2002;15:83–96.
275. Singh D. Female mate value at a glance: relationship of waist-to-hip ratio to health, fecundity and attractiveness. Neuro Endocrinol Lett. 2002;23(Suppl 4):81–91.
276. Marlowe F, Apicella C, Reed D. Men's preferences for women's profile waist-to-hip ratio in two societies. Evol Hum Behav. 2005;26:458–68.
277. Cagnacci A, Zanin R, Cannoletta M, Generali M, Caretto S, Volpe A. Menopause, estrogens, progestins, or their combination on body weight and anthropometric measure. Fertil Steril. 2007;88:1603–8.
278. Freeman EW, Sammel MD, Lin H, Gracia CR. Obesity and reproductive hormone levels in the transition to menopause. Menopause. 2007;17:718–26.
279. Cagnacci A, Zanin R, Cannoletta M, Generali M, Caretto S, Volpe A. Menopause, estrogens, progestins, or their combination on body weight and anthropometric measure. Fertil Steril. 2007;88:1603–8.
280. Ogden CL, Carroll MD, Fryar CD, Flegal KM. Prevalence of childhood and adult obesity in the Unites States, 2011-2012. JAMA. 2014;311:806–14.
281. Vogelezang S, Monnereau C, Gaillard R, Renders CM, Hofman A, Jaddoe VW, Felix JF. Adult adiposity susceptibility loci, early growth and general and abdominal fatness in childhood. The Generation R Study. Int J Obes. 2015;39:1001–9.
282. Shoelson SE, Herrero L, Naaz A. Obesity, inflammation, and insulin resistance. Gastroenterology. 2007;132:2169–80.
283. Dentali F, Squizzato A, Ageno W. The metabolic syndrome as a risk factor for venous and arterial thrombosis. Semin Thromb Hemost. 2009;35:451–7.
284. Pallardo LF, Molina RC. Case of alopecia, in prepuberal obesity syndrome, treated with ACTH. Medicamenta (Madr). 1954;2:121–6.
285. Malaisse W, Lauvaux JP, Franckson JR, Bastenie PA. Diabetes in bearded women (Achard-Thiers-Syndrome): a clinical and metabolic study of 20 cases. Diabetologia. 1966;1:155–61.
286. Lubowe I. Achard-Thiers syndrome. Arch Dermatol. 1971;103:544–5.
287. Gracia-Ramos AE. Morgagni-Stewart-Morel syndrome. Case report and review of the literature. Rev Med Inst Mex Seguro Soc. 2016;54:664–9.

288. Azziz R, Adashi EY. Stein and Leventhal: 80 years on. Am J Obstet Gynecol. 2016;214:247. e1–247.e11.
289. Rotterdam ESHRE/ASRM-Sponsored PCOS consensus workshop group. Revised 2003 consensus on diagnostic criteria and long-term health risks related to polycystic ovary syndrome (PCOS). Hum Reprod. 2004;19:41–7.
290. Ding T, Hardiman PJ, Petersen I, Wang FF, Qu F, Baio G. The prevalence of polycystic ovary syndrome in reproductive-aged women of different ethnicity: a systematic review and meta-analysis. Oncotarget. 2017;8:96,351–8.
291. Spritzer PM, Barone CR, Oliveira FB. Hirsutism in polycystic ovary syndrome: pathophysiology and management. Curr Pharm Des. 2016;22:5603–13.
292. Wong M, Zhao X, Hong Y, Yang D. Semiquantitative assessment of hirsutism in 850 PCOS patients and 2,988 controls in China. Endokrynol Pol. 2014;65(5):365–70.
293. Franik G, Bizoń A, Włoch S, Kowalczyk K, Biernacka-Bartnik A, Madej P. Hormonal and metabolic aspects of acne vulgaris in women with polycystic ovary syndrome. Eur Rev Med Pharmacol Sci. 2018;22:4411–8.
294. Vexiau P, Chaspoux C, Boudou P, et al. Effects of minoxidil 2% vs. cyproterone acetate treatment on female androgenetic alopecia: a controlled, 12-month randomized trial. Br J Dermatol. 2002;146:992–9.
295. Gilbert EW, Tay CT, Hiam DS, Teede HJ, Moran LJ. Comorbidities and complications of polycystic ovary syndrome: an overview of systematic reviews. Clin Endocrinol (Oxf). 2018;89:683–99.
296. O'Brien B, Dahiya R, Kimble R. Hyperandrogenism, insulin resistance and acanthosis nigricans (HAIR-AN syndrome): an extreme subphenotype of polycystic ovary syndrome. BMJ Case Rep. 2020;1:pii e231749.
297. Piacquadio DJ, Rad FS, Spellman MC, Hollenbach KA. Obesity and female androgenic alopecia: a cause and an effect? J Am Acad Dermatol. 1994;30:1028–30.
298. Mirmirani P, Carpenter DM. The impact of obesity on the folliculosebaceous unit. J Am Acad Dermatol. 2014;71:584–5.
299. Yang CC, Hsieh FN, Lin LY, Hsu CK, Sheu HM, Chen W. Higher body mass index is associated with greater severity of alopecia in men with male-pattern androgenetic alopecia in Taiwan: a cross-sectional study. J Am Acad Dermatol. 2014;70:297–302.
300. Hirsso P, Rajala U, Hiltunen L, Jokelainen J, Keinänen-Kiukaanniemi S, Näyhä S. Obesity and low-grade inflammation among young Finnish men with early-onset alopecia. Dermatology. 2007;214:125–9.
301. Arias-Santiago S, Gutiérrez-Salmerón MT, Castellote-Caballero L, Buendía-Eisman A, Naranjo-Sintes. Androgenetic alopecia and cardiovascular risk factors in men and women: a comparative study. J Am Acad Dermatol. 2010;63:420–9.
302. Starka L, Duskova M, Cermakova I, et al. Premature androgenic alopecia and insulin resistance. Male equivalent of polycystic ovary syndrome? Endocr Regul. 2010;39:127–31.
303. Lee CN, Chen W, Hsu CK, Weng TT, Lee JY, Yang CC. Dissecting folliculitis (dissecting cellulitis) of the scalp: a 66-patient case series and proposal of classification. J Dtsch Dermatol Ges. 2018;16:1219–26.
304. Lijesen GK, Theeuwen I, Assendelft WJ, Van Der Wal G. The effect of human chorionic gonadotropin (HCG) in the treatment of obesity by means of the Simeons therapy: a criteria-based meta-analysis. Br J Clin Pharmacol. 1995;40:237–43.
305. Goette DK, Odum RB. Letter: profuse hair loss. Arch Dermatol. 1975;111:930.
306. Griggs J, Almohanna H, Ahmed A, Tosti A. New-onset androgenic alopecia following human chorionic gonadotropic diet and testosterone pellet implantation. Int J Trichology. 2018;10:284–5.
307. Colquitt JL, et al. Surgery for weight loss in adults. Cochrane Database Syst Rev. 2014;8:CD003641.
308. Stein J, Stier C, Raab H, Weinger R. Review article: the nutritional and pharmacological consequence of obesity surgery. Aliment Pharmacol Ther. 2014;40:582–609.

309. Faintuch J, Matsuda M, Cruz ME, et al. Severe protein-calorie malnutrition after bariatric procedures. Obes Surg. 2004;14:175–81.
310. Heber D, Greenway FL, Kaplan LM, Livingston E, .Salvador J, Still C. Endocrine and nutritional management of the post-bariatric surgery patient: an Endocrine Society Clinical Practice Guideline. J Clin Endocrinol Metab 95:4823-4843 (2010)
311. Rennie MJ, Bohe J, Smith K, Wackerhage H, Greenhaff P. Branched amino acids as fuels and ababolic sgnals in human muscle. J Nutr. 2006;136:264S–8S.
312. Janssen I, Fortier A, Hudson R, Ross R. Effects of an energy-restrictive diet with or without exercise on abdominal fat, intermuscular fat, and metabolic risk factors in obese women. Diabetes Care. 2002;25:431–8.
313. Carrodeguas L, Kaidar-Person O, Szomstein S, Antozzi P, Rosenthal R. Preoperative thiamine deficiency in obese population undergoing laparoscopic bariatric surgery. Surg Obes Relat Dis. 2005;1:517–22.
314. Aasheim ET. Wernicke encephalopathy after bariatric surgery: a systematic review. Ann Surg. 2008;248:714–20.
315. WHO. Thiamine deficiency and its prevention and control in major emergencies [online]; 1999. http://whqlibdoc.who.int/hq/1999/WHO_NHD_99.13.pdf
316. Sriram K, Manzanares W, Joseph K. Thiamine in nutrition therapy. Nutr Clin Pract. 2012;27:41–50.
317. Kopelman MD, Thomson AD, Guerrini I, Marshal EJ. The Korsakoff syndrome: clinical aspects, psychology and treatment. Alcohol Alcohol. 2009;44:148–54.
318. Blume CA, Boni CC, Casagrande DS, Rizzolli J, Padoin AV, Mottin CC. Nutritional profile of patients before and after Roux-en-Y gastric bypass: 3-year follow-up. Obes Surg. 2012;22:1676–85.
319. Long AN, Atwell CL, Yoo W, Solomon SS. Vitamin B(12) deficiency associated with concomitant metformin and proton pump inhibitor use. Diabetes Care. 2012;35:e84.
320. Dalcanale L, Oliveira CP, Fainthuch J, et al. Long-term nutritional outcome after gastric bypass. Obes Surg. 2010;20:181–7.
321. Lachner C, Steinle NI, Regenild WT. The neuropsychiatry of vitamin B12 deficiency in elderly patients. J Neuropsychiatry Clin Neurosci. 2012;24:5–115.
322. Daulatabad D, Singal A, Grover C, Chhillar N. Prospective analytical controlled study evaluating serum biotin, vitamin B12, and folic acid in patients with premature canities. Int J Trichology. 2017;9:19–24.
323. Sharma N, Dogra D. Association of epidemiological and biochemical factors with premature graying of hair: a case-control study. Int J Trichology. 2018;10:211–7.
324. Said HM. Intestinal absorption of water-soluble vitamins in health and disease. Biochem J. 2011;437:357–72.
325. Mallory GN, Macgregor AM. Folate status following gastric bypass surgery (the great folate mystery). Obes Surg. 1991;1:69–72.
326. Shane B, Stokstad EL. Vitamin B12-folate interrelationships. Annu Rev Nutr. 1985;5:115–41.
327. von Drygalski A, Andris DA. Anemia after surgery: more than just iron deficiency. Nutr Clin Pract. 2009;234:217–26.
328. Hansen EP, Metzsche C, Henningsen E, Toft P. Severe scurvy after gastric bypass surgery and a poor postoperative diet. J Clin Med Res. 2012;4:135–7.
329. Simmons M. Modern-day scurvy: a case following gastric bypass. Bariatric Nurs Surg Patient Care. 2009;4:139–44.
330. Grethen E, McClintok R, Gupta CE, et al. Vitamin D and hyperparathyroidism in obesity. J Clin Endocrinol Metab. 2011;96:1320–6.
331. Youssef Y, Richards WO, Sekhar N, et al. Risk of secondary hyperparathyroidism after laparoscopic gastric bypass surgery in obese women. Surg Endosc. 2007;21:1393–6.
332. Ross AC, Manson JE, Abrams SA, et al. The 2011 report on dietary reference intakes for calcium and vitamin D from the Institute of Medicine: what clinicians need to know. J Clin Endorcinol Metab. 2011;96:53–8.

333. Hewitt S, Sovik TT, Aasheim ET, et al. Secondary hyperparathyroidism, vitamin D sufficiency, and serum calcium 5 years after gastric bypass and duodenal switch. Obes Surg. 2013;23:384–90.
334. Pereira SE, Saboya CJ, Saunders C, Ramalho A. Serum levels and liver store of retinol and their association with night blindness in individuals with class III obesity. Obes Surg. 2012;22:602–8.
335. Aills L, Blankenship J, Buffington C, Furtado M, Prrott J. ASMBS allied health nutritional guidelines for the surgical weight patient. Surg Obes Relat Dis. 2008;4:S73–108.
336. Slater GH, Ren CJ, Siegel N, et al. Serum fat-soluble vitamin deficiency and abnormal calcium metabolism after malabsorptive bariatric surgery. J Gastrointest Surg. 2004;8:48–55.
337. Strople J, Lovell G, Heubi J. Prevalence of subclinical vitamin K deficiency in cholestatic liver disease. J Pediatr Gastroenterol Nutr. 2009;49:78–84.
338. Ducros V, Pollicand M, Laporte F, Favier A. Quantitative determination of plasma vitamin K1 by high-performance liquid chromatography coupled to isotope dilution tandem mass spectrometry. Anal Biochem. 2010;401:7–14.
339. Watras MM, Patel JP, Arya R. Traditional anticoagulants and hair loss: a role for direct oral anticoagulants? A review of the literature. Drugs Real World Outcomes. 2016;3:1–6.
340. Song A, Fernstrom MH. Nutritional and psychological considerations after bariatric surgery. Aesthet Surg J. 2008;28:195–9.
341. Heber D, Greenway FL, Kaplan LM, Livingston E, Salvador J, Still C. Endocrine and nutritional management of the post-bariatric surgery patient: an Endocrine Society Clinical Practice Guideline. J Clin Endocrinol Metab. 2010;95:4823–43.
342. Castiglioni S, Cazzaniga A, Albisetti W, Maier JA. Magnesium and osteoporosis: current state of knowledge and future research directions. Nutrients. 2013;5:3022–33.
343. Corica F, Allegra A, Ientile R, Buemi M. Magnesium concentrations in plasma, erythrocytes, and platelets in hypertensive and normotensive obese patients. Am J Hypertens. 1997;10:1311–3.
344. Luk CP, Parsons R, Lee YP, Hughes JD. Proton pump inhibitor-associated hypomagnesemia: what do FDA data tell us? Ann Pharmacother. 2013;47:773–80.
345. Walker AF, Marakis G, Christie S, Byng M. Mg citrate found more bioavailable than other Mg preparations in a randomised, double-blind study. Magnes Res. 2003;16:183–91.
346. Ganzoni AM. Intravenous iron-dextran: therapeutic and experimental possibilities. Schweiz Med Wochenschr. 1970;100:301–3.
347. Mechanick JI, Youdim A, Jones DB, et al. Clinical practice guidelines for the perioperative nutritional, metabolic, and nonsurgical support of the bariatric surgery patient—2013 update: cosponsored by American Association of Clinical Endocrinologists, The Obesity Society and American Society of Metabolic & Bariatric Surger. Obesity (Silver Spring). 2013;21(Suppl. 1):S1–27.
348. Shahidzadeh R, Sridhar S. Profound copper deficiency in a patient with gastric bypass. Am J Gastroenterol. 2008;103:2660–2.
349. Franko DL, et al. A longitudinal investigation of mortality in anorexia nervosa and bulimia nervosa. Am J Psychiatry. 2013;2170:917–25.
350. Vaughan ED Jr, Sawyers JL, Scott HW Jr. The Rapunzel syndrome. An unusual complication of intestinal bezoar. Surgery. 1968;63:339–43.
351. Hergüner S, Ozyildirim I, Tanidir C. Is Pica an eating disorder or an obsessive-compulsive spectrum disorder? Prog Neuropsychopharmacol Biol Psychiatry. 2008;32:2010–1.
352. Miao D, Young SL, Golden CD. A meta-analysis of pica and micronutrient status. Am J Hum Biol. 2015;27:84–93.
353. McGehee FT Jr, Buchanan GR. Trichophagia and trichobezoar: etiologic role of iron deficiency. J Pediatr. 1980;97:946–8.
354. Cannalire G, Conti L, Celoni M, Grassi C, Cella A, Bensi G, Capelli P, Biasucci G. Rapunzel syndrome: an infrequent cause of severe iron deficiency anemia and abdominal pain presenting to the pediatric emergency department. BMC Pediatr. 2018;18:125.

218

5 Nutritional Disorders of the Hair and Their Management

355. Hadnagy C, Binder P, Grauzer J, Szöcs K. Trichophagia treated successfully by intravenous iron injections [Article in Hungarian]. Orv Hetil. 1991;132:35–6.
356. Hadnagy C, Grauzer SJ, Binder P, Szöcs K. Iron therapy in mental aberrations (pica) in childhood [Article in German]. Kinderarztl Prax. 1991;59:126–8.
357. Grant JE, Odlaug BL, Kim SW. N-acetylcysteine, a glutamate modulator, in the treatment of trichotillomania: a double-blind, placebo-controlled study. Arch Gen Psychiatry. 2009;66:756–63.
358. Bloch MH, Panza KE, Grant JE, Pittenger C, Leckman JF. N-acetylcysteine in the treatment of pediatric trichotillomania: a randomized, double-blind, placebo-controlled add-on trial. J Am Acad Child Adolesc Psychiatry. 2013;52:231–40.
359. Grant JE, Odlaug BL, Chamberlain SR, Kim SW. Dronabinol, a cannabinoid agonist, reduces hair pulling in trichotillomania: a pilot study. Psychopharmacology (Berl). 2011;218:493–502.
360. Culbert KM, Racine SE, Klump KL. Research review: what have we learned about the causes of eating disorders—a synthesis of sociocultural, psychological and biological research. J Child Psychol Psychiatry. 2015;56:1141–64.
361. Matthews-Ewald MR, Zullig KH, Ward RM. Sexual orientation and disordered eating behaviors among self-identified male and female college students. Eat Behav. 2014;15:441–4.
362. Strumia R. Skin signs in anorexia nervosa. Dermatoendocrinol. 2009;1:268–70.
363. Hediger C, Rost B, Itin P. Cutaneous manifestations in anorexia nervosa. Schweiz Med Wochenschr. 2000;130:565–75.
364. Zucker N, Von Holle A, Thornton LM, Strober M, Plotnicov K, Klump KL, Brandt H, Crawford S, Crow S, Fichter MM, Halmi KA, Johnson C, Kaplan AS, Keel P, LaVia M, Mitchell JE, Rotondo A, Woodside DB, Berrettini WH, Kaye WH, Bulik CM. The significance of repetitive hair-pulling behaviors in eating disorders. J Clin Psychol. 2011;67:391–403.
365. Grillo E, Vano-Galvan S, Diaz-Ley B, Jaén P. Patchy hair loss on the pubis—a case study. Aust Fam Physician. 2013;42:487–9.
366. Achamrah N, Coëffier M, Rimbert A, Charles J, Folope V, Petit A, Déchelotte P, Grigioni S. Micronutrient status in 153 patients with anorexia nervosa. Nutrients. 2017;9:225.
367. Shay NF, Mangian HF. Neurobiology of zinc-influenced eating behavior. J Nutr. 2000;130:1493S–9S.
368. Hambidge KM, Hambidge C, Jacobs M, Baum JD. Low levels of zinc in hair, anorexia, poor growth, and hypogeusia in children. Pediatr Res. 1972;6:868–74.
369. Lask B, Fosson A, Rolfe U, Thomas S. Zinc deficiency and childhood-onset anorexia nervosa. J Clin Psychiatry. 1993;54:63–6.
370. Yamaguchi H, Arita Y, Hara Y, Kimura T, Nawata H. Anorexia nervosa responding to zinc supplementation: a case report. Gastroenterol Jpn. 1992;27:554–8.
371. Birmingham CL, Gritzner S. How does zinc supplementation benefit anorexia nervosa? Eat Weight Disord. 2006;11:e109–11.
372. Seeger G, Braus DF, Ruf M, Goldberger U, Schmidt MH. Body image distortion reveals amygdala activation in patients with anorexia nervosa—a functional magnetic resonance imaging study. Neurosci Lett. 2002;326:25–8.
373. Takano A, Shiga T, Kitagawa N, Koyama T, Katoh C, Tsukamoto E, Tamaki N. Abnormal neuronal network in anorexia nervosa studied with I-123-IMP SPECT. Psychiatry Res. 2001;107:45–50.
374. O'Connor G, Nicholls D. Refeeding hypophosphatemia in adolescents with anorexia nervosa: a systematic review. Nutr Clin Pract. 2013;28:358–64.
375. Kaye W. Neurobiology of anorexia and bulimia nervosa. Physiol Behav. 2008;94:121–35.
376. Dietary Guidelines for Americans 2005. health.gov. 2005. Archived from the original on 1 July 2007. Dietary Guidelines.
377. Young adult drinking. Alcohol alert (68). April 2006. Archived from the original on 13 February 2013. Accessed 18 February 2013.
378. Ryle PR, Thomson AD. Nutrition and vitamins in alcoholism. Contemp Issues Clin Biochem. 1984;1:188–224.

379. Sanvisens A, Zuluaga P, Pineda M, Fuster D, Bolao F, Juncà J, Tor J, Muga R. Folate deficiency in patients seeking treatment of alcohol use disorder. Drug Alcohol Depend. 2017;180:417–22.
380. Narasimha VL, Ganesh S, Reddy S, Shukla L, Mukherjee D, Kandasamy A, Chand PK, Benegal V, Murthy P. Pellagra and alcohol dependence syndrome: findings from a tertiary care addiction treatment centre in India. Alcohol Alcohol. 2019;54:148–51.
381. Shaikh H, Faisal MS, Mewawalla P. Vitamin C deficiency: rare cause of severe anemia with hemolysis. Int J Hematol. 2019;109:618–62.
382. Kopecký A, Benda F, Němčanský J. Xerosis in patient with vitamin A deficiency—a case report. Cesk Slov Oftalmol. 2018;73:222–4.
383. Sharain K, May AM, Gersh BJ. Chronic alcoholism and the danger of profound hypomagnesemia. Am J Med. 2015;128:e17–8.
384. Anty R, Canivet CM, Patouraux S, Ferrari-Panaia P, Saint-Paul MC, Huet PM, Lebeaupin C, Iannelli A, Gual P, Tran A. Severe vitamin D deficiency may be an additional cofactor for the occurrence of alcoholic steatohepatitis. Alcohol Clin Exp Res. 2015;39:1027–33.
385. Shahsavari D, Ahmed Z, Karikkineth A, Williams R, Zigel C. Zinc-deficiency acrodermatitis in a patient with chronic alcoholism and gastric bypass: a case report. J Community Hosp Intern Med Perspect. 2014;31:4.
386. Tanner AR, Bantock I, Hinks L, Lloyd B, Turner NR, Wright R. Depressed selenium and vitamin E levels in an alcoholic population. Possible relationship to hepatic injury through increased lipid peroxidation. Dig Dis Sci. 1986;31:1307–12.
387. Iber FL, Shamszad M, Miller PA, Jacob R. Vitamin K deficiency in chronic alcoholic males. Alcohol Clin Exp Res. 1986;10:679–81.
388. Shibazaki S, Uchiyama S, Tsuda K, Taniuchi N. Copper deficiency caused by excessive alcohol consumption. BMJ Case Rep. 2017;26:pii: bcr-2017-220921.
389. Bahmer FA, Bader M. Skin changes in chronic alcoholism with special reference to the zinc and biotin content of the serum [Article in German]. Z Hautkr. 1987;62:691–5.
390. Bader U, Hafner J, Burg G. Erythroderma and alcohol abuse [Article in German]. Schweiz Med Wochenschr. 1999;129:508–13.
391. Rao GS. Cutaneous changes in chronic alcoholics. Indian J Dermatol Venereol Leprol. 2004;70:79–8.
392. Kostović K, Lipozencić J. Skin diseases in alcoholics. Acta Dermatovenerol Croat. 2004;12:181–90.
393. Christenson B. Queen of Punt. Clin Infect Dis. 2006;42:1344–5.
394. Biondi A, Freni F, Carelli C, Moretti M, Morini L. Ethyl glucuronide hair testing: a review. Forensic Sci Int. 2019;300:106–19.
395. Morini L, Sempio C, Moretti M. Ethyl glucuronide in hair (hEtG) after exposure to alcohol-based perfumes. Curr Pharm Biotechnol. 2018;19:175–9.
396. Luginbühl M, Bekaert B, Suesse S, Weinmann W. Detox shampoos for EtG and FAEE in hair—results from in vitro experiments. Drug Test Anal. 2019;11:870–7.
397. Hayflick L, Moorhead PS. The serial cultivation of human diploid cell strains. Exp Cell Res. 1961;25:585–621.
398. Deutz NE, Bauer JM, Barazzoni R, Biolo G, Boirie Y, Bosy-Westphal A, Cederholm T, Cruz-Jentoft A, Krznarič Z, Nair KS, Singer P, Teta D, Tipton K, Calder PC. Protein intake and exercise for optimal muscle function with aging: recommendations from the ESPEN Expert Group. Clin Nutr. 2014;33:929–36.
399. Food and Nutrition Board, Institute of Medicine. Dietary reference intakes for thiamin, riboflavin, niacin, vitamin B6, folate, vitamin B12, pantothenic acid, biotin, and choline. Washington DC: National Academics Press; 1998.
400. Norman AW, Bouillon R. Vitamin D nutritional policy needs a vision for the future. Exp Biol Med (Maywood). 2010;235:1034–45.
401. Johnson KA, Bernard MA, Funderberg K. Vitamin nutrition in older adults. Clin Geriatr Med. 2002;18:773–99.

402. Wolff JL, Starfield B, Anderson G. Prevalence, expenditures, and complications of multiple chronic conditions in the elderly. Arch Intern Med. 2002;162:2269–76.
403. Diekmann R, Winning K, Uter W, Kaiser MJ, Sieber CC, Volkert D, Bauer JM. Screening for malnutrition among nursing home residents—a comparative analysis of the mini nutritional assessment, the nutritional risk screen, and the malnutrition universal screening tool. J Nutr Health Aging. 2013;17:326–31.
404. Valderas JM, Starfield B, Sibbald B, Salisbury C, Roland M. Defining comorbidity: implications for understanding health and health services. Ann Fam Med. 2009;7:357–63.
405. National Center for Health Statistics. Health, United States, 2014: with special feature of adults aged 55-64. Hyattsville, MD: U.S. Government Printing Office; 2015.
406. Pinkus H. Alopecia: clinicopathologic correlations. Int J Dermatol. 1980;19:245–53.
407. Ebling FJ. Age changes in cutaneous appendages. J Appl Cosmetol. 1985;3:243–50.
408. Kligman AM. The comparative histopathology of male-pattern baldness and senescent baldness. Clin Dermatol. 1988;6:108–18.
409. Trüeb RM, Tobin DH, editors. Aging hair. Berlin Heidelberg: Springer; 2010.
410. Tobin DJ, Paus R. Graying: gerontobiology of the hair follicle pigmentary unit. Exp Gerontol. 2001;36:29–54.
411. Pandhi D, Khanna D. Premature graying of hair. Indian J Dermatol Venereol Leprol. 2013;79:641–53.
412. Mosley JG, Gibbs CC. Premature grey hair and hair loss among smokers: a new opportunity for health education? BMJ. 1996;313:1616.
413. Commo S, Gaillard O, Bernard BA. Human hair greying is linked to a specific depletion of hair follicle melanocytes affecting both the bulb and the outer root sheath. Br J Dermatol. 2004;150:435–43.
414. Tobin DJ, Paus R. Graying: gerontobiology of the hair follicle pigmentary unit. Exp Gerontol. 2001;36:29–54.
415. Harman D. Aging: a theory based on free radical and radiation chemistry. J Gerontol. 1956;11:298–300.
416. Arck PC, Overall R, Spatz K, et al. Towards a "free radical theory of graying": melanocyte apoptosis in the aging human hair follicle is an indicator of oxidative stress induced tissue damage. FASEB J. 2006;20:1567–9.
417. Wood JM, Decker H, Hartmann H, et al. Senile hair greying: H2O2-mediated oxidative stress affects human hair colour by blunting methionine sulfoxide repair. FASEB J. 2009;23:2065–75.
418. Nishimura EK, Jordan SA, Oshima H, et al. Dominant role of the niche in melanocyte stem-cell fate determination. Nature. 2002;416:854–60.
419. Nishimura EK, Granter SR, Fisher DE. Mechanisms of hair graying: incomplete melanocyte stem cell maintenance in the niche. Science. 2005;307:720–4.
420. Hollfelder B, Blankenburg G, Wolfram LJ, Höcker H. Chemical and physical properties of pigmented and non-pigmented hair ('grey hair'). Int J Cosmet Sci. 1995;17:87–9.
421. Jeon SY, Pi LQ, Lee WS. Comparison of hair shaft damage after UVA and UVB irradiation. J Cosmet Sci. 2008;59:151–6.
422. Otsuka H, Nemoto T. Study on Japanese hair. Koshkaischi. 1988;12:192–7.
423. Robbins C, Mirmirani P, Messenger AG, Birch MP, Youngquist RS, Tamura M, Filloon T, Luo F, Dawson TLJ. What women want—quantifying the perception of hair amount: an analysis of hair diameter and density changes with age in Caucasian women. Br J Dermatol. 2012;167:324–32.
424. Birch MP, Messenger JF, Messenger AG. Hair density, hair diameter and the prevalence of female pattern hair loss. Br J Dermatol. 2001;144:297–304.
425. Otsuka H, Nemoto T. Study on Japanese hair. Koshkaischi. 1988;12:192–7.
426. Courtois M, Loussouarn G, Hourseau C, Grollier JF. Aging and hair cycles. Br J Dermatol. 1995;132:86–93.
427. Price VH, Sawaya ME, Headington JT et al. Histology and hormonal activity in senescent thinning in men. Present at SID, Annual Meeting, Washington DC; 2001

428. Sperling LC. Senescent balding ("senile alopecia"). In: Sperling LC, editor. An atlas of hair pathology with clinical correlations. New York: Parthenon Publishing; 2003. p. 35–6.
429. Sinclair R, Chapman A, Magee J. The lack of significant changes in scalp hair follicle density with advancing age. Br J Dermatol. 2005;152:646–9.
430. Whiting DA. How real is senescent alopecia? A histopathologic approach. Clin Dermatol. 2011;29:49–53.
431. Karnik P, Shah S, Dvorkin-Wininger Y, et al. Microarray analysis of androgenetic and senescent alopecia: comparison of gene expression shows two distinct profiles. J Dermatol Sci. 2013;72:183–6.
432. Nagase S, Tsuchiya M, Matsui T, Shibuichi S, Tsujimura H, Masukawa Y, Satoh N, Itou T, Koike K, Tsujii K. Characterization of curved hair of Japanese women with reference to internal structures and amino acid composition. J Cosmet Sci. 2008;59:317–32.
433. Nicolaides N, Rothman S. Studies on the chemical composition of human hair fat. II. The overall composition with regard to age, sex and race. J Invest Dermatol. 1953;21:9–14.
434. Matsumura H, Mohri Y, Binh NT, Morinaga H, Fukuda M, Ito M, Kurata S, Hoeijmakers J, Nishimura EK. Hair follicle aging is driven by transepidermal elimination of stem cells via COL17A1 proteolysis. Science. 2016;351(6273):aad4395.
435. Inomata K, Aoto T, Binh NT, Okamoto N, Tanimura S, Wakayama T, Iseki S, Hara E, Masunaga T, Shimizu H, Nishimura EK. Genotoxic stress abrogates renewal of melanocyte stem cells by triggering their differentiation. Cell. 2009;137:1088–99.
436. Liu N, Matsumura H, Kato T, Ichinose S, Takada A, Namiki T, Asakawa K, Morinaga H, Mohri Y, De Arcangelis A, Geroges-Labouesse E, Nanba D, Nishimura EK. Stem cell competition orchestrates skin homeostasis and ageing. Nature. 2019;568:344–50.
437. Floeth M, Fiedorowicz J, Schäcke H, Hammami-Hausli N, Owaribe K, Trüeb RM, Bruckner-Tuderman L. Novel homozygous and compound heterozygous COL17A1 mutations associated with junctional epidermolysis bullosa. J Invest Dermatol. 1998;111:528–33.
438. Hintner H, Wolff K. Generalized atrophic benign epidermolysis bullosa. Arch Dermatol. 1982;118:375–84.
439. Natsuga K, Watanabe M, Nishie W, Shimizu H. Life before and beyond blistering: the role of collagen XVII in epidermal physiology. Exp Dermatol. 2019;28:1135–41.
440. Harley CB, Futcher AB, Greider CW. Telomeres shorten during ageing of human fibroblasts. Nature. 1990;345:458–60.
441. Rudolph KL, Chang S, Lee HW, et al. Longevity, stress response, and cancer in aging telomerase-deficient mice. Cell. 1999;96:701–12.
442. Kao SH, Liu CS, Wang SY, Wei YH. Ageing-associated large-scale deletions of mitochondrial DNA in human hair follicles. Biochem Mol Biol Int. 1997;42:285–98.
443. Nakauchi Y, Kumon Y, Yamasaki H, et al. Scalp hair loss caused by octreotide in a patient with acromegaly: a case report. Endocr J. 1995;42(3):385–9.
444. Yamada S, Fukuhara N, Nishioka H, et al. Scalp hair loss after transsphenoidal adenomectomy in patients with acromegaly. Clin Endocrinol (Oxf). 2013;79:386–93.
445. Lurie R, Ben-Amitai D, Laron Z. Laron syndrome (primary growth hormone insensitivity): a unique model to explore the effect of insulin-like growth factor 1 deficiency on human hair. Dermatolog. 2004;208:314–8.
446. Rundegren J. Pattern alopecia: what clinical features determine the response to topical minoxidil treatment? (IHRS 2004 abstract B2.4). JDDG. 2004;2:500.
447. CG 210 hair & scalp lotion. Product monograph. Legacy Healthcare.
448. Trüeb RM. Molecular mechanisms of androgenetic alopecia. Exp Gerontol. 2002;37:981–90.
449. Katoulis AC, Liakou AI, Alevizou A, Bonovas S, Bozi E, Kontogiorgi D, Rigopoulos D. Efficacy and safety of a topical botanical in female androgenetic alopecia: a randomized, single-blinded, vehicle-controlled study. Skin Appendage Disord. 2018;4:160–5.
450. McMichael A, Pham A, von Grote E, Meckfessel MH. Efficacy and safety of minoxidil 2% solution in combination with a botanical hair solution in women with female pattern hair loss/androgenic alopecia. J Drugs Dermatol. 2016;15:398–404.

451. Keaney TC, Pham H, von Grote E, Meckfessel MH. Efficacy and safety of minoxidil 5% foam in combination with a botanical hair solution in men with androgenic alopecia. J Drugs Dermatol. 2016;15:406–12.
452. Takeda A, Sato A, Zhang L, Harti S, Cauwen-bergh G, et al. CG210 enables finasteride 1 mg users to further improve hair pattern: a randomized, double-blind, placebo-controlled pilot study. Hair Ther Transplant. 2013;3:107.
453. Cucé LC, Rodrigues CJ, Patriota RCR. Cellium® GC: evaluation of a new natural active ingredient in 210 mg/mL topical solution, through scalp biopsy. Surg Cosmet Dermatol. 2011;3:123–8.
454. Blatt T, Littarru GP. Biochemical rationale and experimental data on the antiaging properties of CoQ(10) at skin level. Biofactors. 2011;37:381–5.
455. Giesen M, Welss T, Wiesche ES, et al. Coenzyme Q10 has anti-aging effects on human hair. Int J Cosmet Sci. 2009;31:154–5.
456. Giesen M, Gruedl S, Holtkoetter O, Fuhrmann G, Koerner A, Petersohn D. Ageing processes influence keratin and KAP expression in human hair follicles. Exp Dermatol. 2011;20:759–61.
457. Choi FD, Sung CT, Juhasz ML, Mesinkovsk NA. Oral collagen supplementation: a systematic review of dermatological applications. J Drugs Dermatol. 2019;18:9–16.
458. Arthur ST, Noone JM, Van Doren BA, Roy D, Blanchette CM. One-year prevalence, comorbidities and cost of cachexia-related inpatient admissions in the USA. Drugs Context. 2014;3:212,265.
459. von Haehling S. Anker SD. Prevalence, incidence and clinical impact of cachexia: facts and numbers-update 2014. J Cachexia Sarcopenia Muscle. 2014;5:261–3.
460. Academy of Nutrition and Dietetics. Nutrition care manual. Chicago, IL: Academy of Nutrition and Dietetics; 2015.
461. Cathcart P, Craddock C, Stebbing J. Fasting: starving cancer. Lancet Oncol. 2017;18(4):431.
462. Saleh AD, Simone BA, Palazzo J, et al. Caloric restriction augments radiation efficacy in breast cancer. Cell Cycle. 2013;12:1955–63.
463. Thissen JP, Ketelslegers JM, Underwood LE. Nutritional regulation of the insulin-like growth factors. Endocr Rev. 1994;15:80–101.
464. Simone BA, Champ CE, Rosenberg AL, Berger AC, Monti DA, Dicker AP, Simone NL. Selectively starving cancer cells through dietary manipulation: methods and clinical implications. Future Oncol. 2013;9:959–76.
465. Blackburn GL, Bistrian BR, Hoag C. Hair loss with rapid weight loss. Arch Dermatol. 1977;113(2):234.
466. Zick SM, Snyder D, Abrams DI. Pros and cons of dietary strategies popular among cancer patients. Oncology (Williston Park). 2018;32:542–7.
467. Dinu M, Abbate R, Gensini GF, et al. Vegetarian, vegan diets and multiple health outcomes: a systematic review with meta-analysis of observational studies. Crit Rev Food Sci Nutr. 2017;57:3640–9.
468. Gröber U, Holzhauer P, Kisters K, Holick MF, Adamietz IA. Micronutrients in oncological intervention. Nutrients. 2016;8:163.
469. Micke O, Bruns F, Glatzel M, Schönekaes K, Micke P, Mücke R. Predictive factors for the use of complementary and alternative medicine (CAM) in radiation oncology. Eur J Integr Med. 2009;1:22–30.
470. Lawenda BD, Kelly KM, Lasas EJ, et al. Should supplemental antioxidant administration be avoided during chemotherapy and radiotherapy? J Natl Cancer Inst. 2008;100:773–83.
471. Gröber U, Mücke R, Adamietz IA, Holzhauer P, Kisters K, Büntzel J, Micke O. Komplementärer Einsatz von Antioxidanzien aund Mikronährstoffen in der Onkologie – Update 2013. Der Onkol. 2013;19:136–43.
472. Moss RW. Should patients undergoing chemotherapy and radiotherapy be prescribed antioxidants? Integr Cancer Ther. 2006;5:63–82.
473. Tong H, Isenring E, Yates P. The prevalence of nutrition impact symptoms and their relationship to quality of life and clinical outcomes in medical oncology patients. Support Care Cancer. 2009;17:83–90.

474. Fearon KC, Voss AC, Hustend DS. Definition of cancer cachexia: effect of weight loss reduced food intake and systemic inflammation on functional status and prognosis. Am J Clin Nutr. 2006;83:1345–50.
475. Bozzetti F. SCRINIO Working Group Screening the nutritional status in oncology: a preliminary report on 1000 outpatients. Support Care Cancer. 2009;17:279–84.
476. Harvie M. Nutritional supplements and cancer: potential benefits and proven harms. Am Soc Clin Oncol Educ Book. 2014:e478–86.
477. Trüeb RM, Jolliffe VML, Régnier AF, et al. Precision medicine and the practice of trichiatry: adapting the concept. Skin Appendage Disord. 2019;5:338–43.
478. McGarvey EL, Baum LD, Pinkerton RC, et al. Psychological sequelae and alopecia among women with cancer. Cancer Pract. 2001;9:283–9.
479. Trüeb RM. Chemotherapy-induced anagen effluvium: diffuse or patterned? Dermatology. 2007;215:1–2.
480. Trüeb RM. Chemotherapy-induced alopecia. Semin Cutan Med Surg. 2009;28:11–4.
481. Baker B, Wilson C, Davis A, et al. Busulphan/cyclophosphamide conditioning for bone marrow transplantation may lead to failure of hair regrowth. Bone Marrow Transplant. 1991;7:43–7.
482. Vowels M, Chan LL, Giri N, et al. Factors affecting hair regrowth after bone marrow transplantation. Bone Marrow Transplant. 1993;12:347–50.
483. Kluger N, Jacot W, Frouin E, et al. Permanent scalp alopecia related to breast cancer chemotherapy by sequential fluorouracil/epirubicin/cyclophosphamide (FEC) and docetaxel: a prospective study of 20 patients. Ann Oncol. 2012;23:2879–84.
484. Miteva M, Misciali C, Fanti PA, Vincenzi C, Romanelli P, Tosti A. Permanent alopecia after systemic chemotherapy: a clinicopathological study of 10 cases. Am J Dermatopathol. 2011;33:345–50.
485. Betticher DC, Delmore G, Breitenstein U, et al. Efficacy and tolerability of two scalp cooling systems for the prevention of alopecia associated with docetaxel treatment. Support Care Cancer. 2013;21:2565–73.
486. Plonka PM, Handjiski B, Popik M, Michalczyk D, Paus R. Zinc as an ambivalent but potent modulator of murine hair growth in vivo preliminary observations. Exp Dermatol. 2005;14:844–53.
487. Tsuruki T, Takahata K, Yoshikawa M. Anti-alopecia mechanisms of soymetide-4, an immunostimulating peptide derived from soy beta-conglycinin. Peptides. 2005;26:707–11.
488. Sieja K, Taleruyk M. Selenium as an element in the treatment of ovarian cancer in women (n = 31) receiving chemotherapy. Gynecol Oncol. 2004;93:320–7.
489. Wang J, Lu Z, Au JLS. Protection against chemotherapy-induced alopecia. Pharm Res. 2006;23:2505–14.
490. Tran D, Sinclair RD, Schwarer AP, et al. Permanent alopecia following chemotherapy and bone marrow transplantation. Austral J Dermatol. 2000;41:106–8.
491. Freites-Martinez A, Shapiro J, Chan D, Fornier M, Modi S, Gajria D, Dusza S, Goldfarb S, Lacouture ME. Endocrine therapy-induced alopecia in patients with breast cancer. JAMA Dermatol. 2018;154:670–5.
492. Kluger N, Jacot W, Frouin E, et al. Permanent scalp alopecia related to breast cancer chemotherapy by sequential fluorouracil/epirubicin/cyclophosphamide (FEC) and docetaxel: a prospective study of 20 patients. Ann Oncol. 2012;23:2879–84.
493. Trüeb RM. Minoxidil for endocrine therapy-induced alopecia in women with breast cancer-saint Agatha's Blessing? JAMA Dermatol. 2018;154:656–8.
494. Mundstedt K, Manthey N, Sachsse S, et al. Changes in self-concept and body image during alopecia induced cancer chemotherapy. Support Care Cancer. 1997;5:139–43.

Value of Nutrition-Based Therapies for Hair Growth, Color, and Quality

6

6.1 Traditional

"Thou shouldst eat to live; not live to eat" is a proverb originally attributed to Socrates, and "Let food be thy medicine" to yet another Ancient Greek, Hippocrates. And yet, there is hardly another field with so much prejudice, misconception, and debate as diet and health, let alone hair health. The fact is that quantity and quality of hair are closely related to the nutritional state of an individual. Whether increasing the content of an already adequate diet with specific nutrients may further promote hair growth and quality has been yet another point of speculations.

6.1.1 Food Based

Despite the enthusiasm for vitamin and mineral supplements, it must be kept in mind that such supplementation is not a substitute for a healthy and balanced diet. Micronutrients in food are typically better absorbed by the body and are associated with fewer potential adverse effects [1]. In fact, research shows that positive health outcomes are more strongly related to dietary patterns and specific food types than to individual micronutrient or nutrient intakes [2].

Traditionally, the ten top foods considered as beneficial for hair health are eggs as source of protein, biotin, and vitamin B12; poultry of high-quality protein and iron with a high degree of bioavailability; salmon of omega-3 fatty acids, protein, vitamin B12, and iron; oysters of zinc; spinach of folate, iron, and vitamins A and C; and beans, lentils, and soybeans of protein iron, zinc, and biotin; soybeans are in addition a source of spermidine, a compound that may prolong the anagen phase of the hair cycle [3]; nuts are a source of vitamin E, B vitamins, zinc, and essential fatty acids: Brazil nuts of selenium; walnuts of zinc and alpha-linolenic acid; pecans, cashews, and almonds of zinc; berries of antioxidants and vitamins, specifically

© Springer Nature Switzerland AG 2020
R. M. Trüeb, *Nutrition for Healthy Hair*,
https://doi.org/10.1007/978-3-030-59920-1_6

strawberries, are rich in vitamin C which aids in collagen production and iron absorption; avocado is rich in vitamin E and essential fatty acids and sweet potatoes in vitamin A.

Other specific nutrients that have been traditionally recommended for hair growth are millet, nutritional yeast, and gelatin.

6.1.2   Millets

Millets are a group of highly variable small-seeded grasses, widely grown around the world as cereal crops or grains. Millets are indigenous to many parts of the world, and may have been consumed by humans for about 7000 years and potentially had a pivotal role in the rise of multi-crop agriculture and settled farming societies [4]. A 100 g serving of raw millet (*Panicum miliaceum or proso millet*) provides 378 calories and is a rich source of amino acids, vitamin B, silica, iron, and linoleic acid. In addition, millet contains miliacin. Miliacin is a triterpenoid known to stimulate keratinocyte metabolism and proliferation [5].

6.1.3   Nutritional Yeast

Nutritional yeast has also played an important role in human diet for thousands of years. Nutritional yeast comes from a species of yeast known as *Saccharomyces cerevisiae*. This fungus is a vital ingredient in bread, beer, and a range of other foods. Traditionally, many people have also consumed a specific type of yeast called nutritional yeast for its alleged health benefits. Nutritional yeast is an excellent source of vitamins, minerals, and high-quality protein. One-quarter of a cup of nutritional yeast contains 60 calories, 8 grams (g) of protein, 3 g of fiber, 11.85 mg of thiamine (vitamin B1), 9.70 mg of riboflavin (vitamin B2), 5.90 mg of vitamin B6, and 17.60 micrograms of vitamin B12. It also contains niacin (vitamin B3), potassium, calcium, and iron. Some research suggests that nutritional yeast can combat hair loss and brittle nails, and may also help reduce acne [6].

6.1.4   Gelatin

Gelatin is a translucent, colorless, flavorless food ingredient, derived from collagen of animal origin. It is also referred to as hydrolyzed collagen, collagen hydrolysate, gelatin hydrolysate, hydrolyzed gelatin, and collagen peptides after it has undergone hydrolysis. It is commonly used as a gelling agent in food, medications, drug, and vitamin capsules. The amino acid content of hydrolyzed collagen is that of the collagen. Hydrolyzed collagen contains 19 amino acids, predominantly glycine, proline, and hydroxyproline, which together represent around 50% of the total amino acid content. Hydrolyzed collagen contains eight out of nine essential amino acids, including glycine and arginine. It contains no tryptophan, and is deficient in isoleucine, threonine, and methionine. Although gelatin is 98–99% protein by dry weight, it has little additional nutritional value. The bioavailability of hydrolyzed collagen was originally demonstrated in mice: orally administered ^{14}C hydrolyzed collagen was digested and more than 90% absorbed within 6 h, with measurable accumulation in the skin [7]. A study in humans found hydrolyzed collagen to be absorbed as small peptides in the blood [8]. Ingestion of hydrolyzed collagen may affect the skin by increasing the density of collagen fibrils and fibroblasts, thereby stimulating collagen production [9]. It has been suggested, based on mouse and in vitro studies, that hydrolyzed collagen peptides have chemotactic properties on fibroblasts [10] or an influence on growth of fibroblasts [11]. Traditionally, oral gelatin has primarily been recommended for the treatment of nail disorders [12]. However, nails do not contain collagen or gelatin, and gelatin is particularly deficient in cystine (<0.1%).

Hydrolyzed collagen, like gelatin, is made from animal by-products from the meat industry, including skin, bones, and connective tissue. Therefore, the consumption of gelatin from particular animals may be forbidden by religious rules or cultural taboos. Also, vegans do not eat foods containing gelatin made from animals.

Finally, some traditional botanicals have been fenugreek, saw palmetto, black cohosh, yam, and soy.

6.1.5   Fenugreek

Fenugreek (*Trigonella foenum-graecum L.*) is an annual plant in the family Fabaceae, with leaves consisting of three small obovate to oblong leaflets. Its seeds and leaves are common ingredients in dishes from the Indian subcontinent. Fenugreek is believed to have been brought into cultivation in the Near East. Charred fenugreek seeds have been recovered from Tell Halal, Iraq (carbon dated to 4000 BC), and desiccated seeds of fenugreek have been recovered from the tomb of Tutankhamun [13]. Fenugreek is one of the oldest medicinal plants with a particular medicinal and nutritional profile. Its description and benefits had been reported in the Ebers Papyrus (earlier in 1500 BC in Egypt) [14]. In Indian subcontinent, fenugreek was being consumed as lactation stimulant and condiment. In ancient Rome, it was purportedly used in labor pain and delivery [15]. In one first-century AD recipe, the Romans flavored wine with fenugreek [16]. Fenugreek dietary supplements are manufactured from powdered seeds into capsules, loose powders, teas, and liquid extracts in many countries, and are used in traditional medicine. Fenugreek seeds contain a substantial amount of fiber; phospholipids; glycolipids; oleic acid; linolenic acid; linoleic acid; choline; vitamins A, B1, B2, and C; nicotinic acid; niacin; and many other functional elements. Different types of glycoside extract of fenugreek have shown androgenic and anabolic effect in (aging) males [17]. It is thought that certain fenugreek compounds inhibit aromatase and 5-alpha-reductase activity, leading to diminished testosterone breakdown. In the context of a randomized, placebo-controlled clinical trial efficacy of a fenugreek seed-containing nutritional supplement against hair loss was evaluated. The results indicated successful treatment of low-to-moderate hair loss in women and men [18].

Pulmonary embolism secondary to fenugreek use has been reported, with testosterone-induced polycythemia being the proposed mechanism for an increased clotting propensity from the testosterone-enhancing herbal supplement [19]. Fenugreek is likely not safe for use during pregnancy as it may have abortifacient effects [20]. Fenugreek may be unsafe for women with hormone-sensitive cancers [21]. Some people are allergic to fenugreek, including those with peanut or chickpea allergies [20]. Because of the high content of coumarin-like compounds in fenugreek, it may interfere with the activity and dosing of oral anticoagulants [20].

6.1.6   Saw Palmetto

Saw palmetto (*Serenoa repens*): Due to the potential sexual and psychological adverse events related to the use of the oral 5α-reductase inhibitors finasteride and dutasteride, there has been a considerable interest in the alternative of botanically derived inhibitors of 5α-reductase, such as saw palmetto (*Serenoa repens*), especially in complementary medicine. Widely advertised on the Web and sold by direct marketing, it is frequently used as self-medication. Saw palmetto is a small palm, growing to a maximum height of around 7–10 ft (2.1–3.0 m) endemic to the subtropical Southeastern United States along the south Atlantic and Gulf Coastal plains and sand hills. It grows in clumps or dense thickets in sandy coastal areas, and as undergrowth in pine woods or hardwood hammocks. It is a fan palm, with the leaves that have a bare petiole terminating in a rounded fan of about 20 leaflets. Saw palmetto extract has been originally researched as a treatment for people with prostate conditions. Rossi et al. [22] performed an open-label study to determine the effectiveness of *Serenoa repens* in treating male androgenetic alopecia compared to oral finasteride. 100 male patients with clinically diagnosed mild-to-moderate androgenetic alopecia were enrolled. One group received 320 mg *Serenoa repens* daily, while the other received 1 mg oral finasteride daily for a total study duration of 24 months (2 years). In order to assess the efficacy of treatments, a score index based on the comparison of the global photographs taken at the beginning and at the end of the treatment was used. The investigators found that *Serenoa repens* could lead to an improvement of androgenetic alopecia, while finasteride was more effective for more than half of patients. Moreover, finasteride acts in both the frontal and the vertex areas, while *Serenoa repens* prevalently in the vertex.

As with finasteride and dutasteride, saw palmetto extract should not be used during pregnancy, since its effects on androgen metabolism can potentially impair fetal genital development [23]. In a case report, a patient on saw palmetto extract had increased bleeding time during surgery that returned to normal after stopping the herb [24]. As a general rule, surgeons should caution patients to discontinue dietary and herbal supplements prior to scheduled surgery.

6.1.7   Black Cohosh

Black cohosh or fairy candle (*Cimicifuga racemosa*) is a species of flowering plant of the family Ranunculaceae that is native to eastern North America from the extreme south of Ontario to central Georgia, and west to Missouri and Arkansas, and was originally used in traditional medicine by Native Americans to treat gynecological and other disorders. Following the arrival of European settlers in the United States who continued the use of fairy candle, the plant appeared in the U.S. Pharmacopeia. Today, its extracts are manufactured as herbal medicines and dietary supplements marketed mainly to women for treating gynecological problems related to estrogen deficiency [25]. Black cohosh contains diverse phytochemicals, such as polyphenols [26, 27] and estrogen-like compounds (phytoestrogens). A meta-analysis of nine placebo-controlled studies published until 2013 confirmed the efficacy of black cohosh-based medicinal products for hot flashes, night sweats, and sleep disturbances associated with these menopausal symptoms [28].

Up to date there are no published data on the effect of black cohosh on hair growth and quality in women, specifically in menopause.

6.1.8   Yam

Yam is the common name for some plant species of the *Dioscoreaceae* family that form edible tubers. They are cultivated in many temperate and tropical world regions, especially Latin America, Africa, Asia, and Oceania, for the consumption of their starchy tubers. Raw yam has only moderate nutrient density, with appreciable content limited to potassium, vitamin B6, manganese, thiamin, dietary fiber, and vitamin C. The protein content of the tubers is lower than other food staples, with the content of yam and potato being around 2% on a fresh-weight basis. As a relatively low-protein food, yam is not a good source of essential amino acids. Yam supplies 118 calories per 100 g. With 54% of glucose per 150 g serving, the yam has a lower glycemic index compared to potato. Yam is an important dietary element for Nigerian and West African people, and an attractive crop in poor farms with limited resources, since it is available all year round, and can be prepared in many ways.

Extracts of *Dioscorea composita* or *Dioscorea villosa* are consumed as supplemental health foods at the time of climacteric. The extracts contain significant amounts of the phytosteroid diosgenin with estrogen-like activity [29]. Tada et al. [30] studied the efficacy and safety of diosgenin against skin aging at the time of climacteric. In vitro, diosgenin enhanced DNA synthesis in a human 3-D skin equivalent model, and increased bromodeoxyuridine uptake and intracellular cAMP level in adult human keratinocytes. The increase of bromodeoxyuridine uptake by diosgenin was blocked by an adenylate cyclase inhibitor, but not by antisense oligonucleotides against estrogen receptor alpha or beta, indicating the involvement of cAMP but not estrogen receptor alpha or beta. In vivo, administration of diosgenin improved epidermal thickness in ovariectomized mice, a climacteric model, without effect on the degree of fat accumulation. In order to examine the safety of diosgenin,

diosgenin and 17-beta-estradiol were administered to breast cancer-burdened mice. The results revealed that while 17-beta-estradiol accelerated tumor growth, diosgenin did not show this effect.

Up to date there are no published data on the effect of yam on hair growth and quality in women, specifically in the climacteric.

6.1.9   Soy

Soy refers to the soybean (*Glycine max*), a species of legume native to East Asia, widely grown for its edible bean, which has numerous uses. Traditional unfermented food uses of soybeans include soy milk, from which tofu is made. Fermented soy foods include soy sauce and fermented bean paste. Defatted soybean meal is a significant and cheap source of protein for many packaged meals. Finally, soybean products, such as textured vegetable protein, are ingredients in many meat and dairy substitutes in the vegan diet. Soy beans contain significant amounts of phytic acid, dietary minerals, and B vitamins, including folate. In addition, soybeans and processed soy foods are among the richest foods in total phytoestrogens, which are present primarily in the form of the isoflavones daidzein and genistein [31]. The effects of soy on diet and health have been topics of intense research for the last 30 years or more. Much of this research has suggested that soy consumption may have beneficial effects on several aspects of human health [32]. Despite the increasing in vitro evidence from topical application exposing potential benefits of soy for skin care [33], little research has been done on the dietary benefits of soy for skin health, let alone the hair.

One study in Taiwanese men suggested an association of androgenetic alopecia with less dietary soy [34]. Draelos et al. [35] reported that hair appearance in postmenopausal women was improved in terms of hair roughness, manageability, and overall appearance after 3 and 6 months of regular soy consumption in comparison to the control subjects maintaining their normal dietary pattern. The mechanisms involved in the beneficial effects of soy have been suggested to be antioxidant functions [36], anti-inflammatory processes [37], reduction in DNA damage [38], suppression of extracellular matrix proteases [39], and upregulation of extracellular matrix components [40].

Allergy to soy is common, and the food is listed with other foods that commonly cause allergic reactions, such as milk, eggs, peanuts, and shellfish. Although it is very difficult to give a reliable estimate of the true prevalence of soy allergy in the general population, to the extent that it does exist, soy allergy may cause urticaria and angioedema.

6.1.10 Marine Complex

The marine complex AminoMar® was originally identified from the fish- and protein-rich diet of the Scandinavian Inuits in the late 1980s. The commercial use of

Viviscal®, specifically for women with thinning hair, was pioneered at the Ablon Skin Institute Research Center in Manhattan Beach, CA. Viviscal® (Lifes2good, Inc., Chicago, IL) is a dietary supplement that contains as its primary active ingredient a combination of proteins, lipids, and glycosaminoglycans (GAGs) derived from a proprietary blend of shark and mollusk powder of marine origin. While there is a paucity of studies examining the dietary benefits of GAGs on hair growth, their impact on skin health and photoaging has been documented [41]. Since the early 1990s, studies have been performed with Viviscal® in promoting hair growth and reducing hair loss summarized in [42]. Ongoing studies are seeking to establish the molecular mechanism by which Viviscal® promotes hair growth.

6.2 Evidence Based

Although testing medical interventions for efficacy had existed since the time of Avicenna's "The Canon of Medicine" in the eleventh century [43], it was only in the twentieth century that this effort evolved to impact almost all fields of health care and policy. In 1967, American physician and mathematician Alvan R. Feinstein published his seminal work "Clinical Judgment" [44], which together with Archie Cochrane's celebrated book "Effectiveness and Efficiency" (1972) [45] led to an increasing acceptance of clinical epidemiology and controlled studies during the 1970s and 1980s and prepared the way for the institutional development of evidence-based medicine (EBM) in the 1990s. EBM seeks to assess the strength of the evidence of risks and benefits of diagnostic tests and treatments, using techniques from science, engineering, and statistics, such as the systematic review of medical literature, meta-analysis, risk-benefit analysis, and randomized controlled trials.

Ultimately, EBM aims for the ideal that healthcare professionals should make conscientious, explicit, and judicious use of the best available evidence gained from the scientific method to clinical decision-making [46].

As EBM guidelines on the treatment of hair loss are scarce, a European consensus group was constituted to develop guidelines for the treatment of the single most frequent cause of hair loss, male and female androgenetic alopecia. It originally conducted a systematic literature review in Medline, Embase, and Cochrane databases until August 2008. 1370 publications were found, 51 added by hand search. 85 publications fulfilled the following inclusion criteria for the guideline: prospective study with a number of patients ≥20 (no minimal patient number required in twin studies), and age ≥12 years, with confirmed diagnosis of androgenetic alopecia (diagnosis either clinically or by further diagnostic evaluations, e.g., trichogram, TrichoScan, biopsy). Objective outcome measure of efficacy described for drug therapy was mean change from baseline hair count in target area or measurement of hair growth/loss in target area by global photography [47, 48].

Not surprisingly, the review revealed excellent evidence levels for the therapeutic use of topical minoxidil and of oral finasteride, and insufficient and lacking evidence for a broad panel of miscellaneous treatments available claiming effectiveness for treatment of male or female androgenetic alopecia, including nutritionals (Table 6.1).

Nevertheless, besides an understanding of the pathologic dynamics of hair loss as they relate to a specific condition such as androgenetic alopecia, insight into a multitude of possible cause relationships underlying hair loss is a prerequisite for

Table 6.1 Overview of miscellaneous treatments with insufficient or lacking evidence for efficacy and proposed mechanisms of action in the treatment of hair loss (from [48])

Promotion of hair regrowth:	• Amino acids • Iron supplements in absence of deficiency • Vitamins (biotin, niacin derivates) • Proanthocyanidines • Millet seed (silic acid, aminoacids, vitamines, minerals) • Marine extract and silicea component • Chinese herbals • Ginkgo biloba • Aloe vera • Ginseng • Bergamot • Hibiscus • Sorphora • Caffeine • Melatonin • Retinoids • Ciclosporine • Electromagnetic/-static field • Low level laser
Improved perifollicular vascularisation:	• Prostaglandins (viprostol, latanoprost) • Aminexil • Glyceroloxyesters and silicium • Minerals • Niacin derivatives • Mesotherapy
DHT-inhibitory activity:	• Saw palmetto • β-sitosterol • Polysorbate 60 • Green tea • *Cimicifuga racemosa*
Anti-inflammatory activity:	• Ketoconazol • Zinc pyrithione • Corticosteroids
Improved hair nutrition:	• Vitamines (biotin, niacin derivates) • Trace elements (zinc, copper)
Others:	• Botulinum toxin

delivering appropriate patient care. It must be borne in mind that hair loss often does not result from a single cause effect, but from a combination of internal and external factors that need to be addressed simultaneously for success, such as smoking, nutritional factors, medications, inflammatory phenomena and scarring, age-related phenomena, and ultimately problems of comorbidities [49–51]. The scientific basis for such an approach is given, but there is need for controlled studies to establish increase in the efficacy of combination regimens including nutritional therapies [52].

Since an important commercial interest lies in the nutritional value of various vitamin and amino acid supplements, an important question that arises is whether increasing the content of an already adequate diet with specific amino acids, vitamins, and/or trace elements may further promote hair growth. Pharmacy aisles and Internet drugstores are full of nutritional supplements promising full, thick, luscious hair for prices that range from suspiciously cheap to dishearteningly exorbitant.

It would appear that unless hair loss is due to a specific nutritional deficiency, there is only so much that nutritional therapies can do to enhance hair growth and quality. However, there are internal and external factors, such as aging and oxidative stress, that influence hair health to such a degree that nutritional therapy can boost hair that is suffering from these problems.

Protein is the main component of hair accounting for between 65 and 95% of the hair by weight. The primary component of the hair fiber is keratin that is made from 18 amino acids (by alphabetical order: alanine, arginine, aspartic acid, cysteine, glutamic acid, glycine, histidine, isoleucine, leucine, lysine, methionine, phenylalanine, proline, serine, threonine, tryptophan, tyrosine, and valine). The most abundant of these is cysteine which gives the hair fiber much of its strength through the linking of the sulfur in cysteine molecules of adjacent keratin proteins together in disulfide bonds.

Ingesting keratin does not help hair growth, as the protein cannot be broken down and absorbed. Therefore, constituent amino acids from which the hair follicle can build up the keratin need to be consumed. Cysteine is catabolized in the gastrointestinal tract and blood plasma, while cystine travels safely through the gastrointestinal tract and blood plasma and is promptly reduced to two cysteine molecules upon cell entry. Originally, the role of cystine in the production of wool was investigated in the 1960s, and it was found that enrichment of even what appeared to be a normal diet with the sulfur-containing amino acids cystine and methionine increased wool production in sheep [53, 54].

The hair follicle exhibits a high rate of metabolism. As a group, B complex vitamins are important for metabolic functions and therefore required to utilize other nutrients like carbohydrate and amino acids (in alphabetical order): biotin (vitamin H), calcium pantothenate (B5), niacinamide (B3), folic acid, and vitamins B6 (pyridoxal phosphate) and B12 (cobalamin).

When considering which dietary supplements could be used for improving hair growth in humans, therefore cystine in combination with B complex vitamins or nutritional yeast, a rich natural source of amino acids and B complex vitamins was taken into consideration.

Starting in the early 1990s, studies on the effect of dietary supplements containing cystine, nutritional yeast, pantothenic acid (CYP complex), and thiamine were performed, showing improvements in the trichogram, in hair swelling as a criterion for hair quality, and in the tensile strength of the hair fiber [55, 56].

Eventually, Lengg et al. [57] performed a double-blind, placebo-controlled study in 30 otherwise healthy women suffering from telogen effluvium and demonstrated by means of the TrichoScan, a GCP-validated tool to measure hair growth [58] (Fig. 6.1a–m), that the CYP complex and thiamine-based dietary supplement increased the anagen hair rate within 6 months of treatment, while placebo did not (Fig. 6.1n).

Also, single studies with combinations of L-cystine with millet extract and pantothenic acid [59], and with low-dose retinol and gelatin [60], showed similar effect on anagen rates.

Ultimately, a meta-analysis of all clinical studies performed with the respective combination of cystine, yeast, and pantothenic acid CYP complex ($n = 180$) demonstrated its efficacy in improving anagen rates versus placebo (Fig. 6.2).

Finally, combining oral CYP and thiamine-based compound with topical minoxidil in the treatment of female androgenetic alopecia was speculated to add an additional benefit. Experiments with labeled thymidine indicated that minoxidil not only induced proliferation of hair epithelial cells near the base of mouse vibrissae follicles in organ culture, but also increased the incorporation of radiolabeled cysteine in the keratogenous zone of follicles [61]. The proof of concept for superiority of combination treatment with CYP complex versus minoxidil monotherapy of female androgenetic alopecia was presented on the occasion of the 8th World Congress for Hair Research, May 14–17, 2014, in Jeju Island, Korea: combined therapy resulted in statistically significant higher proportion of patients with normalized percentage of telogen hairs <15% within 4 months of treatment as compared with minoxidil monotherapy (60% versus 29%, $p = 0.03$).

Interestingly, an experiment performed on C57BL/6 mice who developed hair loss when exposed to cigarette smoke demonstrated that this effect could be prevented by the oral administration of N-acetylcysteine, an analogue and precursor of

Fig. 6.1 (a–m) The TrichoScan represents a method which combines epiluminescence microscopy with automatic digital image to analyze the biological parameters of hair growth: hair density (n/cm²), hair diameter (micrometer), and anagen/telogen ratio. (a–e) Clipping of hair in a defined area identified with a tattoo. (f–j) Dyeing of hair for measurement of hair density, hair diameter, and anagen and telogen rates. (k) Epiluminescence microscopic photography with the PhotoFinder. (l, m) Digital imaging with computer-assisted analysis of hair growth parameters: (l) before treatment (anagen rate: 65%), (m) after 6 months of treatment with CYP complex and thiamine-based dietary supplement (anagen rate: 82%). (n) Double-blinded, placebo-controlled study in healthy women with hair loss using oral combination of cystine, nutritional yeast, pantothenic acid (CYP complex), and thiamine: active compound (verum) led to statistically significant improvement and normalization of mean anagen hair rates within 6 months of treatment, while placebo did not. No placebo effect at 3 months (from Lengg N, Heidecker B, Seifert B, Trüeb RM. Dietary supplement increases anagen hair rate in women with telogen effluvium: results of a double-blind placebo-controlled trial. Therapy 4:59–6 (2007))

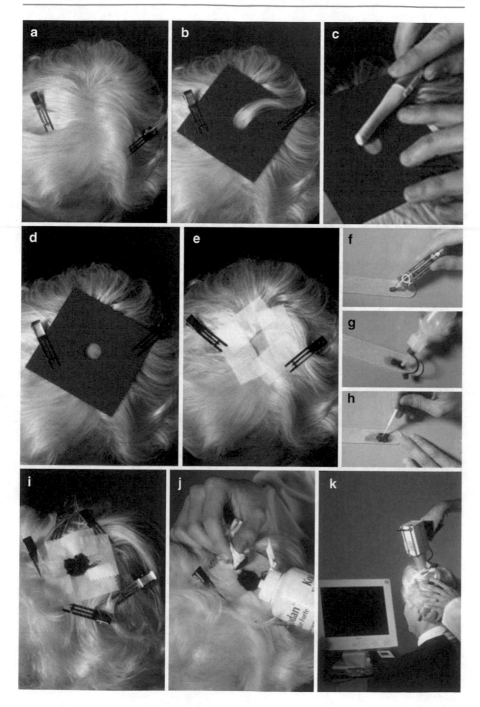

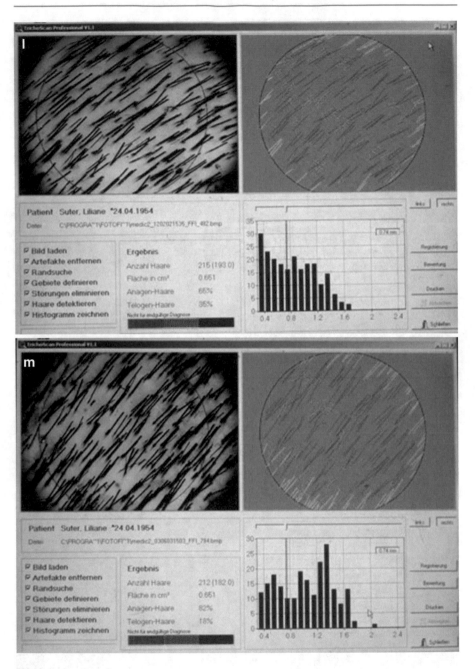

Fig. 6.1 (continued)

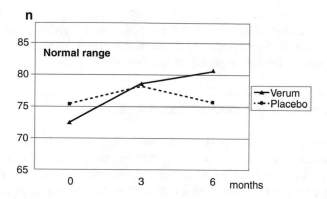

Fig. 6.1 (continued)

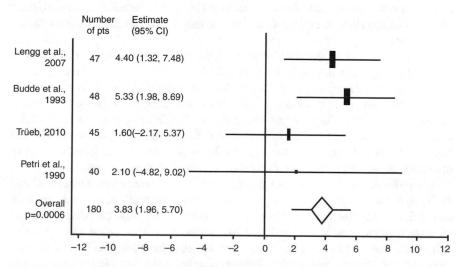

Fig. 6.2 Meta-analysis of clinical studies performed with oral combination of cystine, nutritional yeast, pantothenic acid (CYP complex), and thiamine (Pantogar®) ($n = 180$). Average difference between baseline and close-out anagen rates: verum vs. placebo: 3.83 absolute point improvement in anagen rates. Analysis was carried out using the full analysis set with a fixed-effect model, p-value from the test of overall difference between verum and placebo. Error bars represent standard error of the mean (presented as poster by Andreas Finner, MD, Berlin, Germany, at the 15th EHRS annual meeting, July 6–9, 2011, in Jerusalem, Israel, with permission)

cysteine and reduced glutathione, as well as cystine, the oxidized form of cysteine [62]. The effect was interpreted by the authors as to be possibly related to the glutathione-related detoxification system, an enzymatic antioxidant, while the hair papilla fibroblasts in androgenetic alopecia are understood to have a higher sensitivity to oxidative stress [63].

These observations are in line with the study of Lengg et al., who demonstrated in a regression analysis that efficacy of the combination of cystine, nutritional yeast, pantothenic acid (CYP complex), and thiamine in increasing anagen rates was independent of concomitant androgenetic alopecia or smoking [57].

6.3   From Chinese Medicine and Ayurveda

Finally, there are a number of botanicals with alleged anti-hair loss effects from both traditional Chinese medicine and Ayurvedic medicine (the literal meaning of Ayurveda is "life knowledge") [64]. In the early development of medicine, biologically active plants have played a vital role in providing remedies for pain and diseases. The Materia Medica of Traditional Chinese medicine, Ayurveda, and other systems from other cultures represent an important resource for the development of not only medicinal products, but also nutraceuticals and cosmetics. However, their claims must be critically evaluated in terms of modern-day requirements for safety and efficacy.

The doctrines of traditional Chinese medicine (TCM) are rooted in books such as the Yellow Emperor's Inner Canon (Huangdi Nei Jing), the oldest received work of Chinese medical theory compiled around the first century BC from shorter texts of different medical lineages, and later works. Written in the form of dialogues between the legendary Yellow Emperor and his ministers, it offers explanations on the relation between humans, their environment, and the cosmos; on the contents of the body; on human vitality and pathology; on the symptoms of illness; and on how to make diagnostic and therapeutic decisions in light of all these factors.

With a focus on the enormous Chinese market, pharmaceutical companies have explored the potentials for creating new drugs from the traditional remedies, with as-yet few successful results. Eventually, a "Nature" editorial described TCM as "fraught with pseudoscience," and said that the most obvious reason why it has not delivered many cures is that the majority of its treatments have no logical mechanism of action [65]. Indeed, modern investigative science has not found evidence for traditional Chinese concepts. The effectiveness of Chinese herbal medicine remains poorly researched [66], despite selected instances of systematic reviews published in the Cochrane Library that investigate the efficacy of TCM.

Nevertheless, Asia, Korea, China, and Japan have legally adopted the traditional Oriental medical system along with the Western system. A number of traditional herbal drugs including the polypharmacy type of prescription (combination of multiple herbs) are available and widely dispensed. This polypharmacy type of herbal therapy allegedly exhibits holistic effectiveness by exerting multitargeted effects. The Traditional Oriental Medicine Database (TradiMed 2000 DB) represents a database of traditional Oriental herbal therapy containing specific information such as formulae, chemical information on ingredients, botanical information on herbal materials, and a dictionary of disease classifications. Using the TradiMed 2000 DB, Chang form Seoul National University, Korea, identified more than a dozen herbs with antiaging effects used in traditional Oriental herbal therapy, of which *Polygonum multiflorum* (He Shou Wu) and *Ginseng Radix* (Ren Shen) probably represent the commercially most utilized in hair cosmetics, also on the contemporary Western market. However, the effective constituents of the traditional herbal remedies have not been fully elucidated, though there is a potential to study them systematically with respect to current research trends. As yet, most studies have been in cell cultures and animal models, and thus their relevance to human biology remains unknown.

6.3.1   He Shou Wu

He Shou Wu (*Polygonum multiflorum*, synonym: *Reynoutria multiflora*), also called Fo-Ti, is a species of flowering plant in the buckwheat family *Polygonaceae* native to central and southern China that is also called Chinese knotweed. It is listed in the Chinese Pharmacopoeia, and is one of the most popular traditional Chinese medicines. More than 100 chemical compounds have been isolated from *Polygonum multiflorum*, and the major components have been determined to be stilbenes, quinones, flavonoids, and others. He Shou Wu literally means "Mr. Ho's hair is black." The name refers to the legend of a 58-year-old man named Ho, whose gray hair returned to its black color after taking the herb. He also became more youthful and was able to father several children. Supposedly he lived to become 160, retaining his black hair.

Using a recombinant cell bioassay to measure estrogen bioactivity in herbs, Oerter Klein et al. [67] discovered estrogen activity in extracts of Fo-Ti. The preparations studied had estrogen activity equivalent to 1/300 the activity of 17-beta-estradiol. 2,3,5,4'-Tetrahydroxystilbene-2-O-β-D-glucoside (TSG) is the main component of *Polygonum multiflorum*; however, its role in hair regeneration has as yet not been established [68]. Finally, Sextius et al. [69] showed that *Polygonum multiflorum Radix* extract protects in vitro primary human foreskin melanocytes from the deleterious effects of H_2O_2 exposure, and improves pigmentation within ex vivo human hair follicles, providing in vitro mechanistic evidence for the effect of *Polygonum multiflorum Radix* extract in preventing oxidative stress-induced hair graying, in line with traditional He Shou Wu use.

With respect to menopause and hormonal replacement, the focus tends to be on the issues covered by the Women's Health Initiative [70]. Consequently, many women have become reluctant towards systemic estrogen substitution therapy, and the market for complementary/alternative therapies for hormone replacement has dramatically increased. Women are seeking more natural alternatives to treat menopause-associated issues. However, well-designed randomized clinical trials are lacking, as is the information on long-term safety concerns [71].

6.3.2   Panax Ginseng (Ren Shen)

Ginseng (Radix) is the root of plants of the genus *Panax*, such as Korean ginseng (*P. ginseng*), South China ginseng (*P. notoginseng*), and American ginseng (*P. quinquefolius*). The word "ginseng" derives from Chinese jîn-sim (人蔘). The first character 人 (Modern Standard Mandarin pronunciation: [[ɻə̌n]) means "person," and the second character 蔘 (shēn) "plant root" refers to the root's characteristic anthropomorphic shape (Fig. 6.3). The botanical genus name *Panax*, meaning "all-healing" in Greek, shares the same origin as "panacea," and was adopted for this genus by Carl Linnaeus (1707–1778, Swedish botanist, zoologist, and physician who formalized binomial nomenclature), who was aware of its wide use in Chinese medicine. And yet, there is no substantial evidence that ginseng is effective for treating any specific medical condition [72], and its use has not been approved by the U.S. Food and Drug Administration (as a prescription drug), although commercial ginseng is sold as a dietary supplement in over 35 countries.

One of the original historical texts referring to the use of ginseng as a medicinal herb was the Shen-Nung Pharmacopoeia, written in 196 AD. In his Compendium of Materia Medica (1596), Li Shizhen (1518–1593, Chinese scientific naturalist) described ginseng as a superior tonic. The herb was not used as a cure-all medicine, but rather as a tonic for patients with chronic conditions and those who were in convalescence [73]. The root is most often available in dried form, either whole or sliced.

Fig. 6.3 Panax ginseng. The ginseng root is among the most prized among traditional Chinese herbal remedies based upon a *similia similibus* type of selection for its anthropomorphic form (courtesy of Prof. Alexander Navarini, MD, PhD, Basel, Switzerland)

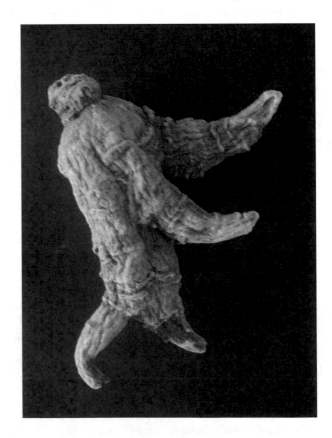

White ginseng is the fresh root which has been peeled and dried without being heated. Drying in the sun bleaches the root to its characteristic yellowish-white color (Fig. 6.3). White ginseng air-dried in the sun may contain less of the therapeutic constituents.

Red ginseng is peeled, heated through steaming at boiling temperature, and then dried. It has a reddish color. Red ginseng is less vulnerable to decay than white ginseng [74].

Ginseng leaf, although not as highly prized, is sometimes also used. Although the roots are used in traditional Chinese medicine, the leaves and stems contain larger quantities of the phytochemicals than the roots [75].

The long history of Ginseng use in traditional Chinese medicine has led to the study of the pharmacological effects of the ginseng compounds. The main active ingredients are ginsenosides and gintonin.

Ginsenosides or panaxosides compose a class of steroid glycosides and triterpene saponins found almost exclusively in the plant genus *Panax ginseng*. Primarily, the ginsenosides likely serve as mechanisms for plant defense. They are naturally bitter tasting and discourage insects and other animals from consuming the plant, and have been found to have both antimicrobial and antifungal properties. Studied in isolation, the ginsenosides exhibit a variety of subtle and difficult-to-characterize biological effects. Many studies suggest that ginsenosides have antioxidant properties. Ginsenosides have been observed to increase internal antioxidant enzymes and act as a free radical scavenger [76]. Based on their similarity to steroid hormones, some ginsenosides have also been shown to be partial agonists of steroid hormone receptors.

Gintonin is the non-saponin glycolipoprotein fraction isolated from ginseng. Lysophospholipid (LPA) receptors are the high-affinity and selective target receptor of gintonin. Gintonin allegedly shows in vivo anti-Alzheimer's efficacy through LPA receptor-mediated non-amyloidogenic pathway and alleviates cognitive functions in elderly human Alzheimer's disease patients [77, 78] through boosting of the hippocampal cholinergic system [79], hippocampal neurogenesis [80], and an anti-depression effect [81].

There has been accumulating evidence suggesting that ginseng may promote hair growth by enhancing proliferation of dermal papilla and preventing hair loss via modulation of various cell signaling pathways [82]. Choi [83] reviewed the molecular mechanisms and the hair growth potential of ginseng and its metabolites. While the role of 5α-reductase enzyme in the hair loss process of androgenetic alopecia is well understood, the emerging biological mechanisms underlying hair follicle proliferation and hair loss may unravel additional targets for designing therapeutics beyond the 5α-reductase inhibitors and minoxidil for the management of hair loss. These targets include WNT/Dickkopf homologue 1 (DKK1), sonic hedgehog (Shh), vascular endothelial growth factor (VEGF), transforming growth factor-beta (TGF-β), matrix metalloproteinases (MMPs), extracellular signal-regulated protein kinase (ERK), and Janus-activated kinase (JAK). Although individual ginsenosides are yet to be investigated for hair growth promotion in human clinical trials, there have been some preliminary studies documenting the potential of Korean red ginseng (KRG) in hair growth promotion.

Oh et al. [84] studied hair growth efficacy and safety of Korean red ginseng in combination with intralesional corticosteroid injection for alopecia areata in human subjects. Patients with alopecia areata were treated with intralesional corticosteroid with or without treatment with Korean red ginseng. Average hair density and hair thickness were significantly increased upon addition of Korean red ginseng with intralesional corticosteroid, suggesting that Korean red ginseng may be considered as a useful complementary supplement for increasing the efficacy of intralesional corticosteroid.

Kim et al. [85] reported the effectiveness of Korean red ginseng in increasing the thickness and density of hair in humans. Specifically, combination treatment with topical minoxidil and oral Korean red ginseng proved to be more effective than topical minoxidil treatment alone for promoting hair growth. Therefore, Korean red ginseng was again expected to be a helpful supplement in the treatment of hair loss [86].

Keum et al. [87] examined the potential of KRG in preventing premature hair follicle dystrophy using a human hair follicle organ culture model. According to this study, human occipital scalp skin specimens were obtained from patients undergoing hair transplantation surgery, and follicular keratinocyte cells (FKC) were cultured in vitro. Treatment of FKCs with 4-hydroxycyclophosphamide (4-HC), a metabolite of chemotherapeutic agent cyclophosphamide, attenuated human hair growth, induced premature catagen development, diminished proliferation, and stimulated apoptosis of hair matrix keratinocytes. Pretreatment with KRG protected against 4-HC-induced hair growth inhibition and premature catagen development partly by blocking 4-HC-induced p53 and Bax/Bcl2 expression.

Finally, Lee et al. [88] identified the gintonin-enriched fraction of Ginseng to promote hair growth in mice in terms of its lysophosphatidic acid receptor ligand activity.

True ginseng plants belong only to the genus *Panax*. Several other plants are sometimes referred to as ginseng, but they are from a different genus or even family. Siberian ginseng (*Eleutherococcus senticosus*) is in the same family, but not genus, as true ginseng. The active compounds in Siberian ginseng are eleutherosides, not ginsenosides. Instead of a fleshy root, Siberian ginseng has a woody root. Eleutheroside A is a saponin and sterol glycoside while other eleutherosides, such as eleutheroside B (syringin), are phenyl propanoid glycosides. There are no definite effects associated with these compounds.

6.3.3   Dong Quai

Dong quai (*Angelica sinensis*), also known as female ginseng, is a herb indigenous to China belonging to the family Apiaceae. The dried root of *A. sinensis* is commonly known as Chinese angelica and is widely used in Chinese traditional medicine in the belief that it benefits women's health [89]. Accordingly, dong quai

(當歸) means that a husband shall return to his wife, which implicitly relates to women's sexual health [90]. The plant's chemical constituents include phytosterols, polysaccharides, ligustilide, butylphthalide, cnidilide, isoenidilide, p-cymene, ferulate, and flavonoids [91].

Kim et al. [92] explored the hair growth effect and the mechanism of *A. sinensis* related to keratinocyte apoptosis-regression during catagen in mice, and found that *A. sinensis* acts through hair cycle pathways associated with apoptosis-mediated regression in catagen. C57BL/6 mice painted with a 70% ethanolic extract of *A. sinensis* showed hair regrowth associated with notably decreased apoptotic cells, along with a significant change in the expression of the respective apoptosis-associated proteins.

Other popular herbal remedies from TCM include Lingzhi (*Ganoderma lucidum*), *Gingko biloba*, and green tea (*Camellia sinensis*).

6.3.4   Lingzhi

The lingzhi mushroom (*Ganoderma lucidum*) is a polypore fungus (bracket fungus) belonging to the genus Ganoderma. In Japan, it is called the reishi mushroom. Its red-varnished, kidney-shaped cap and peripherally inserted stem give it a distinct fanlike appearance (Fig. 6.4a). When fresh, the lingzhi is soft, cork-like, and flat. It lacks gills on its underside, and instead releases its spores via fine pores. Lingzhi is the ancient "mushroom of immortality," revered in China for over 2000 years. Chinese texts have recorded medicinal uses of lingzhi for more than 2000 years. Since both Chinese ling and zhi have multiple meanings, lingzhi has diverse English

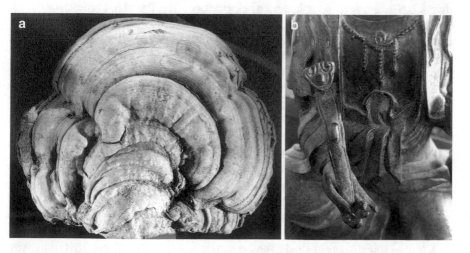

Fig. 6.4 (**a, b**) Lingzhi mushroom (*Ganoderma lucidum*). (**a**) Dried mushroom (private collection). (**b**) In Chinese art, the lingzhi symbolizes great health and longevity, and the goddess of healing Guanyin is sometimes depicted holding a lingzhi mushroom, here as a ruyi scepter with the head fashioned like a lingzhi mushroom (private collection)

translations. Renditions include "[zhi] possessed of soul power," "Herb of Spiritual Potency" or "Mushroom of Immortality," "Divine mushroom," "Magic Fungus," and "Marvelous Fungus" [93]. The Divine Farmer's Classic of Pharmaceutics (Shennong bencao jing) of c.200–250 CE characterizes the red chizhi, (丹芝; "cinnabar mushroom") as "bitter and balanced. It mainly treats binding in the chest, boosts the heart qi, supplements the center, sharpens the wits, and [causes people] not to forget [i.e., improves the memory]. Protracted taking may make the body light, prevent senility, and prolong life so as to make one an immortal" [94]. Stuart and Smith's classic study of Chinese herbology describes the zhi (芝) "in the classics as the plant of immortality, and it is therefore always considered to be a felicitous one. It is said to absorb the earthy vapors and to leave a heavenly atmosphere" [95]. In Chinese art, the stylized lingzhi pictogram is auspicious and symbolizes great health and longevity (Fig. 6.4b).

Ganoderma lucidum contains diverse phytochemicals, including triterpenes (ganoderic acids), which have a molecular structure similar to that of steroid hormones, polysaccharides (such as beta-glucan), coumarin, mannitol, and alkaloids [96]. Because of its bitter taste, lingzhi is traditionally prepared as a hot water extract product from thinly sliced or pulverized lingzhi added to the boiling water which is then reduced to a simmer, covered, and left for 2 h. Commercially manufactured and sold lingzhi is also processed into tablets or capsules to be directly ingested.

6.3.5   Gingko biloba

Also known as the maidenhair tree, *Gingko biloba* is the only living species in the division *Ginkgophyta*, with all others being extinct. It is found in fossils dating back 270 million years. Native to China, the tree was already cultivated early in human history. It has various uses as a source of food and in traditional medicine. Ginkgos are large trees, normally reaching a height of 20–35 m (66–115 ft), with some in China reaching over 50 m (160 ft). The leaves are unique among seed plants, being fan shaped with veins radiating out into the leaf blade, sometimes bifurcating, but never anastomosing to form a network. A combination of resistance to disease, insect-resistant wood, and ability to form aerial roots and sprouts makes ginkgos long-lived, with some specimens claimed to be more than 2500 years old. In 2020, a study in China of gingko trees up to 667 years old showed little effects of aging, finding that the trees continued to grow with age and displayed no genetic evidence of senescence [97]. Extreme examples of the ginkgo's tenacity may be seen in Hiroshima, Japan, where six trees growing between 1 and 2 km (0.62–1.24 mi) from the 1945 atom bomb explosion were among the few living things in the area to survive the blast.

Chinese scientists published a draft genome of Ginkgo biloba in 2016 [98]. The tree has a large genome of 10.6 billion DNA nucleobase "letters" (the human genome has three billion) and about 41,840 predicted genes which enable a considerable number of antibacterial and chemical defense mechanisms.

Extracts of ginkgo leaves contain phenolic acids; proanthocyanidins; flavonoid glycosides, such as myricetin, kaempferol, isorhamnetin, and quercetin; and the terpene trilactones, ginkgolides, and bilobalides. The leaves also contain unique ginkgo biflavones, as well as alkylphenols and polyprenols [99].

The first use of gingko as a medicine was recorded in the late fifteenth century in China, and among Western countries, its first registered medicinal use was in Germany in 1965. It has been used in the traditional treatment of Alzheimer's disease [100]. Despite its widespread and popular use, controlled studies do not support the extract's efficacy for most of the indicated conditions [101].

One Japanese study of 1993 [102] investigated the effects of a 70% ethanolic extract from leaves of Ginkgo biloba (GBE) on hair regrowth in normal and high butter diet-pretreated C3H strain mice which were shaved on the back. GBE showed a promoting effect on the hair regrowth. GBE had inhibitory effects on blood platelet aggregation, thrombin activity, and fibrinolysis. GBE inhibited the increase of serum and triglyceride level in high-cholesterol-diet-treated rats. These results suggested that GBE promotes hair regrowth via increase of blood flow to the skin. As yet, no clinical study on its efficacy in treating hair loss in humans has been conducted.

6.3.6   Green Tea

Green tea is made from *Camellia sinensis* leaves and buds that have not undergone the same withering and oxidation process (fermentation) used to make the oolong teas and black teas. *Camellia sinensis* is a species of evergreen shrubs in the flowering plant family *Theaceae*. White tea, yellow tea, green tea, oolong, dark tea (including pu-erh tea), and black tea are all harvested from one or the other, but are processed differently to attain varying levels of oxidation. Green tea originated in China, and its consumption has its legendary origins in China during the reign of the legendary Emperor Shennong. A book written by Lu Yu (733–804, Chinese tea master and writer) during the Tang dynasty (618–907 AD), *The Classic of Tea*, is considered important in green tea history. Loose leaf green tea has been the most popular form of tea in China since at least the Southern Song dynasty (1127–1279). While Chinese green tea was originally steamed, as still in Japan, during the Ming dynasty (1368–1644) it was processed by being pan-fired in a dry wok. The *Kissa Yojoki* (Book of Tea), written in 1211 by Eisai (1141–1215), a Japanese Zen Buddhist priest, credited with bringing green tea from China to Japan, describes how drinking green tea may affect the vital organs. The generic name *Camellia* is taken from the Latinized name of Rev. Georg Kamel, SJ (1661–1706), a Jesuit lay brother, pharmacist, and missionary to the Philippines. Carl Linnaeus chose his name in 1753 for the genus to honor Kamel's contributions to botany, although Kamel neither discovered nor named this plant.

Regular green tea is 99.9% water, provides 1 calorie per 100 mL serving, and is devoid of significant nutrient content. It contains phytochemicals, such as polyphenols and caffeine. The polyphenols found in green tea include epigallocatechin gallate (EGCG), epicatechin gallate, epicatechins, and flavanols. Other components include three kinds of flavonoids: kaempferol, quercetin, and myricetin. The mean content of flavonoids and catechins in a cup of green tea is higher than that in the same volume of other food and drink items that are traditionally considered to promote health, and yet human clinical research has not provided conclusive evidence of any significant health effects from regular green tea consumption. Although green tea may enhance mental alertness due to the caffeine, there is only weak and inconclusive evidence that green tea has any effect on the risk of cancer, specifically stomach cancer [103], and non-melanoma skin cancers [104], or cardiovascular diseases [105], and there is no evidence that it benefits weight loss [106].

Studies on the cosmetic applications of plant extracts have increasingly found the attention of the scientific community in view of a current trend to natural treatments in skin and hair care. Specifically, green tea, due to its rich composition and complex biological actions, has gained an important role among both dietary supplements and cosmetic applications. Accordingly, cosmetic preparations containing green tea extracts have been taken into consideration for androgenetic alopecia and hair loss, regardless of gender. In several studies tea polyphenols, essential oils, and caffeine present in tea plant leaves inhibit the activity of 5α-reductase, which results in a decreased dihydrotestosterone formation [107]. The former compounds were also found to stimulate hair roots and extend the hair growth phase (anagen phase) [108]. Therefore, constituents of green tea have become ingredients of interest for hair and scalp care, particularly for individuals having excessive greasy hair [109].

Fischer et al. [110] demonstrated that external application of caffeine in a concentration of 0.001% and 0.005% led to a significant stimulation of human hair follicle growth in an in vitro study. They concluded that caffeine may reduce smooth muscle tension near the hair follicle, thereby increasing the delivery of nutrients through the microcirculation of hair follicle papillae.

Kwon et al. [111] evaluated the efficacy of one of the main catechins present in green tea extract—EGCG—on human hair growth. The study revealed that EGCG stimulated hair growth in hair follicle ex vivo culture and proliferation of cultured human dermal papilla cells. Moreover, it was shown that epigallocatechin-3-gallate promoted hair growth in vivo dermal papillae of human scalps. The growth stimulation of DPCs by EGCG in vitro may be mediated through the upregulations of phosphorylated Erk and Akt and by an increase in the ratio of Bcl-2/Bax. Similar results were also obtained in in vivo dermal papillae of human scalps. It was concluded that EGCG stimulates hair growth through dual proliferative and anti-apoptotic effect.

Kim et al. [112] examined the usefulness of apoptotic fragment assay for investigating the radiation response of hair follicles and evaluating radioprotective agents in mice. The extent of changes following 100 cGy (1000 cGy/min) irradiation of mice was studied at 0, 2, 4, 8, 12, 16, or 20 h after exposure. The maximal frequency was found 12 h after exposure. The mice that received 50, 100, 200, 400, or 800 cGy of gamma rays were examined 12 h after irradiation. Measurements performed after gamma-ray irradiation showed a dose-related increase in apoptotic cells in each mouse studied. The frequency of radiation (100 cGy)-induced apoptosis in hair follicles was reduced by pretreatment with green tea.

Finally, green tea hair tonics were closed-patch tested and clinically evaluated in 20 volunteers for 28 days by using a Sebumeter®. Hair tonic base with glycerin and butylene glycol (total 4%) incorporated with green tea extract gained the highest consumers' preference. All of the products were stable and none caused skin irritation. Green tea hair tonic (2%) significantly ($p \leq 0.024$) lowered scalp sebum for 21 and 28 days following the application, suggesting that this topical therapy of scalp greasiness is safe and efficient [113].

In summary, the abovementioned experiments point to a potential practical usefulness of green tea extract in formulating cosmetics, which improve hair growth and condition.

6.3.7   Shou Wu Chih

Shou Wu Chih is a Chinese patent medicine containing *Polygonum multiflorum, Angelica sinensis,* and other herbal ingredients that is reputed to act as a tonic and to turn gray hair black. It is a liquid tonic formula for men and women sold in glass bottles produced in Guangzhou, Guangdong, China, under the brand name Yang Cheng, and exported to other nations, including the United States. It is claimed by the manufacturers that it increases the energy level and it tonifies, warms, and invigorates the blood; nourishes the liver and kidneys (and hence the hair which is connected to the kidneys in traditional Chinese medicine); and benefits the eyes. It is composed of *Polygonum multiflorum* (25%), *Angelica sinensis* (25%), *Polygonatum sibiricum* (20%), *Rehmannia glutinosa* (10%), *Ligusticum wallichii* (10%), *Angelica glabra Makino* (7%), *Villous amomum,* a type of cardamom (2%), and clove (1%).

In a study of 5α-reductase inhibitory activities of several traditional Chinese herbs, extract of *Ganoderma lucidum, Polygonum multiflorum, Cacumen platycladi* (Ce Bai Ye), and *Cynomorium songaricum* (Suoyang) tested positive. In addition, *Cacumen platycladi* extract demonstrated hair growth-promoting activity in the in vivo androgen-sensitive mouse model via inhibiting the 5α-reductase activity, decreasing dihydrotestosterone levels, and in turn suppressing the expression of 5α-reductase [114].

6.3.8   Ayurveda

Ayurveda is a system of medicine from the Indian subcontinent with its historical roots dating back to 6000 BC when it originated as an oral tradition. The first recorded medical texts of Ayurveda evolved from the Vedas. In the Atharva Veda, first written mention is made of diseases and their treatments. Later, from the sixth century BC to the seventh century AD there was a systematic development of the science in the so-called Samhita period, during which a number of classical works with evidence of an organized medical care were produced by several authors. After the eighth century AD no book of distinction was written, and the literature from then on up to the sixteenth century consisted mainly of commentaries on the original texts [115].

Ayurveda is one of the few systems of medicine developed in ancient times that is still practiced today. All early societies have had collections of remedies for common conditions that evolved through trial and error, accident, or inspiration; were purely empirical; and were not based on any logical understanding. As such, Ayurveda is prone to the criticism that its conceptual basis is obsolete, and that its contemporary practitioners have not taken account of the developments of modern medicine. During the period of colonial British rule of India (1793–1947), the practice of Ayurveda was neglected by the British Indian Government, in favor of Western medicine. Only after Indian independence, there was again focus on Ayurveda and other traditional medical systems. Today, Ayurveda is regarded as part of the Indian national healthcare system, with state hospitals for Ayurveda established across the country.

Ayurvedic doctors regard physical existence, mental existence, and personality as their own units, with each being able to influence the others. This is a holistic approach that is fundamental to Ayurveda. Contemporary Ayurveda tends to stress attaining vitality by building a healthy metabolic system. Ayurveda follows the concept that natural cycles, such as waking, sleeping, working, and meditation, are important for health. Hygiene, including regular bathing, cleaning of teeth, tongue scraping, skin care, and eye washing, is also of central importance. Ultimately globalized in countries beyond India, Ayurvedic therapies have become part of general wellness programs, and of alternative medical practice.

Ayurvedic therapies are typically based on complex herbal compounds, minerals, and metal substances. Plant-based treatments in Ayurveda may be derived from roots, leaves, fruits, bark, or seeds. In the nineteenth century, William Dymock and co-authors [116] summarized hundreds of plant-derived medicines along with their uses, microscopic structure, chemical composition, toxicology, prevalent myths and stories, and relation to commerce in British India. Animal products used in Ayurveda include milk, bones, and gallstones. In addition, fats are prescribed both for consumption and for external use. Consumption of minerals, including sulfur, arsenic, lead, copper sulfate, and gold, is traditionally also prescribed.

Many of the medicinal plants have come under scientific scrutiny starting in the middle of the nineteenth century, and some have even been proven to be pharmacologically effective, such as *Psoralea corylifolia* (antileucoderma), *Rauwolfia serpentina* (antihypertensive), *Commiphora wightii* (hypolipidemic), *Boswellia serrata* (anti-inflammatory), and *Curcuma longa* (anti-inflammatory) [117]. Nevertheless, for most others there is no scientific evidence that any are effective as currently practiced both in India and in the Western world. In India, research in Ayurveda is undertaken by the Ministry of AYUSH, an abbreviation for the Department of Ayurveda, Yoga and Naturopathy, Unani, Siddha, and Homoeopathy, through a national network of research institutes [118]. The Indian Government supports research and teaching in Ayurveda, and helps to institutionalize traditional medicine so that it can be studied in major agglomerations of India. Starting in the 1960s,

Ayurveda has been advertised as an alternative medicine in the Western world. Due to different laws and medical regulations in the rest of the world, the unregulated practice and commercialization of Ayurveda have raised ethical and legal issues.

A number of Indian medicinal plants have been recommended in the Ayurvedic system for promoting hair growth. Hair is a powerful metaphor in Hindu mythology. Tracing back the importance and significance of human hair to the dawn of civilization on the Indian subcontinent, we find that all Vedic gods, Shiva (the destroyer or transformer), Vishnu (the preserver), and Brahma (the creator), are depicted with long hair. The same is true of the Hindu avatars (incarnations of deities), Rama and Krishna, the epic heroes of the Ramayana and the Mahabharata (and Bhagavad Gita) [119]. Hair was not merely an organ of attraction and look, but was also important socially. Specifically, scanty hair was considered as a setback in both the male and the female. In the Rigveda, a woman prays for the growth of hair on her body as well as on her father''s scalp:

> *"imāni trīṇi viṣṭapā tānīndra bi rohaya śirastatasyorbarāmādidaṃ mā upodare.*
> *asau ca yā na urbarādimāṃ tanwaṃ mama atho tatasya yacchirah sarva tā romasā kr̥dhi."*
> [5]O Indra, cause to sprout again three places, these which I declare,– My father's head, his cultured field, and this the part below my waist.
> [6]Make all of these grow crops of hair, you cultivated field of ours, my body, and my father's head." (R̥igveda. VIII.80.5, 6).

Originally, the research division of Hindustan Lever (Mumbai, India) had devised a system for screening plant extracts that may promote hair growth based on the premise that transport of nutrients to the hair papilla would be facilitated by strengthening the hair vascular system. For this purpose, the chicken chorioallantoic membrane assay was developed, a model for angiogenesis. The presumption was that if any of the traditional plants promoted angiogenesis, this would aid blood supply to the hair papilla. Among the botanicals with positive results in the assay were *Hedychium spicatum* (spiked ginger lily), *Hemidesmus indicus* (Indian sarsaparilla), *Nardostachys jatamansi* (spikenard), and *Saussurea lappa* (Kuth root) [117].

With expansion of knowledge on the pathologic dynamics of hair loss on the biochemical and cellular levels, other mechanisms of action have come into the focus of the more modern in vitro efficacy assessments, such as inflammation, apoptosis, oxidative stress, and 5α-reductase activity, culminating in the in vivo efficacy assessments in animal models.

Examples are the study of the effect of *Cuscuta reflexa Roxb* (giant dodder) on androgen-induced alopecia in albino mice [120]; of hair growth-promoting activity of *Eclipta alba* (false daisy) in male albino rats [121] and in pigmented C57/BL6 mice [122]; and of the development and evaluation of a polyherbal formulation of the traditionally acclaimed herbs for hair growth promotion, *Cuscuta reflexa (Roxb.)*, *Citrullus colocynthis (Schrad.)* (Colocynth), and *Eclipta alba (Hassk.)*, in rats [123].

As yet, the respective clinical studies on hair growth and shedding have not been performed in humans. The potential of Ayurvedic medicine needs to be explored further with modern scientific validation approaches for better therapeutic leads and global acceptance. Therapeutic efficacy of Ayurvedic herbs may be enhanced with high quality and proper standardization of products, which is achieved by identity, purity, safety, drug content, and physical and biological properties [124].

References

1. Rautiainen S, Manson JE, Lichtenstein AH, Sesso HD. Dietary supplements and disease prevention: a global overview. Nat Rev Endocrinol. 2016;12:407–20.
2. Marra MV, Boyar AP. Position of the American Dietetic Association: nutrient supplementation. J Am Diet Assoc. 2009;109:2073–85.
3. Rinaldi F, Marzani B, Pinto D, Ramot Y. A spermidine-based nutritional supplement prolongs the anagen phase of hair follicles in humans: a randomized, placebo-controlled, double-blind study. Dermatol Pract Concept. 2017;7:17–21.
4. Cherfas J. Millet: how a trendy ancient grain turned nomads into farmers. National Public Radio. The Salt; 2015. Accessed 4 May 2018.
5. Keophiphath M, Courbière C, Manzato L, Lamour I, Gaillard E. Miliacin encapsulated by polar lipids stimulates cell proliferation in hair bulb and improves telogen effluvium in women. J Cosmet Dermatol. 2020;19:485–93.
6. Weber G, Adamczyk A, Freytag S. Treatment of acne with a yeast preparation [Article in German]. Fortschr Med. 1989;107:563–6.
7. Oesser S, Adam M, Babel W, Seifert J. Oral administration of 14C labelled gelatine hydrolysate leads to an accumulation of radioactivity in cartilage of mice (C57/BL). J Nutr. 1999;129:1891–5.
8. Iwai K, Hasegawa T, Taguchi Y, Morimatsu F, Sato K, Nakamura Y, Higashi A, Kido Y, Nakabo Y, Ohtsuki K. Identification of food-derived collagen peptides in human blood after oral ingestion of gelatine hydrolysates. J Agric Food Chem. 2005;53:6531–6.
9. Matsuda N, Koyama Y, Hosaka Y, Ueda H, Watanabe T, Araya T, Irie S, Takehana K. Effects of ingestion of collagen peptide on collagen fibrils and glycosaminoglycans in the dermis. J Nutr Sci Vitaminol. 2006;52:211–5.
10. Postlethwaite AE, Seyer JM, Kang AH. Chemotactic attraction of human fibroblasts to type I, II, and III collagens and collagen-derived peptides. Proc Natl Acad Sci U S A. 1978;75:871–5.
11. Shigemura Y, Iwai K, Morimatsu F, Iwamoto T, Mori T, Oda C, Taira T, Park EY, Nakamura Y, Sato K. Effect of prolyl-hydroxyproline (Pro-Hyp), a food-derived collagen peptide in human blood, on growth of fibroblasts from mouse skin. J Agric Food Chem. 2009;57:444–9.
12. Patiri C. Experience with gelatin treatment of nail growth disorders [Article in German]. Z Haut Geschlechtskr. 1971;46:523–6.
13. Zohary D, Hopf M, Weiss E. Domestication of plants in the old world: the origin and spread of domesticated plants in southwest Asia, Europe, and the Mediterranean Basin. 4th ed. New York: Oxford University Press; 2012. p. 122.
14. Betty R. The Many healing virtues of fenugreek. Spice India. 2008:17–9.
15. Ahmada A, Alghamdia S, Mahmood K, Afzal M. Fenugreek a multipurpose crop: potentialities and improvements. Saudi J Biol Sci. 2016;23:300–10.
16. Curry A. A 9,000-year love affair. Natl Geogr. 2010;231:46.
17. Mansoori A, Hosseini S, Zilaee M, Hormoznejad R, Fathi M. Effect of fenugreek extract supplement on testosterone levels in male: a meta-analysis of clinical trials. Phytother Res. 2020;34:1550–5. [Online ahead of print].
18. Schulz C, Bielfeldt S, Reimann J. Fenugreek + micronutrients: efficacy of a food supplement against hair loss. Cosmetic Med. 2006;27:1430–4031.
19. Nguyen SM, Ko NK, Sattar AS, Ipek EG, Ali S. Pulmonary embolism secondary to testosterone-enhancing herbal supplement use. Cureus. 2017;9:e1545.

20. Ouzir M, El Bairi K, Amzazi S. Toxicological properties of fenugreek (Trigonella foenum graecum). Food Chem Toxicol. 2016;96:145–54.
21. Fenugreek. National Center for Complementary and Integrative Health; 2016. Accessed 6 Feb 2017.
22. Rossi A, Mari E, Scarno M, Garelli V, Maxia C, Scali E, Iorio A, Carlesimo M. Comparitive effectiveness of finasteride vs Serenoa repens in male androgenetic alopecia: a two-year study. Int J Immunopathol Pharmacol. 2012;25:1167–73.
23. Saw Palmetto. Natural standard: the authority on integrative medicine. Natural Standard Accessed 29 Oct 2014
24. Cheema P, El-Mefty O, Jazieh AR. Intraoperative haemorrhage associated with the use of extract of Saw Palmetto herb: a case report and review of literature. J Intern Med. 2001;250:167–9.
25. Leach MJ, Moore V. Black cohosh (Cimicifuga spp.) for menopausal symptoms. Cochrane Database Syst Rev. 2012;9:CD007244.
26. Viereck V, Emons G, Wuttke W. Black cohosh: just another phytoestrogen? Trends Endocrinol Metab. 2005;16:214–21.
27. Nuntanakorn P, Jiang B, Yang H, Cervantes-Cervantes M, Kronenberg F, Kennelly EJ. Analysis of polyphenolic compounds and radical scavenging activity of four American Actaea species. Phytochem Anal. 2007;18:219–28.
28. Henneicke-von Zepelin HH. 60 years of Cimicifuga racemosa medicinal products: clinical research milestones, current study findings and current development. Wien Med Wochenschr. 2017;167:147–59.
29. Mirkin G. Estrogen in yams. JAMA. 1991;265:912.
30. Tada Y, Kanda N, Haratake A, Tobiishi M, Uchiwa H, Watanabe S. Novel effects of diosgenin on skin aging. Steroids. 2009;74:504–11.
31. Thompson LU, Boucher BA, Liu Z, Cotterchio M, Kreiger N. Phytoestrogen content of foods consumed in Canada, including isoflavones, lignans, and coumestan. Nutr Cancer. 2006;54:184–201.
32. Soy Isoflavones. Micronutrient Information Center, Linus Pauling Institute, Oregon State University, Corvallis; 2016. Accessed 23 May 2016.
33. Huang ZR, Hung CF, Lin YK, Fang JY. In vitro and in vivo evaluation of topical delivery and potential dermal use of soy isoflavones genistein and daidzein. Int J Pharm. 2008;364:36–44.
34. Lai CH, Chu NF, Chang CW, Wang SL, Yang HC, Chu CM, Chang CT, Lin MH, Chien WC, Su SL, Chou YC, Chen KH, Wang WM, Liou SH. Androgenic alopecia is associated with less dietary soy, lower [corrected] blood vanadium and rs1160312 1 polymorphism in Taiwanese communities. PLoS One. 2013;8:e79789.
35. Draelos Z, Blair R, Tabor A. Oral soy supplementation and dermatology. Cosmet Dermatol. 2007;20:202–4.
36. Rüfer CE, Kulling SE. Antioxidant activity of isoflavones and their major metabolites using different in vitro assays. J Agric Food Chem. 2006;54:2926–31.
37. Trompezinski S, Denis A, Schmitt D, Viac J. Comparative effects of polyphenols from green tea (EGCG) and soybean (genistein) on VEGF and IL-8 release from normal human keratinocytes stimulated with the proinflammatory cytokine TNFalpha. Arch Dermatol Res. 2003;295:112–6.
38. Liu Z, Lu Y, Lebwohl M, Wei H. PUVA (8-methoxy-psoralen plus ultraviolet A) induces the formation of 8-hydroxy-2′-deoxyguanosine and DNA fragmentation in calf thymus DNA and human epidermoid carcinoma cells. Free Radic Biol Med. 1999;27:127–33.
39. Kähäri VM, Saarialho-Kere U. Matrix metalloproteinases in skin. Exp Dermatol. 1997;6:199–213.
40. Südel KM, Venzke K, Mielke H, Breitenbach U, Mundt C, Jaspers S, Koop U, Sauermann K, Knussman-Hartig E, Moll I, Gercken G, Young AR, Stäb F, Wenck H, Gallinat S. Novel aspects of intrinsic and extrinsic aging of human skin: beneficial effects of soy extract. Photochem Photobiol. 2005;81:581–7.

41. Di Cerbo A, Laurino C, Palmieri B, Iannitti T. A dietary supplement improves facial photoaging and skin sebum, hydration and tonicity modulating serum fibronectin, neutrophil elastase 2, hyaluronic acid and carbonylated proteins. J Photochem Photobiol B. 2015;144:94–103.

42. Hornfeldt CS, Holland M, Bucay VW, Roberts WE, Waldorf HA, Dayan SH. The safety and efficacy of a sustainable marine extract for the treatment of thinning hair: a summary of new clinical research and results from a panel discussion on the problem of thinning hair and current treatments. J Drugs Dermatol. 2015;14:s15–22.

43. Akhondzadeh S. Avicenna and evidence based medicine. Avicenna J Med Biotechnol. 2014;6:1–2.

44. Feinstein AR. Clinical judgement. Philadelphia: Williams & Wilkins; 1967.

45. Cochrane AL. Effectiveness and efficiency: random reflections on health services. London: Nuffield Provincial Hospitals Trust; 1972.

46. Sackett DL, Rosenberg WM, Gray JA, Haynes RB, Richardson WS. Evidence based medicine: what it is and what it isn't. BMJ. 1996;312:71–2.

47. Blumeyer A, Tosti A, Messenger A, et al. Evidence-based (S3) guideline for the treatment of androgenetic alopecia in women and in men. J Dtsch Dermatol Ges. 2011;9(Suppl. 6):S1–S57.

48. Kanti V, Messenger A, Dobos G, Reygagne P, Finner A, Blumeyer A, Trakatelli M, Tosti A, Del Marmol V, Piraccini BM, Nast A, Blume-Peytavi U. Evidence-based (S3) guideline for the treatment of androgenetic alopecia in women and in men—short version. J Eur Acad Dermatol Venereol. 2018;32:11–22.

49. Van Weel C, Schellevis FG. Comorbidity and guidelines: conflicting interests. Lancet. 2006;367:550–1.

50. Mangin D, Heath I, Jamoulle M. Beyond diagnosis: rising to the multimorbidity challenge. BMJ. 2012;344:e3526.

51. Jakovljević M, Ostojić L. Comorbidity and multimorbidity in medicine today: challenges and opportunities for bringing separated branches of medicine closer to each other. Psychiatr Danub. 2013;25(Suppl 1):18–28.

52. Rajput RJ. Controversy: is there a role for adjuvants in the management of male pattern hair loss? J Cutan Aesthet Surg. 2010;3:82–6.

53. Gillespie JM, Reis PJ. Dietary regulated biosynthesis of high-sulfur wool proteins. Biochem J. 1966;98:669–77.

54. Reis PJ, Tunks DA, Sharry LF. Plasma amino acid patterns in sheep receiving abomasal infusions of methionine and cystine. Aust J Biol Sci. 1973;26:635–44.

55. Petri H, Perchalla P, Tronnier H. Die Wirksamkeit einer medikamentösen Therapie bei Haarstrukturschäden und diffusen Effluvien—vergleichende Doppelblindstudie. Schweiz Rundsch Med Prax. 1990;79:1457–62.

56. Budde J, Tronnier H, Rahlfs VW, Frei-Kleiner S. Systemische Therapie von diffusem Effluvium und Haarstrukturschäden. Hautarzt. 1993;44:380–4.

57. Lengg N, Heidecker B, Seifert B, Trüeb RM. Dietary supplement increases anagen hair rate in women with telogen effluvium: results of a double-blind placebo-controlled trial. Therapy. 2007;4:59–6.

58. Hoffmann R. TrichoScan, a GCP-validated tool to measure hair growth. J Eur Acad Dermatol Venereol. 2008;22(1):132–4.

59. Gehring W, Gloor M. Das Phototrichogramm als Verfahren zur Beurteilung haarwachstumsfördernder Präparate am Beispiel einer Kombination von Hirsefruchtextrakt, L-Cystin und Calciumpanthotenat. Zeitschrift für Hautkrankheiten H+G. 2000;7(/8):419–23.

60. Hertel H, Gollnick H, Matthies C, Baumann I, Orfanos CE. [Low dosage retinol and L-cystine combination improve alopecia of the diffuse type following long-term oral administration]. [Article in German]. Hautarzt. 1989;40:490–5.

61. Buhl AE, Waldon DJ, Kawabe TT, Holland JM. Minoxidil stimulates mouse vibrissae follicles in organ culture. J Invest Dermatol. 1989;92:315–20.

62. D'Agostini F, Fiallo P, Pennisi TM, De Flora S. Chemoprevention of smoke-induced alopecia in mice by oral administration of L-cystine and vitamin B6. J Dermatol Sci. 2007;46:189–98.

63. Upton JH, Hannen RF, Bahta AW, Farjo N, Farjo B, Philpott MP. Oxidative stress-associated senescence in dermal papilla cells of men with androgenetic alopecia. J Invest Dermatol. 2015;135:1244–52.
64. Thas JJ. Siddha medicine—background and principles and the application for skin diseases. Clin Dermatol. 2008;26:62–78.
65. [No authors listed] Hard to swallow. Nature 2007;448: 105–106.
66. Shang A, Huwiler K, Nartey L, Jüni P, Egge M. Placebo-controlled trials of Chinese herbal medicine and conventional medicine comparative study. Int J Epidemiol. 2007;36:1086–92.
67. Oerter Klein K, Janfaza M, Wong JA, Chang RJ. Estrogen bioactivity in Fo-Ti and other herbs used for their estrogen-like effects as determined by a recombinant cell bioassay. J Clin Endocrinol Metabol. 2003;88:4077–9.
68. Chen L, Duan H, Xie F, Gao Z, Wu X, Chen F, Wu W. Tetrahydroxystilbene glucoside effectively prevents apoptosis induced hair loss. Biomed Res Int. 2018;2:1380146.
69. Sextius P, Betts R, Benkhalifa I, Commo S, Eilstein J, Massironi M, Wang P, Michelet JF, Qiu J, Tan X, Jeulin S. Polygonum multiflorum Radix extract protects human foreskin melanocytes from oxidative stress in vitro and potentiates hair follicle pigmentation ex vivo. Int J Cosmet Sci. 2017;39:419–25.
70. Rossouw JE, Anderson GL, Prentice RL, et al. Risks and benefits of estrogen plus progestin in healthy postmenopausal women: principal results from the Women's Health Initiative randomized controlled trial. JAMA. 2002;288:321–33.
71. Russell L, Hicks GS, Low AK, Shepherd JM, Brown CA. Phytoestrogens: a viable option? Am J Med Sci. 2002;324:185–8.
72. Asian ginseng. National Center for Complementary and Integrative Health, US National Institutes of Health, Bethesda, MD; September 2016. Accessed 10 Feb 2017.
73. Mahady GB, Fong HS, Farnsworth NR. Botanical dietary supplements. Boca Raton: CRC Press; 2001. p. 207–15.
74. Fulder S. The book of ginseng. 2nd ed. Rochester, VT: Healing Arts Press; 1993. p. 300.
75. Wang H, Peng D, Xie J. Ginseng leaf-stem: bioactive constituents and pharmacological functions. Chin Med. 2009;4(20):20.
76. Lü JM, Yao Q, Chen C. Ginseng compounds: an update on their molecular mechanisms and medical applications. Curr Vasc Pharmacol. 2009;7:293–302.
77. Hwang SH, Shin EJ, Shin TJ, Lee BH, Choi SH, Kang J, Kim HJ, Kwon SH, Jang CG, Lee JH, Kim HC, Nah SY. Gintonin, a ginseng-derived lysophosphatidic acid receptor ligand, attenuates Alzheimer's disease-related neuropathies: involvement of non-amyloidogenic processing. J Alzheimers Dis. 2012;31:207–23.
78. Moon J, Choi SH, Shim JY, Park HJ, Oh MJ, Kim M, Nah SY. Gintonin administration is safe and potentially beneficial in cognitively impaired elderly. Alzheimer Dis Assoc Disord. 2017;32:85–7.
79. Kim HJ, Shin EJ, Lee BH, Choi SH, Jung SW, Cho IH, Hwang SH, Kim JY, Han JS, Chung C, Jang CG, Rhim H, Kim HC, Nah SY. Oral administration of gintonin attenuates cholinergic impairments by scopolamine, amyloid-β protein, and mouse model of Alzheimer's disease. Mol Cells. 2015;38:796–805.
80. Kim HJ, Kim DJ, Shin EJ, Lee BH, Choi SH, Hwang SH, Rhim H, Cho IH, Kim HC, Nah SY. Effects of gintonin-enriched fraction on hippocampal cell proliferation in wild-type mice and an APPswe/PSEN-1 double Tg mouse model of Alzheimer's disease. Neurochem Int. 2016;101:56–65.
81. Kim HJ, Park SD, Lee RM, Lee BH, Choi SH, Hwang SH, Rhim H, Kim HC, Nah SY. Gintonin attenuates depressive-like behaviors associated with alcohol withdrawal in mice. J Affect Disord. 2017;215:23–9.
82. Park GH, Park KY, Cho HI, Lee SM, Han JS, Won CH, Chang SE, Lee MW, Choi JH, Moon KC, et al. Red ginseng extract promotes the hair growth in cultured human hair follicles. J Med Food. 2015;18:354–62.
83. Choi BY. Hair-growth potential of ginseng and its major metabolites: a review on its molecular mechanisms. Int J Mol Sci. 2018;19(9):pii:E2703.

84. Oh GN, Son SW. Efficacy of Korean red ginseng in the treatment of alopecia areata. J Ginseng Res. 2012;36:391–5.

85. Kim JH, Yi SM, Choi JE, Son SW. Study of the efficacy of Korean red ginseng in the treatment of androgenic alopecia. J Ginseng Res. 2009;33:223–8.

86. Ryu HJ, Yoo MG, Son SW. The efficacy of 3% minoxidil vs. combined 3% minoxidil and Korean red ginseng in treating female pattern alopecia. Int J Dermatol. 2014;53:e340–2.

87. Keum DI, Pi LQ, Hwang ST, Lee WS. Protective effect of korean red ginseng against chemotherapeutic drug-induced premature catagen development assessed with human hair follicle organ culture model. J Ginseng Res. 2016;40:169–75.

88. Lee NE, Park SD, Hwang H, Choi SH, Lee RM, Nam SM, Choi JH, Rhim H, Cho IH, Kim HC, Hwang SH, Nah SY. Effects of a gintonin-enriched fraction on hair growth: an in vitro and in vivo study. J Ginseng Res. 2020;44:168–77.

89. Dietz BM, Hajirahimkhan A, Dunlap TL, Bolton JL. Botanicals and their bioactive phytochemicals for women's health. Pharmacol Rev. 2016;68:1026–73.

90. Mazaro-Costa R, Andersen ML, Hachul H, Tufik S. Medicinal plants as alternative treatments for female sexual dysfunction: utopian vision or possible treatment in climacteric women? J Sex Med. 2010;7:3695–714.

91. Chen XP, Li W, Xiao XF, Zhang LL, Liu CX. Phytochemical and pharmacological studies on Radix Angelica sinensis. Chin J Nat Med. 2013;11:577–87.

92. Kim MH, Choi YY, Cho IH, Hong J, Kim SH, Yang WM. Angelica sinensis induces hair regrowth via the inhibition of apoptosis signaling. Am J Chin Med. 2014;42:1021–34.

93. Lin Z. Ganoderma (Lingzhi) in traditional Chinese medicine and Chinese culture. Adv Exp Med Biol. 2019;1181:1–13.

94. The Divine Farmer's Materia Medica. A translation of the Shen Nong Ben Cao Jing. Translated by Yang. Shouzhong: Blue Poppy Enterprises; 1998. p. 17–8.

95. Stuart GA, Smith FP. Chinese Materia Medica, Pt. 1, vegetable kingdom, vol. 274: Presbyterian Mission Press; 1911. p. 271.

96. Paterson R, Russell M. Ganoderma—a therapeutic fungal biofactory. Phytochemistry. 2006;67:1985–2001.

97. Hunt K. Some trees can live for more than 1,000 years and scientists may have figured out why. CNN; 2020. Accessed 19 Jan 2020.

98. Guan R, Zhao Y, Zhang H, Fan G, Liu X, Zhou W, Shi C, Wang J, Liu W. Draft genome of the living fossil Ginkgo biloba. GigaScience. 2016;5:49.

99. van Beek TA, Montoro P. Chemical analysis and quality control of Ginkgo biloba leaves, extracts, and phytopharmaceuticals. J Chromatogr A. 2009;1216:2002–32.

100. dos Santos-Neto LL, de Vilhena T, Maria A, Medeiros-Souza P, de Souza GA. The use of herbal medicine in Alzheimer's disease—a systematic review. Evid Based Complement Alternat Med. 2006;3:441–5.

101. Committee on Herbal Medicinal Products. Assessment report on Ginkgo biloba L., folium (PDF). European Medicines Agency.

102. Kobayashi N, Suzuki R, Koide C, Suzuki T, Matsuda H, Kubo M. Effect of leaves of Ginkgo biloba on hair regrowth in C3H strain mice [Article in Japanese]. Yakugaku Zasshi. 1993;113:718–24.

103. Hou IC, Amarnani S, Chong MT, Bishayee A. Green tea and the risk of gastric cancer: epidemiological evidence. World J Gastroenterol. 2013;19:3713–22.

104. Caini S, Cattaruzza MS, Bendinelli B, Tosti G, Masala G, Gnagnarella P, Assedi M, Stanganelli I, Palli D, Gandini S. Coffee, tea and caffeine intake and the risk of non-melanoma skin cancer: a review of the literature and meta-analysis. Eur J Nutr. 2017;56:1–12.

105. Tang J, Zheng JS, Fang L, Jin Y, Cai W, Li D. Tea consumption and mortality of all cancers, CVD and all causes: a meta-analysis of eighteen prospective cohort studies. Br J Nutr. 2015;114:673–83.

106. Jurgens TM, Whelan AM, Killian L, Doucette S, Kirk S, Foy E. Green tea for weight loss and weight maintenance in overweight or obese adults. Cochrane Database Syst Rev. 2012:CD008650. https://doi.org/10.1002/14651858.CD008650.pub2.

107. Mahmood T, Akhtar N. Moldovan C. A comparison of the effects of topical green tea and lotus on facial sebum control in healthy humans. Hippokratia. 2013;17:64–7.
108. Majewska K, Older D, Pawełczyk A, Zaprutko T, Żwawiak J, Zaprutko L. Aktywne kosmetyki wśród produktów spożywczych. Homines Hominibus. 2010;6:65–96.
109. Koch W, Zagórska J, Marzec Z, Kukula-Koch W. Applications of tea (Camellia sinensis) and its active constituents in cosmetics. Molecules. 2019;24:4277.
110. Fischer TW, Hipler UC, Elsner P. Effect of caffeine and testosterone on the proliferation of human hair follicles in vitro. Int J Dermatol. 2007;46:27–35.
111. Kwon OS, Han JH, Yoo HG, Chung JH, Cho KH, Eun HC, Kim KH. Human hair growth enhancement in vitro by green tea epigallocatechin-3-gallate (EGCG). Phytomedicine. 2007;14:551–5.
112. Kim SH, Kim SR, Lee HJ, Oh H, Ryu SY, Lee YS, Kim TH, Jo SK. Apoptosis in growing hair follicles following gamma-irradiation and application for the evaluation of radioprotective agents. In Vivo. 2003;17:211–4.
113. Nualsri C, Lourith N, Kanlayavattanakul M. Development and clinical evaluation of green tea hair tonic for greasy scalp treatment. J Cosmet Sci. 2016;67:161–6.
114. Zhang B, Zhang RW, Yin XQ, Lao ZZ, Zhang Z, Wu QG, Yu LW, Lai XP, Wan YH, Li G. Inhibitory activities of some traditional Chinese herbs against testosterone 5α-reductase and effects of Cacumen platycladi on hair re-growth in testosterone-treated mice. J Ethnopharmacol. 2016;177:1–9.
115. Narayanaswamy V. Origin and developments of Ayurveda (a brief history). Ancient Sci Life. 1981;1:1–7.
116. Dymock W, et al. Pharmacographia Indica, A history of principal drugs of vegetable origin in British India, vol. 1: K. Paul, Trench, Trübner & Company, London; 1890.
117. Dev S. Ancient-modern concordance in ayurvedic plants: some examples. Environ Health Perspect. 1999;107:783–9.
118. Research in Ayurveda—About CCRAS. Central Council for Research in Ayurveda and Siddha. Department Of AYUSH, Ministry of Health and Family Welfare. Archived from the original on 30 May 2014.
119. Trüeb RM. From hair in India to hair India. Int J Trichology. 2017;9:1–6.
120. Pandit S, Chauhan NS, Dixit VK. Effect of Cuscuta reflexa Roxb on androgen-induced alopecia. J Cosmet Dermatol. 2008;7:199–204.
121. Roy RK, Thakur M, Dixit VK. Hair growth promoting activity of Eclipta alba in male albino rats. Arch Dermatol Res. 2008;300:357–64.
122. Datta K, Singh AT, Mukherjee A, Bhat B, Ramesh B, Burman AC. Eclipta alba extract with potential for hair growth promoting activity. J Ethnopharmacol. 2009;124:450–6.
123. Roy RK, Thakur M, Dixit VK. Development and evaluation of polyherbal formulation for hair growth-promoting activity. J Cosmet Dermatol. 2007;6:108–12.
124. Mukherjee PK, Harwansh RK, Bahadur S, Banerjee S, Kar A, Chanda J, Biswas S, Ahmmed SM, Katiyar CK. Development of ayurveda—tradition to trend. J Ethnopharmacol. 2017;197:10–24.

Safety and Efficacy of Nutrition-Based Interventions for Hair

7

Nutritional or dietary supplements are manufactured products intended to supplement the diet when taken orally. Supplements can provide nutrients either extracted from food sources or of synthetic origin, individually or in combination, in order to increase the quantity of their consumption. The classes of nutrient compounds include the nutritionally essential vitamins, essential minerals, amino acids, essential fatty acids, and substances that have not been confirmed as being essential to life, but are marketed as having a beneficial biological effect, such as plant pigments and polyphenols. The natural products are manufactured using intact sources or extracts from plants, animals, algae, fungi, or bacteria, or in the instance of probiotics, live bacteria. They include such examples as *Ginkgo biloba*, curcumin, cranberry, St. John's wort, ginseng, resveratrol, glucosamine, and collagen. Animal sources can also serve for supplement ingredients, as for example collagen from chickens or fish, and keratin from pigs. In fact, also rhinoceros horn (Fig. 7.1) and pangolin scales, whose use to cure a variety of ailments is highly praised in the traditional medicine systems in Asia, are composed largely of keratin. However, ingesting keratin does not help hair growth, as the protein cannot be broken down and absorbed. In other words, there is no evidence to support the plethora of claims about the healing properties of the horns and scales, and one would do just as well chewing on the fingernails. While most of the latter have a long history of use in herbalism and various forms of traditional medicine, concerns exist about their actual efficacy, safety, and consistency of quality.

7.1 Bioavailability

Nutrients that the body requires do not come ready to use from food; rather they are packaged in a variety of forms. Therefore, whole food must be broken down for absorption and metabolism to meet the body's need. This involves a series of successive events that include digestion, absorption, transport, and metabolism. When digestion is complete, food will be changed into simple end products that are ready

© Springer Nature Switzerland AG 2020
R. M. Trüeb, *Nutrition for Healthy Hair*,
https://doi.org/10.1007/978-3-030-59920-1_7

257

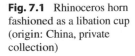

Fig. 7.1 Rhinoceros horn
fashioned as a libation cup
(origin: China, private
collection)

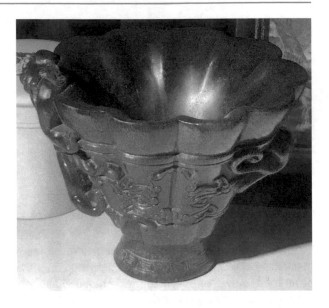

for absorption: carbohydrate foods into the simple sugars glucose, fructose, and galactose; fats into fatty acids and glycerides; and protein into single amino acids, while the vitamins and minerals are liberated. Of the micronutrients, vitamins and minerals require little or no digestion, with the exception of vitamin A, biotin, and vitamin B12.

For many of the nutrients, in particular vitamins and minerals, the point of absorption becomes the vital gatekeeper that determines how much of a given nutrient becomes available at the cellular level. A nutrient's bioavailability depends on (1) the amount of nutrient present in the gastrointestinal tract, (2) the form in which the nutrient is present, and (3) the competition among nutrients for common absorptive sites. For example, the phytic acid found in grain products decreases the bioavailability of iron in the respective enriched grain products, also divalent cations, such as iron, zinc, and copper compete for binding to transporter molecules during absorption throughout the gastrointestinal tract. Finally, the interaction with hydrochloric acid in the stomach increases the bioavailability of vitamin B12, calcium, iron, zinc, and magnesium.

Bioavailability of orally administered nutritional supplements, such as vitamins, minerals, trace elements, and their combinations, is also subject to a number of influences. The most straightforward approach to this issue is to determine the fraction of an oral dose that reaches the systemic circulation. For micronutrients, however, this approach has to consider the physiological plasma concentration as well as the mechanisms that regulate intestinal absorption and distribution of micronutrients between functional and storage compartments in response to the demand. The rate of exchange between these compartments has an impact on the delivery of such compounds into the plasma compartment as well as on the plasma clearance. In nutritional science, the term bioavailability encompasses the sum of impacts that may reduce or foster the metabolic utilization of a nutrient. In practice, bioavailability can be assessed by the rate by which deficiency symptoms are cured [1].

For non-metabolizable supplemental nutrients, bioavailability is effectively equivalent to absorbability. Methods for measuring absorbability include balance, serum concentration, tracer methods, urine increment, evoked physiological responses, and in vitro methods [2].

The balance method refers to the difference between what goes in at the mouth and what comes out in the feces. It refers in this case not to total body balance, but to intestinal balance. Moreover, its endpoint is subject to the influence of bacterial action on the nutrient concerned in the colon.

The measurement of serum concentration reflects the rise in the serum concentration of the nutrient as it is introduced into the circulation during its absorption. Analogous to the pharmacokinetic measure used for drugs, it yields an area under the curve, as well as the other standard pharmacokinetic measures. Monitoring the area under the plasma concentration–time curve after oral administration is an inadequate tool for bioavailability determination if there are substantial impacts of homeostatic mechanisms on the plasma concentration of a micronutrient.

When intrinsic labeling of a source is possible, the tracer methods are generally the most accurate and precise. The method has a very high sensitivity because the normal background for the tracer, particularly if radioactive, is usually very low.

The urine increment method is based on the fact that as the serum concentration of the nutrient rises, some of the nutrient spills over into the urine. The method is less sensitive than the measurement of serum concentration, and it adds another layer of biological variability (renal clearance).

The evoked physiological responses or effect of the nutrient on target systems is intuitively attractive, inasmuch as the method directly addresses the reason for taking the nutritional supplement in the first place. Their limitation lies in the fact that the biological response will be a function not only of the bioavailability of the nutrient tested, but also of the need status of the individual recipient. Examples are the increment in serum 25-hydroxycholecalciferol produced by a given dose of vitamin D being an inverse function of both the basal 25-hydroxycholecalciferol status and the dose itself, and variation in the hemoglobin response to oral iron which can vary from 1 g hemoglobin/week in patients with iron-deficiency anemia to nil in individuals who are iron replete.

Factors influencing the measured endpoints of the various methods include (1) source factors such as pharmaceutic formulation, (2) subject factors such as mucosal surface and the need status of the absorbing subject, and (3) co-ingested factors such as other food constituents.

Finally, most natural antioxidants such as alpha-tocopherol, ascorbic acid, and others are biologically unstable; have variable solubility in water; and are poorly distributed to target tissue sites. Because of these shortcomings, the early enthusiasm for prophylactic applications of dietary supplements such as antioxidants and phytochemicals has stagnated. This is partially due to a lack of basic awareness of appropriate drug delivery systems for effective nutritional supplementation. Currently, there are some challenging works to improve their bioavailability using delivery systems such as liposomal formulations to promote their therapeutic value [3].

Experience has shown that bioavailability is difficult to predict only from the knowledge of the chemistry of the source, or from the results of in vitro testing. Direct measurements of bioavailability are essential to assure regulators, prescribers, and the consumer that the source delivers what it promises [2]. Ultimately, it is fundamental to investigate into the bioavailability of specific nutrients with the claim of effects on hair growth and quality, with special attention to their distribution and mechanisms of transport, in tandem with in vitro efficacy assessment, as a prerequisite to the final clinical efficacy studies.

7.2   In Vitro Efficacy Assessment

The fundamental approach to in vitro efficacy assessment of nutrients is based on the knowledge of the bioavailability of the actives, and the cellular and tissular physiology of the hair follicle. This enables to define relevant parameters of efficacy in relation to the circulating concentration of the actives found after ingestion as determined from the bioavailability studies.

7.2.1   2-D Assays

In vitro, two-dimensional (2-D) cultures of normal human epidermal keratinocytes (NHEKs) have been established as an important tool for investigating general aspects of skin physiology. NHEKs and hair follicle-associated keratinocytes can be functionally differentiated in vivo. Nevertheless, scatterplot analysis of DNA microarray data revealed a good correlation of the gene expression profile of these two cell types, with only a limited number of genes differentially expressed between them [4]. Moreover, with regard to more basic functions like proliferation and general control of metabolic activity, keratinocytes from the hair follicle and epidermal skin layer can be expected to behave in a similar way. Measuring the metabolic activity and proliferation of NHEKs is therefore considered to be a preliminary robust surrogate model and readout for hair follicle functionality, and is useful indirectly as a simplified indicator for potential enhanced hair growth.

To mimic the reduced activity of keratinocytes believed to be associated with telogen effluvium, Hengl et al. from Merz Pharmaceuticals GmbH [5] established a growth-limiting in vitro system using NHEKs cultivated in different growth-impacting media, including minimal growth medium (MGM) lacking cystine, thiamine, calcium D-pantothenate, folic acid, and biotin. Metabolic activity and proliferation were determined after the cells had been incubated with their respective test media. A cell number-dependent increase in metabolic activity with a linear relationship could be detected in keratinocytes cultivated in either MGM, basal medium, or growth medium (Fig. 7.2a). However, time-dependent analysis of metabolic activity (Fig. 7.2b) demonstrated only a small increase in the metabolic

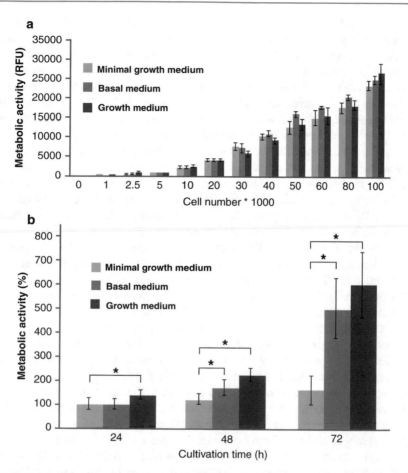

Fig. 7.2 (**a, b**) Metabolic activity of NHEKs cultivated in three different media. (**a**) Cell number-dependent metabolic activity of NHEKs cultivated for 24 h. (**b**) Metabolic activity of NHEKs over time. Compared with NHEKs grown in basal or growth media, the use of MGM reduced the proliferation of NHEKs significantly, representing a valid in vitro model for NHEKs under growth-limiting conditions (from [5])

activity of cells cultivated in MGM, whereas keratinocytes cultivated in basal and growth medium showed nearly a twofold increase after 48 h and up to a four- to fivefold increase after 72 h. Taken together, compared with NHEKs grown in basal or growth media, the use of MGM reduced the proliferation of NHEKs significantly, representing a valid in vitro model for NHEKs under growth-limiting conditions.

Based on expected systemic bioavailability, Hengl et al. established in a second step an in vitro correlate (P-IC) of the commercial hair growth formulation Panto(vi)gar® consisting of L-cystine, thiamine, folic acid (an assumed metabolite of the PABA in Panto(vi)gar®), and calcium D-pantothenate for in vitro analysis. The effects of the four components of the oral formulation on the metabolic activity and proliferation of NHEKs were tested in a dose-dependent manner as individual compounds and as a combination (P-IC) using supplemented MGM. L-Cystine and thiamine showed a clear positive impact on metabolic activity and proliferation of NHEKs in a dose-dependent manner compared with MGM alone (Fig. 7.2a, b). Of the individual components tested, L-cystine was observed to have the largest effect on metabolic activity (50 μM L-cystine: threefold increase versus MGM) and prolif-eration (50 μM L-cystine, threefold increase versus MGM). Thiamine also had a notable effect on the metabolic activity of NHEKs, while calcium D-pantothenate and folic acid were demonstrated to have no significant impact (Fig. 7.3a, b). Further to the effects of the individual components, a significant effect on metabolic activ-ity, proliferation, and DNA synthesis was demonstrated for the P-IC combination (Fig. 7.3a–c). Addition of L-cystine, especially at concentrations of 5 μM or greater (i.e., in 1/10 P-IC or P-IC), with other P-IC components appeared to facilitate the increased DNA synthesis capacity, with P-IC resulting in 40% more DNA synthesis than the individual L-cystine dose equivalent (50 μM).

Finally, Hengl et al. assessed the capacity of the ingredients of the respective oral formulation, again both separately and in combination, to modulate the effects of UV radiation (UVR) in growth-limited NHEKs in vitro (Fig. 7.4a, b).

The hair and scalp, like the rest of the skin, are exposed to a variety of noxious environmental factors, including ultraviolet radiation (UVR). While the conse-quences of sustained UVR on unprotected skin are well appreciated, mainly aging and photocarcinogenesis, the effects of UVR on the hair are less understood. However, clinical and morphologic observations, as well as theoretical consider-ations, suggest that UVR has some negative effects [6]: Camacho et al. [7] origi-nally reported a specific type of telogen effluvium, characterized by frontovertical hair shedding and an increase of telogen hairs by trichogram, that occurs 3–4 months after sunburn of the scalp in those with hairstyles that left areas of scalp uncovered during prolonged periods of sun exposure. The pathogenesis of this type of telogen effluvium is not clear; however, it has been shown that UV-B light negatively affects the viability of upper hair follicles [8], perhaps directly by the energy delivered to absorbing structures within cells (e.g., DNA) or indirectly via oxygen radicals and activation of cell surface growth factor and cytokine receptors. In addition, it has been proposed that the columns of cells in the hair shaft act as an efficient fiber-optic-type system, transmitting UV light down into the hair follicle. Morphologically, the keratinocytes within the hair shaft are arranged in compressed linear columns that resemble the coaxial bundles of commercial fiber-optic strands. Thus, hair fol-licular melanocytes located in the region of the hair matrix may function as UV biosensors and respond to photic inputs [9]. Finally, in a study of organ-cultured human anagen hair follicles in vitro, the effects of UV irradiation at the molecular level were reported to be a differentially modified hair growth cycle and promotion of cell death, among other events [10]. In summary, it can be concluded that depend-ing on the quantity of UVR exposure, it is conceivable that photodamage may also occur in the hair follicle.

In MGM, NHEKs showed a UVR dose-dependent decrease in metabolic activity 24 h after irradiation (Fig. 7.4a). Analysis of induction of apoptosis revealed a maxi-mal induction of caspase activity 14 h after irradiation (Fig. 7.4b).

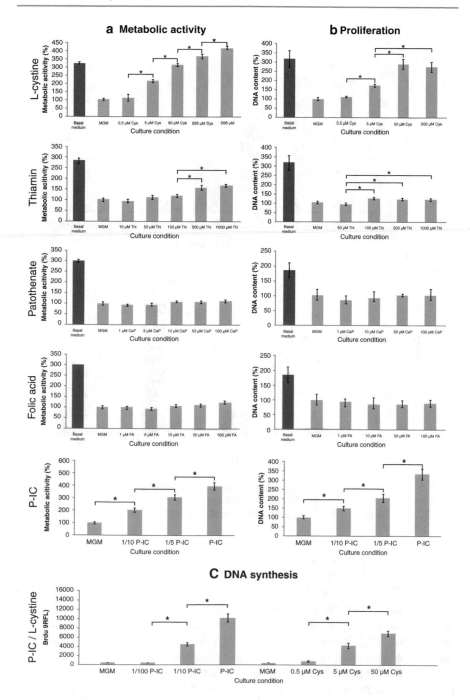

Fig. 7.3 (**a–c**) Impact of the oral formulation, both separately (L-cystine, thiamine, pantothenate, folic acid) and as combination (P-IC), on (**a**) metabolic activity, (**b**) proliferation of NHEKs cultivated in the respective media. (**c**) Impact of P-IC and L-cystine on DNA synthesis measured via BrdU incorporation (from [5])

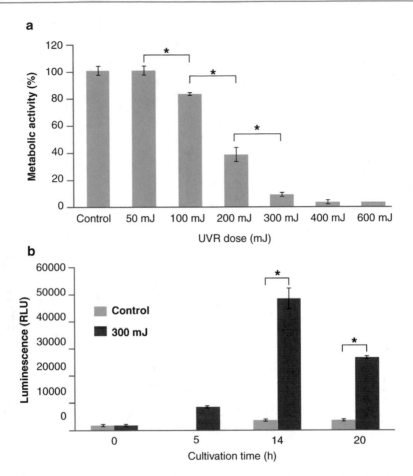

Fig. 7.4 (**a, b**) UVR under limited growth conditions. (**a**) Metabolic activity of NHEKs in MGM, measured 24 h post-UVR in dependence of UVR dose (mJ) as indicated. (**b**) Apoptosis of NHEKs over time (h) following UVR compared with control, nonirradiated cells, measured by caspase activity (from [5])

Microscopic analysis and caspase activity revealed that P-IC and $10 \times$ P-IC significantly ($p < 0.05$) reduced the amount of UV-induced apoptosis of NHEKs cultured in MGM alone (Fig. 7.5a–e). Also, the negative impact of UV irradiation on metabolic activity was attenuated by the addition of P-IC to MGM, as demonstrated by reduction of only 12–18% in metabolic activity observed for nonirradiated, P-IC-treated NHEKs compared with the 72% reduction observed in UV-irradiated cells versus nonirradiated cells cultured in MGM alone (Fig. 7.5f).

When P-IC was compared with the UV-filtering reference compound, PABA (Fig. 7.6a), the prevention of the effects of UVR with P-IC was greater than that with PABA, as demonstrated by the greater metabolic activity and lower degree of apoptosis observed in irradiated cells treated with P-IC compared with those treated with PABA only (Fig. 7.6b, c). Treatment with P-IC resulted in only 30% of the level of apoptosis observed in the presence of PABA (Fig. 7.6c).

These data confirm and extend previous findings [11, 12] on the relevance of L-cystine for metabolic activity and proliferation of human keratinocytes. Importantly, the UV irradiation analysis indicated that P-IC may be protective against the negative impact of solar UVR. In daily life, the hair and scalp are challenged constantly by solar UVR. Previous studies have established UV-protective benefits of other cystine derivatives [13]. Notably, thiol compounds can act as direct scavengers of radicals and UV-induced reactive oxygen species [13]. Moreover, oral administration of L-cystine and vitamin B6 prevented hair loss in C57BL/6 mice exposed to cigarette smoke, another environmental factor that both is genotoxic and generates oxidative stress [14].

Ultimately, Bahta et al. [15] cultured dermal hair papilla cells (DPCs) from both balding and non-balding human scalps and demonstrated that balding DPCs grew slower in vitro than non-balding DPCs. Loss of proliferative capacity of balding DPCs was associated with changes in cell morphology, expression of senescence-associated beta-galactosidase and markers of oxidative stress and DNA damage, as well as decreased expression of proliferating cell nuclear antigen and Bmi-1. This suggests that balding DPCs are particularly sensitive to environmental stressors such as cigarette smoke [16] and UVR [6]. These findings, along with the existing

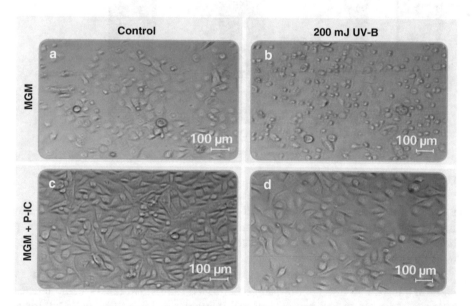

Fig. 7.5 (**a–f**) The effects of the in vitro correlate (P-IC) of the oral formulation on UV radiation (200 mJ UV-B) of keratinocytes. (**a–d**) Microscopic analysis of impact on cell density and morphology of NHEKs cultivated in (**a, b**) MGM and in (**c, d**) MGM + P-IC. (**e**) Apoptosis of NHEKs post-UVR. (**f**) Metabolic activity of NHEKs post-UVR. Both the amount of UV-induced apoptosis and the negative impact of UV irradiation on metabolic activity of NHEKs were attenuated by the addition of P-IC to MGM (from [5])

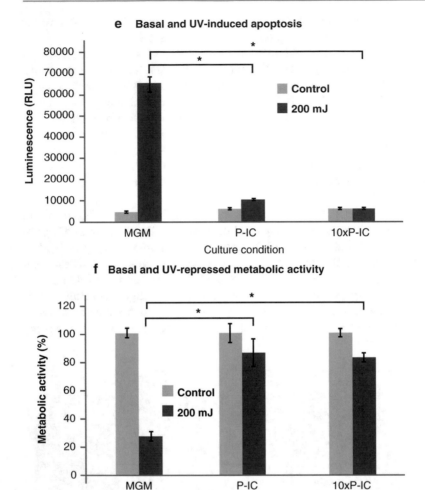

Fig. 7.5 (continued)

unmet needs in the management of androgenetic alopecia beyond minoxidil and finasteride, suggest that further pathogenic pathways contributing to hair loss may be relevant and represent opportunities for further therapeutic strategies to include nutritional therapy.

Follow-up studies using hair follicle-derived keratinocytes would be helpful to confirm and extend these preliminary data. Since the hair follicle-specific phenotype also depends on organotypic cell-cell interactions, in addition to 2-D cultivation, 3-D cultivation of hair follicle cells would provide a valuable additional in vitro model.

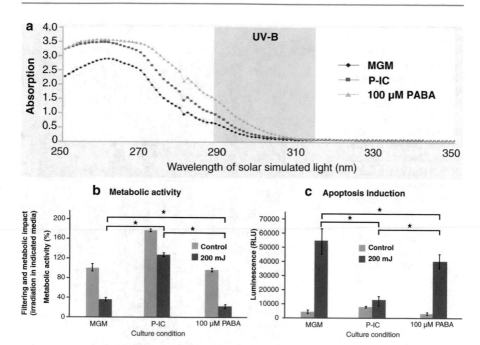

Fig. 7.6 (**a–c**) When the in vitro correlate P-IC was compared with the UV-filtering reference compound, PABA, (**a**) the prevention of the effects of UVR with P-IC was greater than that with PABA, as demonstrated by (**b**) the greater metabolic activity and (**c**) lower degree of apoptosis observed in irradiated cells treated with P-IC compared with those treated with PABA only

7.2.2   3-D Assays

While two-dimensional monolayer cell culture models are widely used for screening purposes or to understand physiological pathways on a cellular level, physiological properties and differentiation processes are in vivo the result of three-dimensional (3-D) interactions within organs or mini-organs such as the hair follicle. Associated processes like differentiation or morphogenesis can be simulated in vitro by using 3-DA culture models.

Again, Hengl et al. were interested in a 3-D culture system mimicking more closely the in vivo situation of the human hair follicle [17]. Therefore they evaluated the application of in vitro heterotypic spheroids as a hair follicle model using human dermal papilla cells (dP) and hair follicle-associated keratinocytes (FK). The analysis of the initial spheroid formation process was performed by observing cell type-specific migration/distribution patterns by automated live-cell fluorescence microscopy. After spheroid formation the cell type-specific distribution in the 3-D spheroid model was examined by light sheet-based fluorescence microscopy (LSM). To mimic situations of telogen effluvium they again used MGM which allows the analysis of the effect of the hair growth-promoting formulation by again adding its in vitro correlate (P-Ic). MGM-cultivated cells failed to form a spheroid whereas P-Ic supplementation restored the capability to form a stable spheroid (Fig. 7.7).

Fig. 7.7 3-D assay: modeling the hair follicle with in vitro heterotypic spheroids using human dermal papilla cells and hair follicle-associated keratinocytes. To mimic situations of telogen effluvium minimal growth medium (MGM) is used which allows the analysis of the effect of the hair growth-promoting formulation by adding an in vitro correlate (P-Ic) to the medium. MGM-cultivated cells fail to form a spheroid, whereas P-Ic supplementation restores the capability to form a stable spheroid

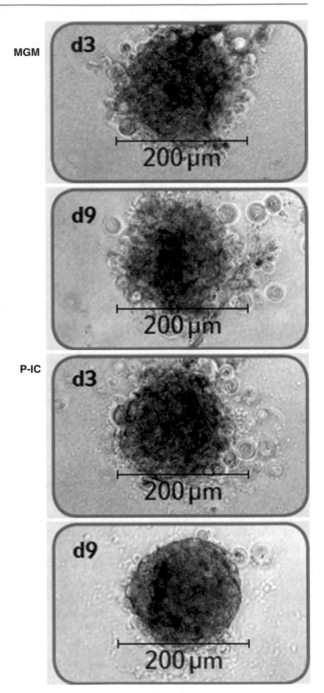

Thus, the established model was again successfully used to investigate the in vitro efficacy of the particular nutritional hair growth-promoting formulation. Further studies will help to gain a better understanding of the mode of action of well-established hair growth-promoting formulations and enable to identify new compounds for hair growth promotion.

7.2.3 Whole-Hair Follicle Culture

Alternatively, taking advantage of the ability of human hair follicle to grow in vitro while maintaining most of the characteristic features of normal hair follicle in vivo, the culture of whole-hair follicles [18] has been introduced originally by Philpott and Kealey [19] for the study of human hair growth. For this purpose, human anagen hair follicles were isolated by microdissection from human scalp skin by cutting the follicle at the dermo-subcutaneous fat interface using a scalpel blade. Intact hair follicles were then removed from the fat using watchmakers' forceps. Isolated hair follicles maintained to be free floating in supplemented Williams E medium originally showed a significant increase in length over 4 days. The increase in length was attributed to the production of a keratinized hair shaft, and was not associated with loss of hair follicle morphology. Furthermore, [methyl-3H]thymidine autoradiography confirmed that in vitro the in vivo pattern of DNA synthesis was maintained, and [35S]methionine labeling of keratins showed that their patterns of synthesis do not change with maintenance. Later, serum was found to inhibit hair follicle growth in vitro, while follicles that are maintained in serum-free medium grow for up to 10 days, suggesting that in vitro the hair follicles are able to regulate their own growth, possibly by the production of relevant growth factors. This proved useful for the study of the autocrine/paracrine mechanisms that operate in the hair follicle. Using this system, Philpott et al. identified transforming growth factor-beta (TGF-beta) as a negative regulator of hair follicle growth, and showed that physiological levels of insulin-like growth factor-I (IGF-I) can support the same rates of hair follicle growth as supraphysiological levels of insulin. In the absence of insulin hair follicles showed premature entry into a catagen-like state that was prevented by physiological levels of IGF-I. Finally, the hair follicle was demonstrated to be an aerobic glycolytic, glutaminolytic tissue, providing in-depth insights into the metabolism of the hair follicle [20].

Using this system, Collin et al. from L'Oréal Research, Clichy, France [21], studied (i) taurine uptake by isolated human hair follicles; (ii) its effects on hair growth and survival rate; and (iii) its protective potential against transforming growth factor (TGF)-beta1. They showed that taurine was taken up by the connective tissue sheath, proximal outer root sheath, and hair bulb; promoted hair survival in vitro; and prevented TGF-beta1-induced deleterious effects on hair follicle, in terms of inhibition of in vitro hair growth and a master switch of fibrotic program.

Taurine is a naturally occurring 2-aminoethanesulfonic acid produced by methionine and cysteine metabolism. It has been implicated in a wide array of physiological phenomena including inhibitory neurotransmission [22], feedback inhibition of neutrophil/macrophage respiratory burst, adipose tissue regulation [23], and calcium homeostasis [24].

A review published in 2008 found no documented reports of negative or positive health effects associated with the amount of taurine used in energy drinks, concluding, "The amounts of guarana, taurine, and ginseng found in popular energy drinks are far below the amounts expected to deliver either therapeutic benefits or adverse events" [25]. Taurine has an observed safe level of supplemental intake in normal healthy adults at up to 3 g/day [26].

Munkhbayar et al. [27] investigated the effect of arachidonic acid on hair growth by using in vitro and in vivo models. In the MTT assay (a colorimetric assay for assessing cell metabolic activity), arachidonic acid was found to enhance the viability of human dermal papilla cells (hDPCs) and promote the expression of several factors responsible for hair growth, including fibroblast growth factor-7 (FGF-7) and FGF-10. Western blotting identified the role of arachidonic acid in the phosphorylation of various transcription factors (ERK, CREB, and AKT) and increased expression of Bcl-2 in hDPCs. In the ex vivo hair follicle culture, arachidonic acid significantly promoted hair shaft elongation, with increased proliferation of matrix keratinocytes. Finally, arachidonic acid was found to promote hair growth by induction and prolongation of anagen phase in telogen-stage C57BL/6 mice.

Arachidonic acid is an omega-6 polyunsaturated fatty acid involved in the regulation of many cellular processes, including cell survival, angiogenesis, and mitogenesis. Arachidonic acid supplementation of the diets of healthy adults appears to offer no toxicity or significant safety risk. Arachidonic acid supplementation in daily doses of 1000–1500 mg for 50 days has been well tolerated during several clinical studies, with no significant side effects reported. All common markers of health, including serum lipids [28], immunity [29], and platelet aggregation [30], appear to be unaffected with this level and duration of use.

7.3   Clinical Efficacy

In vivo efficacy assessment or clinical efficacy studies are essentially the gold standard for any product with the claim of enhancing hair growth and/or quality. It is important to keep in mind that clinical effects on hair lag the biological effects induced by the particular active. Clinical efficacy studies must therefore be carried out over a relatively long time (at least 6 months), and conducted in a randomized, placebo-controlled manner in a sufficient number of test subjects to observe significant effects.

The clinical efficacy studies in promoting hair growth in androgenetic alopecia originally performed with topical minoxidil [31–33] and subsequently with oral finasteride [34] have set the current standards for the assessment of products with the claim of promoting hair growth.

Standardized global photographic assessment (Fig. 7.8) has successfully been established as a method for objectively monitoring cosmetically significant hair

Fig. 7.8 Standardized global photographic assessment

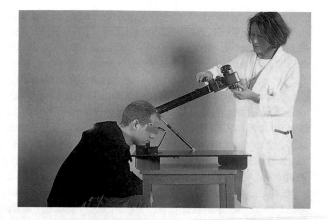

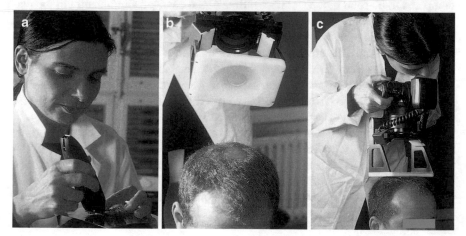

Fig. 7.9 (a–c) Phototrichogram (courtesy of Dr. M. Wyss, Zurich, Switzerland)

growth. For clinical study purposes the method is used in tandem with the phototrichogram technique (Fig. 7.9). While the latter yields a quantitative measure of the hair number (n), hair density (n/cm²), ratio of anagen to telogen phase hairs (%), hair thickness (μm), and linear hair growth rate (mm/day) within a defined area of the scalp, the former reflects the overall clinical changes in the patient over time in a standardized manner.

While describing the changes in hair diameter and density in relation to age, Robbins et al. [35] proposed a new metric relative scalp coverage for the perception of the amount of hair on one's head. This metric is defined as a two-dimensional parameter as the average of fiber cross-sectional area multiplied by the number of hair fibers per square centimeter. Robbins et al. further proposed that when additional relevant parameters are taken into account for relative scalp coverage, it will provide a multidimensional parameter involving diameter, density, fiber curvature, and color.

In addition, measurements of tensile break stress and torsion pendulum testing for assessment of behavioral properties of hair are important for efficacy assessment of hair cosmetics [36], and may also be relevant for the clinical efficacy of nutritionals for hair quality.

For example, silicon administered as *choline-stabilized orthosilicic acid* (ch-OSA) was shown to improve hair tensile strength, including elasticity and break load. The effect of ch-OSA on hair was investigated in a randomized, double-blind, placebo-controlled study. Forty-eight women with fine hair were given 10 mg silicon/day in the form of ch-OSA beadlets ($n = 24$) or a placebo ($n = 24$), orally for 9 months. Hair morphology and tensile properties were evaluated before and after treatment. Urinary silicon concentration increased significantly in the ch-OSA-supplemented group but not in the placebo group. The elastic gradient decreased in both groups but the change was significantly smaller in the ch-OSA group (-4.52%) compared to placebo group (-11.9%). Break load changed significantly in the placebo group (-10.8%) but not in the ch-OSA-supplemented group (-2.20%). Break stress and elastic modulus decreased in both groups but the change was smaller in the ch-OSA group. The cross-sectional area increased significantly after 9 months compared to baseline in ch-OSA-supplemented subjects but not in the placebo group. The change in urinary silicon excretion was significantly correlated with the change in cross-sectional area. Oral intake of ch-OSA had a positive effect on tensile strength including elasticity and break load and resulted in thicker hair [37].

The proper selection of study subjects is of major significance: they have to be recruited so as to form strictly homogeneous groups. Besides the clinical hair parameters that will be studied, it is crucial to consider the test person's gender, hormonal status, age, nutritional and health status, lifestyle (smoking [16], solar exposure [6]), and environment (climate, pollution, season). Not taking these variables into account while selecting the test subjects may result in hiding the efficacy of the product in question.

In 823 otherwise healthy women with telogen effluvium during an observational period of 6 years Kunz et al. [38] demonstrated the existence of an overall annual periodicity in the growth and shedding of hair, manifested by a maximal proportion of telogen hairs in July (Fig. 7.10).

Taking a scalp hair telogen-phase duration of approximately 100 days into account, one would expect shedding of these hairs by autumn. The authors pointed out that existence of seasonal fluctuations in hair growth and shedding complicates the assessment of pharmacological effects. Awareness of these fluctuations has potentially serious implications for investigations on hair growth-promoting agents. Depending on the stage of periodicity in growth and shedding of hair for a particular subject, the heterogeneity of included subjects relating to the season may be enough to distort clinical efficacy results of an investigational agent. In the active stage of seasonal telogen effluvium, the involved hair follicles would probably fail to respond to the therapeutic agent, which may cause a false-negative result. In the recovery stage, the increased amounts of spontaneous hair regrowth might be interpreted falsely as a positive result.

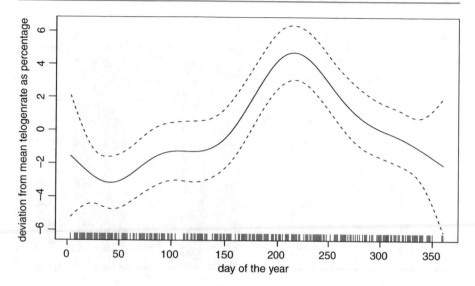

Fig. 7.10 Seasonal hair growth and shedding: fluctuations in frontal telogen rates ($n = 823$) in relation to the day of the year. From [38]

In her inaugural dissertation, Hotzenköcherle Trüeb [39] demonstrated the impact of seasonality of hair growth and shedding on study results through inhomogeneous inclusion of study subjects in relation to the season. In a preceding double-blind placebo-controlled study combining epiluminescence microscopy and digital imaging, efficacy of a specific oral hair growth-promoting nutrient based on L-cystine, nutritional yeast, vitamin B5 (CYP complex), and thiamine for treating telogen effluvium in otherwise healthy women was demonstrated [40], and this independent of patient age. Therefore, an open-label pilot study with the same product was performed in five women aged between 64 and 84 years, which confirmed the former results with increase and normalization of anagen rates within 3 months of treatment (unpublished data) (Fig. 7.11). To further verify the efficacy of the product in women aged 60 years and above, Hotzenköcherle Trüeb performed a double-blind placebo-controlled study in 36 patients for a duration of 6 months. Unexpectedly, placebo showed similar improvement of hair growth as compared to active compound. A further sub-analysis of patient data demonstrated that the result was falsified through inhomogeneous inclusion of study patients in relation to the season, with a cluster of patients on placebo profiting from the spontaneous recovery phase of seasonal hair growth and shedding (Fig. 7.12a–d). Hotzenköcherle Trüeb demonstrated that the impact of seasonality of hair growth and shedding on clinical trials with hair growth-promoting agents should always be taken into consideration, especially in studies with small numbers of patients and study durations <12 months, since heterogeneity of patient inclusion may be enough to distort clinical efficacy results.

Patient Nº	Initials	Sex	Age	T0 % Anagen	T0 Haircount	T3mo % Anagen	T3mo Haircount
1	EZ	Female	83	67	125	86	137
2	IE	Female	76	68	155	77	128
3	VH	Female	78	61	93	78	89
4	DC	Female	71	64	128	77	135
5	NS	Female	64	71	140	81	175

Fig. 7.11 Increase in anagen rates in women aged 60 years and older with telogen effluvium within 3 months of treatment with oral combination of L-cystine, nutritional yeast, pantothenic acid, and thiamine

Finally, assessment of in vivo molecular parameters is another notable approach to determine the biological effects of nutritional supplements in human intervention studies. Molecular changes can be detected much earlier than the clinical changes, and they provide a mechanistic understanding of the modes of action of the respective nutrient. Such studies have been performed with success on human skin to determine the efficacy of specific nutritional supplementation on UVR-induced gene expression [41]. A disadvantage, however, is the requirement of bioptic material.

7.4   Safety Issues

The last decades have witnessed an unprecedented growth in the use of nutritional therapies in all areas of health, including the hair. While a limited number of studies have substantiated some benefit of nutritional treatments for enhancement of hair growth and quality, the rampant use of some nutritionals and unawareness on the part of consumers, pharmacists, and the prescribing physician may carry some specific health risks.

7.4.1   Hypervitaminosis A

Vitamin A is an important hormonelike growth factor for growth and development of epithelial and other cells, and for the maintenance of the immune system and a

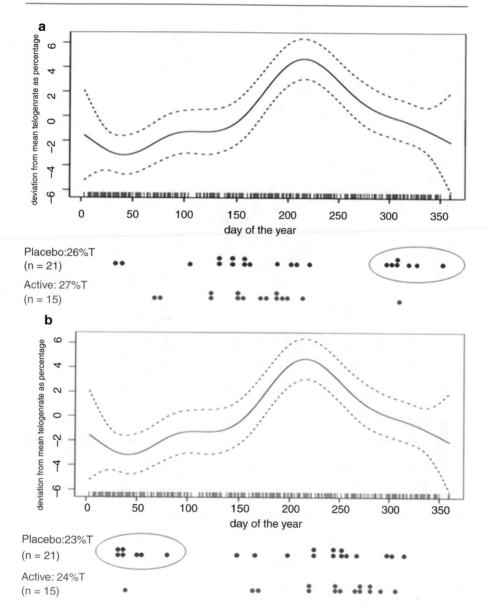

Fig. 7.12 (**a–d**) Inhomogeneous inclusion of study patients in relation to periodicity of hair growth and shedding: (**a**) at inclusion, (**b**) at 3 months, (**c**) at 6 months. Ellipse highlights cluster of patients in the placebo group that profited from seasonal hair growth within first 3 months of treatment. (**d**) Improvement of anagen rates after 3 and 6 months of treatment with active and placebo (from Hotzenköcherle Trüeb. Inaugural Dissertation, University of Zurich 2015, with permission)

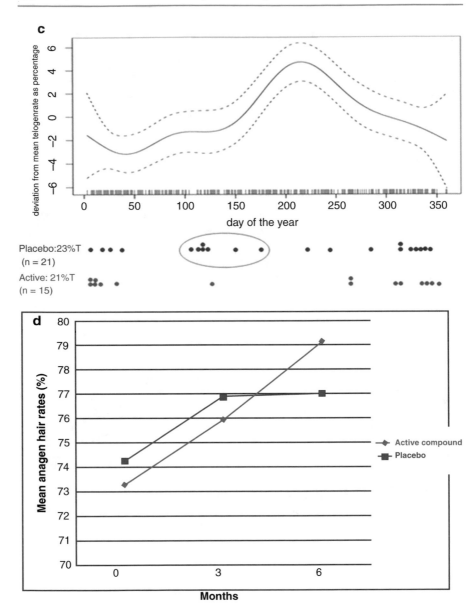

Fig. 7.12 (continued)

good vision. Deficiency disorders include night blindness, xeropthalmia, keratomalacia, impaired immunity, and follicular hyperkeratosis (phrynoderma). Therefore, vitamin A supplementation has been dermatologically recommended for the treatment of follicular hyperkeratosis (keratosis pilaris), usually in doses of 3 x 50,000 IU per day, and vitamin A has been included in some nutritional hair growth formulations.

Excess vitamin A, which is most common with high-dose vitamin A supplements, may cause birth defects and therefore should not exceed recommended daily values depending on age, sex, pregnancy, and lactation. Since vitamin A is fat soluble, disposing of any dietary takes longer than with the water-soluble vitamins, allowing for toxic levels to accumulate. Acute toxicity occurs at doses of 25,000 IU/kg of body weight, and chronic toxicity at 4000 IU/kg of body weight daily for >6 months. Symptoms of vitamin A toxicity include nausea, irritability, anorexia, vomiting, blurry vision, headaches, muscle and abdominal pain and weakness, drowsiness, and altered mental status. Vitamin A in doses of >50,000 IU daily may actually cause hair loss, a typical side effect of the synthetic retinoids acitretin and isotretinoin for treatment of dermatologic conditions, such as psoriasis and acne. Excessive intake of foods with a high content of β-carotene may cause a harmless orange skin (carotinosis) discoloration that is reversible upon discontinuation, while excessive intake of β-carotene supplements may promote oxidative damage and cell division.

7.4.2   Selenosis

Although correlative epidemiological studies have connected selenium deficiency as measured by blood levels to a number of chronic diseases, such as cancer, diabetes, and HIV/AIDS, randomized, blinded, controlled prospective trials failed to confirm that selenium supplementation reduces the incidence of any disease, nor has a meta-analysis of selenium supplementation studies detected a decrease in overall mortality [42–44]. Nevertheless, selenium has become a popular ingredient in many multivitamins and other dietary supplements, which typically contain 55 or 70 μg/serving. Selenium-specific supplements may contain up to 200 μg/serving, while the US Recommended Dietary Allowance (RDA) for teenagers and adults is 55 μg/day.

Although selenium is an essential trace element, it is toxic if taken in excess. Exceeding the tolerable upper intake level of 400 micrograms per day can lead to selenosis. Signs and symptoms of selenosis include garlic odor on the breath, gastrointestinal disorders, hair loss, sloughing of nails, fatigue, irritability, and neurological damage.

7.4.3   Iron Overload

Also, a caveat should be spoken against uncritical iron supplementations, since there is the possibility that increased iron storage could enhance oxidative injury by inducing the Fenton's reaction, with the prospective of increasing the risk of cardiovascular disease and cancer [45].

In an attempt to demonstrate the prooxidative capacity of oral iron supplementation, King et al. [46] performed a study on women with low iron stores (plasma ferritin < or = 20 microg/L) receiving a daily iron supplement for 8 weeks at a level commonly used to treat poor iron status. They measured increased lipid peroxidation by ethane exhalation rates and plasma malondialdehyde. The women served as their own control as pre- and post-supplementation periods were compared. After 6 weeks of iron supplementation, serum ferritin almost doubled and body iron more than doubled, hemoglobin levels increased slightly, and other indicators of iron status became normal. However, plasma malondialdehyde and breath ethane exhalation rates increased by more than 40% between baseline and 6 weeks of supplementation. These increases correlated significantly with plasma iron and ferritin levels. The authors concluded that the increased indicators of lipid peroxidation with duration of supplementation and as iron status improved suggest that providing daily nearly 100 mg iron may not be a totally innocuous regimen for correcting iron depletion.

7.4.4   Zinc Overload

Zinc is an essential mineral perceived by the public today as being of exceptional biologic and public health importance. A variety of zinc compounds are commonly used in medicine and cosmetology, such as zinc carbonate and zinc gluconate as dietary supplements, zinc chloride in deodorants, and zinc pyrithione in anti-dandruff shampoos. Zinc is included in most single-tablet over-the-counter daily vitamin and mineral supplements. Oral preparations include zinc sulfate, zinc carbonate, and zinc gluconate (with enhanced gastrointestinal tolerance). Zinc is believed to possess antioxidant properties, and protect against accelerated aging, while respective studies differ as to its effectiveness. Zinc helps speed up the healing process of wounds, and is also alleged to be beneficial to the body's immune system. Dermatological uses of oral zinc include skin ulcerations, acne, and alopecia areata.

Although zinc is an essential requirement for good health, excess zinc can be harmful. Excessive absorption of zinc suppresses copper and iron absorption. There is evidence of induced copper deficiency in those taking 100–300 mg of zinc daily, resulting in anemia refractory to iron. Zinc overload has been recognized as the second most common etiology of copper myelopathy [47]. The Recommended Dietary Allowance (RDA) is 8 mg/day for women and 11 mg/day for men. Zinc deficiency is relatively uncommon, since the daily requirement per day is usually obtained in a normal diet. Zinc supplements should only be ingested when there is zinc deficiency or increased zinc necessity, such as following bariatric surgery. Patients receiving zinc supplements on a long-term basis should receive 1–2 mg of copper for each 15 mg of zinc [48].

7.4.5   Biotin

There have been no reported cases of toxicity from high doses of biotin, in particular when used for the treatment of the rare inborn errors of biotin metabolism in doses up to 30 mg daily, specifically holocarboxylase synthetase deficiency and biotinidase deficiency.

Nevertheless, the U.S. FDA has recently issued an alert, stating that biotin administrated in high doses can interfere with biotin-streptavidin reaction-based diagnostic laboratory tests [49], including thyroid function tests and others [50]. Biotin interference may pose a particular problem for patients in cardiac emergency situations, where intake of high doses of biotin may interfere with troponin testing resulting in falsely low test results. The recommendation has been that the daily recommended dosage of biotin should not exceed 0.03 mg/day. At this level, it does not interfere with any laboratory tests. Since biotin is only effective at doses of 5 mg daily for brittle nails, 10 mg daily in holocarboxylase deficiency in pregnancy, and 10–40 mg daily in biotinidase deficiency, awareness and a comprehensive patient history regarding nutritional supplements are mandatory while performing biotin-streptavidin reaction-based diagnostic laboratory tests. In any case of high-dose biotin supplementation, patients should wait at least 8 h before blood is drawn for the respective laboratory examination.

7.4.6 Vitamin B6

Vitamin B6 either alone or together with other vitamins of the B complex is popularly combined with cystine or cysteine in nutrients for hair growth promotion. Although vitamin B6 is a water-soluble vitamin and therefore excreted in the urine, doses of pyridoxine in excess of the dietary upper limit (UL) of 100 mg/day over sustained periods of time may cause damage to the dorsal root ganglia, resulting in painful and ultimately irreversible neurological problems. Sensory neuropathy develops at doses of pyridoxine in excess of 1000 mg per day, but adverse effects can occur with less. Doses over 200 mg are not considered safe [51]. In fact symptoms have been reported among women even taking lower doses of vitamin B6 [52].

7.4.7 Vitamin D Toxicity

Hypervitaminosis D is a state of vitamin D toxicity. The harm from vitamin D3 in larger doses is demonstrated in that very high doses have been used as a rodenticide, where it causes hypercalcemia leading to death, typically only days after ingestion of the high dose [53]. In humans, hypervitaminosis D symptoms appear several months after administration of excessive doses of vitamin D.

Excess of vitamin D causes hypercalcemia, which can result in metastatic calcification of soft tissues, the heart, and the kidneys, and in hypertension. Symptoms of vitamin D toxicity may include dehydration, decreased appetite, vomiting, diarrhea or constipation, irritability, fatigue, and muscle weakness. Acute overdose requires between 15,000 μg/d (600,000 IU per day) and 42,000 μg/d (1,680,000 IU per day) over a period of several days to months.

Based on risk assessment, a safe upper intake level of 250 µg (10,000 IU) per day in healthy adults has been suggested by nongovernment authors [54, 55]. However, no government has a UL higher than 4000 IU. The recommended dietary allowance is 15 µg/d (600 IU per day; 800 IU for those over 70 years).

Excessive exposure to sunlight poses no risk in vitamin D toxicity through over-production of vitamin D precursor, cholecalciferol, regulating vitamin D production. During ultraviolet exposure, the concentration of vitamin D precursors produced in the skin reaches an equilibrium, and any further vitamin D that is produced is degraded [56]. This process is less efficient with increased melanin pigmentation in the skin. Endogenous production with full body exposure to sunlight is comparable to taking an oral dose between 250 and 625 µg (10,000 and 25,000 IU) per day. Possible ethnic differences in physiological pathways for ingested vitamin D may confound across the board recommendations for vitamin D levels. Studies on the South Asian population uniformly point to low 25(OH)D levels, despite abundant sunshine [57]. Measuring melanin content to assess skin pigmentation showed an inverse relationship with serum 25(OH)D [58].

It is possible that some of the symptoms of vitamin D toxicity are actually due to vitamin K depletion. Accordingly, physicians would be able to treat patients with doses of vitamin D that possess greater therapeutic value than those currently being used while avoiding the risk of adverse effects by administering vitamin D together with vitamin K [59].

Finally, a mutation of the CYP24A1 gene can lead to a reduction in the degradation of vitamin D resulting in hereditary hypercalcemia [60].

Complex regulatory mechanisms control metabolism. Recent epidemiologic evidence suggests that there is a narrow range of vitamin D levels in which vascular function is optimized. Levels above or below this range increased mortality [61]. Evidence suggests that dietary vitamin D may be carried by lipoprotein particles into cells of the artery wall and atherosclerotic plaque, where it may be converted to active form by monocyte-macrophages [62–64]. This raises questions regarding the effects of vitamin D intake on atherosclerotic calcification and cardiovascular risk as it may be causing vascular calcification [65].

7.4.8 Shark Cartilage

Shark cartilage is a dietary supplement made from the dried and powdered cartilage of a shark and marketed as a treatment or preventive for various conditions, including cancer, based on the misconception that sharks do not get cancer, a myth popularized by the 1992 book "Sharks Don't Get Cancer. How Shark Cartilage Could Save Your Life" written by I. William Lane and Linda Comac and published by Avery Publishing in the United States. Yet, there is no scientific evidence that shark cartilage is useful in treating or preventing cancer or other diseases [66]. Shark cartilage is not a defined single product. Native shark cartilage is harvested as the tough elastic cartilage from different shark species and contains proteins, proteoglycans, glycosaminoglycans, minerals, carbohydrate, and lipid. Depending on harvest conditions, preparations are often contaminated by other shark tissues, such as shark liver containing squalamine, and by heavy metals and bacterial contaminants [67]. Specifically, sharks are long-lived apex predators that bioaccumulate environmental methylmercury and marine toxins from dietary exposures. Shark fins and cartilage also contain β-N-methylamino-l-alanine (BMAA) [68], an ubiquitous cyanobacterial toxin linked to neurodegenerative diseases, such as Alzheimer's disease and amyotrophic lateral sclerosis [69].

7.4.9 Toxicities from Chinese Herbs and Ayurveda

Traditional Chinese herbal remedies are readily available in most Chinese neighborhoods. Some of these items are imported illegally, claim therapeutic benefit without medical evidence, and may contain toxic ingredients. For most, efficacy and toxicity are based on traditional knowledge rather than laboratory analysis and testing. Since the earliest records of TCM, the toxicity of certain substances has been described in all Chinese Materia Medica. Since TCM has become popularized in the Western world, there have been increasing concerns about the potential toxicity of traditional Chinese medicinals, including plants, animal parts, and minerals, as well as over the illegal trade of endangered species, such as the rhinoceros and the pangolin, and the welfare of specially farmed animals including bears for their bile.

Traditional herbal medicines can contain extremely toxic chemicals and heavy metals, and naturally occurring toxins. Botanical misidentification or mislabeling of plant material can play a role for toxic reactions. Some plant descriptions in traditional herbal medicine have changed over time, which may lead to unintended intoxication by using wrong plants. Another problem is also the contamination of herbals with microorganisms, and fungal toxins, such as aflatoxin, pesticides, and heavy metals, including lead, mercury, arsenic, copper, cadmium, and thallium [70]. Unprofessional processing, which differs from safe traditional preparation, represents yet another potential source for herbal poisoning. Unwanted effects of herbal products may also develop by the interaction of herbs with conventional drugs upon concomitant intake [71]. Finally, adulteration of some herbal medicine preparations with conventional drugs, such as corticosteroids, phenylbutazone, phenytoin, and glibenclamide, which may cause serious adverse effects has been reported [72].

Chinese herbal medicine has been a major cause of acute liver failure in China [73].

Overconsumption of He Shou Wu (*Polygonum multiflorum*) can lead to toxicity-induced hepatitis [74].

Ginseng generally has a good safety profile and the incidence of adverse effects is minor when used over a short term [75]. Concerns exist when ginseng is used chronically, potentially causing side effects such as headaches, insomnia, and digestive problems. Other side effects may include feeling anxious, fluctuations in blood pressure, breast pain, and vaginal bleeding. Inconsistent manufacturing practices have led to analyses showing that some ginseng products may be contaminated with toxic metals or unrelated filler compounds, such as rice or wheat.

There is evidence that dong quai (*A. sinensis*) may affect the muscles of the uterus [76]. Women who are pregnant or planning on becoming pregnant should not use *A. sinensis,* because it may induce a miscarriage. One case of gynecomastia has been reported following consumption of dong quai root powder pills [77].

Wanachiwanawin et al. [78] reported a case of pseudoparasitos due to consumption of *Ganoderma lucidum*. A 49-year-old male patient with non-Hodgkin lymphoma and a history of consumption of powdered lingzhi extract as a dietary supplement and herbal medicine presented with chronic watery diarrhea. Stool examination demonstrated spores of *G. lucidum* with resemblance with intestinal helminth ova and coccidia. After discontinuation of mushroom ingestion, the diarrheal symptoms improved and fecal examination subsequently showed no *Ganoderma* spores.

Kim et al. [79] reported on incidental *Podostroma cornu-damae* (poison fire coral) poisoning. In this case report, two patients made tea with the fungus and drank it over a 2-week period. Both patients presented with bicytopenia (leukopenia and thrombocytopenia), and one patient had desquamation of the palms and soles. *Podostroma cornu-damae* is a rare, deadly fungus that can be easily mistaken for the Lingzhi mushroom (*Ganoderma lucidum*). Several poisonings have been reported in Japan resulting from the consumption of the fungus. In 1999, one of a group of five people from Niigata prefecture died 2 days after consuming about 1 g (0.035 oz) of fruit body that had been soaked in sake. The symptoms associated with consumption in these cases included stomach pains, changes in perception, decrease in the number of leukocytes and thrombocytes, peeling skin, hair loss, and shrinking of the cerebellum, resulting in speech impediment and problems with voluntary movement [80]. In another instance, an autopsy revealed multiple-organ failure, including acute kidney failure, liver necrosis, and disseminated intravascular coagulation [81]. Saikawa et al. [80] discovered the chemical components of the macrocyclic trichothecene group of mycotoxins in the fruit body of this fungus, including satratoxin H 12'-18'-diacetate, satratoxin H 12'-acetate, satratoxin H 13'-acetate, satratoxin H, roridin E, and verucarin J. Upon consumption, the toxins inhibit ribosomal protein, DNA and RNA synthesis, mitochondrial functions, and cell division.

The use of *Ginkgo biloba* leaf extracts may have adverse effects, particularly for individuals with blood circulation disorders and those taking anticoagulants, although studies have found that ginkgo has little or no effect on the anticoagulant properties or pharmacodynamics of warfarin in healthy subjects [82]. Additional side effects include increased risk of bleeding, gastrointestinal discomfort, nausea, vomiting, diarrhea, headaches, dizziness, heart palpitations, and restlessness [83].

According to a systemic review, the effects of ginkgo on pregnant women may include increased bleeding time, and it should be avoided during lactation because of inadequate safety evidence [84].

Ginkgo biloba leaves also contain ginkgolic acids [85] which are highly allergenic, long-chain alkylphenols such as bilobol or adipostatin A [86]. Bilobol is a substance related to anacardic acid from cashew nut shells and urushiols present in poison ivy [87]. Individuals with a history of strong allergic reactions to poison ivy, mangoes, cashews, and other alkylphenol-producing plants are more likely to experience allergic reaction when consuming ginkgo-containing preparations, combinations, or extracts thereof.

Overconsumption of *Ginkgo biloba* seeds can deplete vitamin B6 [88, 89].

Several case reports on hepatotoxicity after the intake of green tea derivatives containing *Camellia sinensis* have been published, also from treatment of hair loss with oral green tea extracts. Verhelst et al. [90] reported a patient with an acute hepatitis after intake of an oral green tea derivative claiming protection against hair loss, showing a histological image compatible with drug-induced hepatitis. Other important causes of hepatitis were excluded. After cessation of this nutritional additive there was a rapid and sustained recovery. In 2018, a scientific panel for the European Food Safety Authority reviewed the safety of green tea consumption over a low-moderate range of daily EGCG intake from 90 to 300 mg per day, and with exposure from high green tea consumption estimated to supply up to 866 mg EGCG per day. Dietary supplements containing EGCG may supply up to 1000 mg EGCG and other catechins per day. The panel concluded that EGCG and other catechins from green tea in low-moderate daily amounts are generally regarded as safe, but in some cases of excessive consumption of green tea or use of high-EGCG supplements, liver toxicity may occur [91, 92].

On 17 June 2011, at Charles de Gaulle airport in Paris, France, radioactive cesium of 1038 becquerels per kilogram was measured in tea leaves imported from Shizuoka Prefecture, Japan, as a result of the Fukushima Daiichi nuclear disaster on 11 March, which was more than twice the restricted amount in the European Union of 500 becquerels per kilogram. The government of France announced that they rejected the leaves, which totaled 162 kg (357 lb) [93].

Some traditional Indian herbal medicinal products contain harmful levels of heavy metals, including lead [94]. A 1990 study on Ayurvedic medicines in India found that 41% of the products tested contained arsenic, and that 64% contained lead and mercury [95]. A 2004 study found toxic levels of heavy metals in 20% of Ayurvedic preparations made in South Asia and sold in the Boston area, and concluded that Ayurvedic products posed serious health risks and should be tested for heavy metal contamination [96]. A 2008 study of more than 230 products found that approximately 20% of remedies (and 40% of rasa shastra medicines) purchased over the Internet from US and Indian suppliers contained lead, mercury, or arsenic [97]. A report in the August 27, 2008, issue of the Journal of the American Medical Association found that nearly 21% of 193 ayurvedic herbal supplements bought online, produced in both India and the United States, contained lead, mercury, or arsenic [98]. A 2015 study of users in the United States found elevated blood lead levels in 40% of those tested, leading physician and former U.S. Air Force flight surgeon Harriet Hall to say, "Ayurveda is basically superstition mixed with a soupçon of practical health advice. And it can be dangerous" [99, 100].

References

1. Schümann K, Classen HG, Hages M, Prinz-Langenohl R, Pietrzik K, Biesalski HK. Bioavailability of oral vitamins, minerals, and trace elements in perspective. Arzneimittelforschung. 1997;47(4):369–80.
2. Heaney RP. Factors influencing the measurement of bioavailability, taking calcium as a model. J Nutr. 2001;13:1344S–8S.
3. Shoji Y, Nakashima H. Nutraceutics and delivery systems. J Drug Target. 2004;12:385–91.
4. Nakano M, Kamada N, Suehiro K, Oikawa A, Shibata C, Nakamura Y, Matsue H, Sasahara Y, Hosokawa H, Nakayama T, Nonaka K, OOhara O. Establishment of a new three-dimensional human epidermal model reconstructed from plucked hair follicle-derived keratinocytes. Exp Dermatol. 2016;25:903–6.
5. Hengl T, Herfert J, Soliman A, Schlinzig K, Trüeb RM, Abts HF. Cystine-thiamin-containing hair-growth formulation modulates the response to UV radiation in an in vitro model for growth-limiting conditions of human keratinocytes. J Photochem Photobiol B. 2018;189:318–25.
6. Trüeb RM. Is androgenetic alopecia a photoaggravated dermatosis? Dermatology. 2003;207:343–8.
7. Camacho F, Moreno JC, Garcia-Hernandez MJ. Telogen alopecia from UV rays. Arch Dermatol. 1996;132:1398–9.
8. Müller-Röver S, Rossiter H, Paus R, Handjiski B, Peters EMJ, Murphy JE, Mecklenburg L, Kupper TS. Overexpression of Bcl-2 protects from ultraviolet B-induced apoptosis but promotes hair follicle regression and chemotherapy-induced alopecia. Am J Pathol. 2000;156:1395–405.
9. Iyengar B. The hair follicle: a specialised UV receptor in the human skin? Biol Signals Recept. 1998;7:188–94.
10. Lu Z, Fischer TW, Hasse S, Sugawara K, Kamenisch Y, Krengel S, Funk W, Berneburg M, Paus R. Profiling the response of human hair follicles to ultraviolet radiation. J Invest Dermatol. 2009;129:1790–804.
11. Obrigkeit DT, Jugert FK, Merk HF, Kubicki J. Xenobiotics in vitro: the influence of L-cystine, pantothenate, and miliacin on metabolic and proliferative capacity of keratinocytes. Cutan Ocul Toxicol. 2006;25:13–22.
12. Steenvoorden DP, Beijersbergen van Henegouwen GM. Cysteine derivatives protect against UV-induced reactive intermediates in human keratinocytes: the role of glutathione synthesis. Photochem Photobiol. 1997;66:665–71.
13. van den Broeke L, Beyersbergen Van Henegouwen G. Thiols as potential UV radiation protectors: an in vitro study. J Photochem Photobiol B: Biol. 1993;17:279–86.
14. D'Agostini F, Fiallo P, Pennisi TM, De Flora S. Chemoprevention of smoke-induced alopecia in mice by oral administration of L-cystine and vitamin B6. J Dermatol Sci. 2007;46:189–98.
15. Bahta AW, Farjo N, Farjo B, Philpott MP. Premature senescence of balding dermal papilla cells in vitro is associated with p16(INK4a) expression. J Invest Dermatol. 2008;128:1088–94.
16. Trüeb RM. Association between smoking and hair loss: another opportunity for health education against smoking? Dermatology. 2003;206:189–91.
17. Hengl T, Krischok S, Riegel K, Ansari N, Stelzer E, Abts HF. A 3-D heterotypic hair-follicle spheroid model for the investigation of diminished hair-growth and hair-growth promoting compounds (Poster 229). 10th World Congress of Hair Research Oct 31–Nov 3; 2017.
18. Philpott MP, Sanders DA, Kealey T. Whole hair follicle culture. Dermatol Clin. 1996;14:595–607.
19. Philpott MP, Green MR, Kealey T. Human hair growth in vitro. J Cell Sci. 1990;97:463–71.
20. Philpott MP, Sanders D, Westgate GE, Kealey T. Human hair growth in vitro: a model for the study of hair follicle biology. Dermatol Sci. 1994;7(Suppl):S55–72.

21. Collin C, Gautier B, Gaillard O, Hallegot P, Chabane S, Bastien P, Peyron M, Bouleau M, Thibaut S, Pruche F, Duranton A, Bernard BA. Protective effects of taurine on human hair follicle grown in vitro. Int J Cosmet Sci. 2006;28:289–98.
22. Olive MF. Interactions between taurine and ethanol in the central nervous system. Amino Acids. 2002;23:345–57.
23. Tsuboyama-Kasaoka N, Shozawa C, Sano K, Kamei Y, Kasaoka S, Hosokawa Y, Ezaki O. Taurine (2-aminoethanesulfonic acid) deficiency creates a vicious circle promoting obesity. Endocrinology. 2006;147:3276–84.
24. Foos TM, Wu JY. The role of taurine in the central nervous system and the modulation of intracellular calcium homeostasis. Neurochem Res. 2002;27:21–6.
25. Clauson KA, Shields KM, McQueen CE, Persad N. Safety issues associated with commercially available energy drinks. J Am Pharm Assoc. 2008;48:e55–63.
26. Shao A, Hathcock JN. Risk assessment for the amino acids taurine, L-glutamine and L-arginine. Regul Toxicol Pharmacol. 2008;50:376–99.
27. Munkhbayar S, Jang S, Cho A, Choi S, Yup Shin C, Chul Eun H, Han Kim K, Kwon O. Role of arachidonic acid in promoting hair growth. Ann Dermatol. 2016;28:55–64.
28. Nelson GJ, Schmidt PC, Bartolini G, Kelley DS, Phinney SD, Kyle D, Silbermann S, Schaefer EJ. The effect of dietary arachidonic acid on plasma lipoprotein distributions, apoproteins, blood lipid levels, and tissue fatty acid composition in humans. Lipids. 1997;32:427–33.
29. Kelley DS, Taylor PC, Nelson GJ, MacKey BE. Arachidonic acid supplementation enhances synthesis of eicosanoids without suppressing immune functions in young healthy men. Lipids. 1998;33:125–30.
30. Nelson GJ, Schmidt PC, Bartolini G, Kelley DS, Kyle D. The effect of dietary arachidonic acid on platelet function, platelet fatty acid composition, and blood coagulation in humans. Lipids. 1997;32:421–5.
31. Olsen EA, Weiner MS, Delong ER, et al. Topical minoxidil in early male pattern baldness. J Am Acad Dermatol. 1985;13:185–92.
32. De Villez RL, Jacobs JP, Szpunar CA, Warner ML. Androgenetic alopecia in the female. Treatment with 2% topical minoxidil solution. Arch Dermatol. 1994;3:303–7.
33. Olsen EA, Dunlap FE, Funicella T, et al. A randomized clinical trial of 5% topical minoxidil versus 2% topical minoxidil and placebo in the treatment of androgenetic alopecia in men. J Am Acad Dermatol. 2002;47:377–85.
34. Kaufman KD, Olsen EA, Whiting D, et al. Finasteride in the treatment of men with androgenetic alopecia. Finasteride Male Pattern Hair Loss Study Group. J Am Acad Dermatol. 1998;39:578–89.
35. Robbins C, Mirmirani P, Messenger AG, Birch MP, Youngquist RS, Tamura M, Filloon T, Luo F, Dawson TLJ. What women want—quantifying the perception of hair amount: an analysis of hair diameter and density changes with age in Caucasian women. Br J Dermatol. 2012;167:324–32.
36. Davis MG, Thomas JH, van de Velde S, Boissy Y, Dawson TL Jr, Iveson R, Sutton K. A novel cosmetic approach to treat thinning hair. Br J Dermatol. 2011;165(Suppl 3):24–30.
37. Wickett RR, Kossmann E, Barel A, Demeester N, Clarys P, Vanden Berghe D, Calomme M. Effect of oral intake of choline-stabilized orthosilicic acid on hair tensile strength and morphology in women with fine hair. Arch Dermatol Res. 2007;299:499–505.
38. Kunz M, Seifert B, Trüeb RM. Seasonality of hair shedding in healthy women complaining of hair loss. Dermatology. 2009;219:105–10.
39. Hotzenköcherle Trüeb B. Impact of seasonality of hair growth and shedding on clinical trials with hair growth promoting agents. Inaugural Dissertation, University of Zurich; 2015.
40. Lengg N, Heidecker B, Seifert B, Trüeb RM. Dietary supplement increases anagen hair rate in women with telogen effluvium: results of a double-blind placebo-controlled trial. Therapy. 2007;4:59–65.
41. Krutmann J. Pre- and probiotics for human skin. Clin Plast Surg. 2012;39:59–64.

42. Vinceti M, Filippini T, Del Giovane C, Dennert G, Zwahlen M, Brinkman M, Zeegers M, Horneber M, D'Amico R. Selenium for preventing cancer. Cochrane Database Syst Rev. 2018;1:CD005195.
43. Mao S, Zhang A, Huang S. Selenium supplementation and the risk of type 2 diabetes mellitus: a meta-analysis of randomized controlled trials. Endocrine. 2014;47(3):758–63.
44. Stone CA, Kawai K, Kupka R, Fawzi WW. Role of selenium in HIV infection. Nutr Rev. 2010;68:671–81.
45. Yoshimura K, Nakano H, Yokoyama K, Nakayama M. High iron storage levels are associated with increased DNA oxidative injury in patients on regular hemodialysis. Clin Exp Nephrol. 2005;9:158–63.
46. King SM, Donangelo CM, Knutson MD, Walter PB, Ames BN, Viteri FE, King JC. Daily supplementation with iron increases lipid peroxidation in young women with low iron stores. Exp Biol Med. 2008;233:701–7.
47. Jaier SR, Winston GP. Copper deficiency myelopathy. J Neurol. 2010;257:869–81.
48. Mechanick JI, Youdim A, Jones DB, et al. Clinical practice guidelines for the perioperative nutritional, metabolic, and nonsurgical support of the bariatric surgery patient—2013 update: cosponsored by American Association of Clinical Endocrinologists, The Obesity Society and American Society of Metabolic & Bariatric Surger. Obesity (Silver Spring). 2013;21(Suppl. 1):S1–27.
49. Gifford JL. Biotin interference. Underrecognized patient safety risk in laboratory testing. Can Fam Physician. 2018;64:370.
50. Elston MS, Sehgal S, Du Toit S, Yarndley T, Conaglen JV. Factitious Graves' disease due to biotin immunoassay interference—a case and review of the literature. J Clin Endocrinol Metab. 2016;101:3251–5.
51. Katan MB. How much vitamin B6 is toxic? Ned Tijdschr Geneeskd. 2005;149:2545–6.
52. Dalton K, Dalton MJT. Characteristics of pyridoxine overdose neuropathy syndrome. Acta Neurol Scand. 1987;76:8–11.
53. Suzanne E, Arjo WM, Bulkin S, Nolte DL. Efficacy of cholecalciferol baits for pocket gopher control and possible effects on non-target rodents in Pacific Northwest forests. Vertebrate pest conference; 2006. USDA. Archived from the original on 2012-09-14. Accessed 27 Aug 2019. "0.15% cholecalciferol bait appears to have application for pocket gopher control." Cholecalciferol can be a single high-dose toxicant or a cumulative multiple low-dose toxicant (2006)
54. Hathcock JN, Shao A, Vieth R, Heaney R. Risk assessment for vitamin D. Am J Clin Nutr. 2007;85(1):6–18.
55. Vieth R. Vitamin D toxicity, policy, and science. J Bone Miner Research. 2007;22:V64–8.
56. Holick MF. Environmental factors that influence the cutaneous production of vitamin D. Am J Clin Nutr. 1995;61(3 Suppl):638S–45S.
57. Vitamin D status in India—its implications and remedial measures. www.JAPI.org. Accessed 22 Jan 2018.
58. Gozdzik A, Barta JL, Wu H, Wagner D, Cole DE, Vieth R, Whiting S, Parra EJ. Low wintertime vitamin D levels in a sample of healthy young adults of diverse ancestry living in the Toronto area: associations with vitamin D intake and skin pigmentation. BMC Public Health. 2008;8:336.
59. Masterjohn C. Vitamin D toxicity redefined: vitamin K and the molecular mechanism. Med Hypotheses. 2007;68:1026–34.
60. Carpenter TO. CYP24A1 loss of function: clinical phenotype of monoallelic and biallelic mutations. J Steroid Biochem Mol Biol. 2017;173:337–40.
61. Hsu JJ, Tintut Y, Demer LL. Vitamin D and osteogenic differentiation in the artery wall. Clin J Am Soc Nephrol. 2008;3:1542–7.
62. Haddad JG, Matsuoka LY, Hollis BW, Hu YZ, Wortsman J. Human plasma transport of vitamin D after its endogenous synthesis. J Clin Invest. 1993;91:2552–5.
63. Hsu JJ, Tintut Y, Demer LL. Vitamin D and osteogenic differentiation in the artery wall. Clin J Am Soc Nephrol. 2008;3:1542–7.

References 287

64. Speeckaert MM, Taes YE, De Buyzere ML, Christophe AB, Kaufman JM, Delanghe JR. Investigation of the potential association of vitamin D binding protein with lipoproteins. Ann Clin Biochem. 2010;47:143–50.
65. Demer LL, Tintut Y. Vascular calcification: pathobiology of a multifaceted disease. Circulation. 2008;117(22):2938–48.
66. Ostrander GK, Cheng KC, Wolf JC, Wolfe MJ. Shark cartilage, cancer and the growing threat of pseudoscience. Cancer Res. 2004;64:8485–91.
67. Institute of Medicine (US) and National Research Council (US) Committee on the Framework for Evaluating the Safety of Dietary Supplements. Washington (DC): Dietary supplements: a framework for evaluating safety. National Academies Press (US); 2005
68. Hammerschlag N, Davis DA, Mondo K, Seely MS, Murch SJ, Glover WB, Divoll T, Evers DC, Mash DC. Cyanobacterial neurotoxin BMAA and mercury in sharks. Toxins (Basel). 2016;8:pii:E238.
69. Chiu AS, Gehringer MM, Welch JH, Neilan BA. Does α-amino-β-methylaminopropionic acid (BMAA) play a role in neurodegeneration? Int J Environ Res Public Health. 2011;8:3728–46.
70. Genuis SJ, Schwalfenberg G, Siy AK, Rodushkin I. Toxic element contamination of natural health products and pharmaceutical preparations. PLoS One. 2012;7(11):e49676.
71. Efferth T, Kaina B. Toxicities by herbal medicines with emphasis to traditional Chinese medicine. Curr Drug Metab. 2011;12:989–96.
72. Ernst E. Adulteration of Chinese herbal medicines with synthetic drugs: a systematic review. J Intern Med. 2002;252(2):107–13.
73. Zhao P, Wang C, Li W, Chen G, Liu X, Wang X, Wang B, Yu L, Sun Y, Liang X, Yang H, Zhang F. Causes and outcomes of acute liver failure in China. PLoS One. 2013;8:e80991.
74. Jung KA, Min HJ, Yoo SS, Kim HJ, Choi SN, Ha CY, Kim HJ, Kim TH, et al. Drug-induced liver injury: twenty five cases of acute hepatitis following ingestion of polygonum multiflorum Thunb. Gut Liver. 2011;5:493–9.
75. Kim Y-S, Woo Y-Y, Han C-K, Chang I-M. Safety analysis of panax ginseng in randomized clinical trials: a systematic review. Medicines. 2015;2:106–26.
76. Hong M, Yu L, Ma C, Zhu Q. Effect of extract from Shenghua decoction on myoelectric activity of rabbit uterine muscle in the latest period of pregnancy [article in Chinese]. Zhongguo Zhong Yao Za Zhi. 2003;28:1162–4.
77. Goh SY, Loh KC. Gynaecomastia and the herbal tonic Dong Quai. Singapore Med J. 2001;42:115–6.
78. Wanachiwanawin D, Piankijagum A, Chaiprasert A, Lertlaituan P, Tungtrongchitr A, Chinabutr P. Ganoderma lucidum: a cause of pseudoparasitosis. Southeast Asian J Trop Med Public Health. 2006;37:1099–102.
79. Kim HN, Do HH, Seo JS, Kim HY. Two cases of incidental Podostroma cornu-damae poisoning. Clin Exp Emerg Med. 2016;3:186–9.
80. Saikawa Y, Okamoto H, Inui T, Makabe M, Okuno T, Suda T, Hashimoto K, Nakata M. Toxic principles of a poisonous mushroom Podostroma cornu-damae. Tetrahedron. 2001;57:8277–81.
81. Koichi M, Haruo T, Toshihiro Y, Masami O, Sadao N, Koichiro K. Case report: food poisoning to death by Podostroma cornu-damae, its case history and autopsy findings (in Japanese). Acta Criminol Med Legal Jap. 2003;69:14–20.
82. Jiang X, Williams KM, Liauw WS, Ammit AJ, Roufogalis BD, Duke CC, Day RO, McLachlan AJ. Effect of ginkgo and ginger on the pharmacokinetics and pharmacodynamics of warfarin in healthy subjects. Br J Clin Pharmacol. 2005;59:425–32.
83. Medline Plus Herbs and Supplements: Ginkgo (Ginkgo biloba L.). National Institutes of Health. Archived from the original on 17 May 2008. Accessed 10 April 2008.
84. Dugoua JJ, Mills E, Perri D, Koren G. Safety and efficacy of ginkgo (Ginkgo biloba) during pregnancy and lactation. Can J Clin Pharmacol. 2006;13:e277–84.
85. He X, Bernart MW, Nolan GS, Lin L, Lindenmaier MP. High-performance liquid chromatography-electrospray ionization-mass spectrometry study of ginkgolic acid in the leaves and fruits of the ginkgo tree (Ginkgo biloba). J Chromatogr Sci. 2000;38:169–73.

86. Tanaka A, Arai Y, Kim SN, Ham J, Usuki T. Synthesis and biological evaluation of bilobol and adipostatin A. J Asian Nat Prod Res. 2011;13(4):290–6.
87. Schötz K. Quantification of allergenic urushiols in extracts of Ginkgo biloba leaves, in simple one-step extracts and refined manufactured material(EGb 761). Phytochem Anal. 2004;15:1–8.
88. Kobayashi D. Food poisoning by Ginkgo seeds through vitamin B6 depletion (article in Japanese). Yakugaku Zasshi. 2019;139:1–6.
89. Wada K, Ishigaki S, Ueda K, Sakata M, Haga M. An antivitamin B6, 4′-methoxypyridoxine, from the seed of Ginkgo biloba L. Chem Pharm Bull. 1985;33:3555–7.
90. Verhelst X, Burvenich P, Van Sassenbroeck D, Gabriel C, Lootens M, Baert D. Acute hepatitis after treatment for hair loss with oral green tea extracts (Camellia Sinensis). Acta Gastroenterol Belg. 2009;72:262–4.
91. EFSA Panel on Food Additives and Nutrient Sources added to Food. Scientific opinion on the safety of green tea catechins. EFSA J. 2018;16:e05239.
92. Lambert JD, Sang S, Yang CS. Possible controversy over dietary polyphenols: benefits vs risks. Chem Res Toxicol. 2007;20:583–5.
93. 日本からの緑茶に基準超えるセシウム パリの空港で検出." (Japanese); 2011. Asahi Shimbun. Accessed 10 June 2011.
94. Ernst E. Heavy metals in traditional Indian remedies. Eur J Clin Pharmacol. 2002;57:891–6.
95. Dargan P, Gawarammana I, Archer J, House I, Shaw D, Wood D. Heavy metal poisoning from Ayurvedic traditional medicines: an emerging problem? Int J Environ Health. 2008;2:463.
96. Saper RB, Kales SN, Paquin J, et al. Heavy metal content of Ayurveda herbal medicine products. JAMA. 2004;292:2868–73.
97. Saper RB, Phillips RS, et al. Lead, mercury, and arsenic in US- and Indian-manufactured medicines sold via the internet. JAMA. 2008;300:915–23.
98. Szabo L. Study finds toxins in some herbal medicines. USA Today. Archived from the original on 8 October 2012; 2008.
99. Ayurveda: ancient superstition, not ancient wisdom. Skeptical Inquirer. Accessed 1 Feb 2018.
100. Breeher L, Mikulski MA, Czeczok T, Leinenkugel K, Fuortes LJ. A cluster of lead poisoning among consumers of Ayurvedic medicine. Int J Occup Environ Health. 2015;21(4):303–7.

Concluding Remarks

8

"Knowledge is in the end based on acknowledgement."

Ludwig Wittgenstein (1889–1951)

In national surveys from 1999 to 2012, 52% of US adults reported use of at least one supplement product, and 10% reported use of at least four such products [1]. The reasons of such practice are varied, with the most common being general improvements in health and well-being. Many of the most commonly indicated reasons for use have little connection to specific, measurable health goals, and are more likely driven by individual perceptions of efficacy than by external scientific evidence [2].

The popularity of supplements has varied over time and differs according to age and gender. Supplement users are more likely than nonusers to be female, white, well educated, and of higher socioeconomic status. A significant upward trend in the use of dietary supplements since the 1990s resulted in a more widespread awareness of and interest in these products. Understanding patterns of supplement use is helpful in encouraging communication about nutritional supplementation between patients and healthcare providers.

Two notable trends in recent years are distinguishable. First, there is the acceptance of dietary supplements as part of the mainstream health scene. Second, the marketing strategy for multivitamin products appears to have broadened from supplying recommended daily allowances of nutrients that may be deficient in the diet to preventing specific chronic health conditions [3].

In a survey conducted in 2008, 75% of dermatologists said that they use dietary supplements at least occasionally. The product most commonly reported to be used was a multivitamin, but over 25% said that they used omega-3 fatty acids and over 20% said that they used some botanical supplements. Regular dietary supplement use was reported by 59% of dermatologists. 66% of dermatologists reported recommending dietary supplements to their patients. The primary reason given for recommending dietary supplements to patients was for benefits for skin, hair, or nails [4].

© Springer Nature Switzerland AG 2020
R. M. Trüeb, *Nutrition for Healthy Hair*,
https://doi.org/10.1007/978-3-030-59920-1_8

And yet, medical schools and residency programs have continued to neglect comprehensive nutritional education. Nutrition education focuses on the uncommon specific nutrient-deficiency diseases, despite the emerging recognition that diet is important in the prevention and treatment of chronic health issues. There are two main reasons why the lack of commitment to nutrition education is problematic. First, the public considers the physician to be among the most trusted sources for nutrition-related information, and second, poor nutrition is an important cause of morbidity and mortality. Nutrition-related issues are estimated to account for more than 25% of visits to primary care providers [5]. Still, physicians often lack the confidence and competence to counsel their patients about nutrition in a professional manner. Moreover, familiarity breeds conclusions and sometimes a certain degree of contempt for alternatives [6]. Deficiencies in nutrition education help explain this disturbing mismatch between the skills of physicians and the needs of patients [7]. Moreover, physician knowledge of dietary supplement regulation and adverse event reporting is poor [8].

Academic medicine has notoriously resisted the concept that nutritional therapy might have health benefits of any significance. Part of this resistance arises from the fact that the potential benefits of nutritionals have been advocated by outsiders, who took their message directly to the public bypassing the establishment, and part from the fact that the concept of a deficiency disorder did not fit in well with the prevailing biomedical paradigms of disease. This resistance is evident in several ways: (1) by uncritical acceptance of either overvalued or even unsubstantiated reports of toxicity of nutritional supplements; (2) by a scornful and dismissive tone of discussion about nutrient supplementation in the standard textbooks of medicine; and (3) by skepticism towards any claim of efficacy of a nutritional, as opposed to the established medicinal therapies, and ignorism [9].

Moreover, what are scientists, physicians, and the general public to make of the many nil findings from the randomized controlled trials (RCTs) with vitamin and other nutritional supplements? Misleading study outcomes may be due to flaws in the study design and performance. Most RCTs of supplements are designed to test the hypothesis that supplementation, irrespective of the nutrient status, is protective, while treatment may not have been effective in these trials because nutrient intake among the participants was already at optimum levels. A basic principle of nutrition is that nutrient level has a nonlinear, Gaussian distribution in relation to physiological function. The nutritional state of the individual is usually not considered in trial inclusion criteria, and trial volunteers are often healthy behavior-seeking individuals who are unlikely to have low nutrient intake. In fact, the public health may be better served by initially conducting trials in individuals with insufficient nutrition from either specific deficiency disorders such as iron deficiency or the complex nutritional disorders such as the eating disorders and bariatric surgery, before testing the effectiveness in those with adequate nutrient levels [10].

Other factors to be considered in RCTs for hair are seasonality of hair growth and shedding [11], and the placebo effect. Both necessitate studies of a sufficient duration (at least 6 months). The therapeutic effect of a nutrient may be delayed, generally becoming evident not before 3 months. This delayed effect distinguishes active from the placebo effect, which typically is seen early and decays over time [12]. The placebo effect is about more than just the pill. It is about the cultural meaning of the treatment. Homeopathy is a perfect example of the value in ceremony. The effects of color, packaging, brand name, cost, and route of administration are all of significance. The more elaborate the ritual, the more effective the placebo. An injection is a much more dramatic intervention than just taking a pill. For example, intravenous vitamin B5 and biotin for treatment of telogen effluvium in women have been reported to be more effective than the respective oral or intramuscular way of administration [13]. Finally, both what the doctor says and what the doctor believes himself have an effect on treatment outcome, even if the doctor says nothing, what he or she knows or assumes leaks out, in mannerisms, affect, eyebrows, and nervous smiles.

Finally, it has been assumed that industry sponsorship of nutrition research may bias research reports, systematic reviews, and dietary guidelines. Chartres et al. [14] performed a systematic review and meta-analysis of reports that evaluated primary research studies or reviews and quantitatively compared food industry-sponsored studies with those that had no or other sources of funding. The objective was to determine whether food industry sponsorship is associated with effect sizes, statistical significance of results, and conclusions of nutrition studies with findings that are favorable to the sponsor and, secondarily, to determine whether nutrition studies differ in their methodological quality depending on whether they are industry sponsored. The study examined 12 reports and found that 8, which included 340 studies, could be combined in a meta-analysis. Although industry-sponsored studies were more likely to have conclusions favorable to industry than nonindustry-sponsored studies, the difference was not significant. There was also insufficient evidence to assess the quantitative effect of industry sponsorship on the results and quality of nutrition research.

8.1   Guidance for Supplementation

Ultimately, targeted supplementation for healthy hair based on knowledge of quantity, quality, and combination of nutrients in relation to age, sex, occupation, environmental exposure, and health status is warranted in the high-risk groups for whom nutritional requirements may not be met through diet alone, including individuals at certain life stages, and those with specific risk factors (Box 8.1).

Box 8.1 Key Points on Nutritional Supplements for Hair Growth and Quality
General Guidance for Supplementation

Micronutrients in food are typically better absorbed by the body and are associated with fewer potential adverse effects. Therefore, positive health outcomes are more strongly related to dietary patterns and specific food types than to individual micronutrient or nutrient intakes.

It would appear that unless hair loss is due to a specific nutritional deficiency, there is only so much that nutritional therapies can do to enhance hair growth and quality. However, there are a number of factors, such as inborn errors of metabolism, life cycle needs, dietary habits, lifestyle, environmental toxins, age, and comorbidities, that influence hair health to such a degree that nutritional therapy may boost hair that is suffering from these problems.

Accelerating economic development and modernization of agricultural, food processing, and food formulation techniques globally reduced single-nutrient-deficiency diseases. In response, nutrition science shifted to the research on the role of nutrition in complex noncommunicable chronic health conditions. Additional complexity may arise in nutritional recommendations for general well-being versus treatment of specific conditions.

Most of what we know about the effect of nutrition on hair stems from observations in those lacking nutrition, specifically deficiencies of protein and calories, biotin, essential fatty acids, iron, and zinc. Healthy hair requires a complexity of nutrients and a ready supply of oxygen, but comparatively few authoritative studies have trialed ingredients to maintain or promote hair growth and quality.

Targeted supplementation for healthy hair is based on knowledge of quantity, quality, and combination of nutrients in relation to age, sex, occupation, environmental exposure, and health status.

Guidance for Supplementation in a Healthy Population by Life Stage
The human life cycle spans four stages of growth and development: infancy, childhood, adolescence, and adulthood, with the nutritional needs and patterns depending on the age group. Nutritional needs fluctuate with age and with situations that occur throughout the life cycle, including pregnancy and lactation.

Pregnancy and Lactation: Protein, calories, copper, iodine, iron, magnesium, calcium, phosphorus, manganese, molybdenum, selenium, zinc, chromium (usually supplied in prenatal vitamins), biotin, vitamin D, folic acid.

Infancy: Vitamin K, for breastfed infants vitamin D until weaning and iron from age 4–6 months; for the first 6 months of life the protein requirements of an infant are 1.52 g/kg/day.

Childhood: During the first 3 years of life, children need between 80 and 120 kcal/kg/day to support normal growth. There has been much debate over the need of dietary supplements for infants and children. In fact, excessive supplementation is not uncommon, and toxicity is a danger. Fortification of cereals and breads with iron have significantly reduced the frequency of iron-deficiency anemia. Excess amounts of vitamin A and D are of special concern in children.

Adolescence: Teenagers' eating habits are considerably influenced by their rapid growth, increasing self-consciousness, and peer pressure. Due to their larger appetite and the amounts of food consumed, boys usually fare better than girls with regard to their overall nutrition. In contrast, girls may tend to restrict their food and have an inadequate nutrient intake because they are under a greater social pressure for thinness (see anorexia and bulimia).

Adulthood: After physical maturity is established, energy requirements decrease, protein needs of an adult are 0.8 g/kg/day, and some may benefit from supplemental vitamin B12, vitamin D, calcium, folic acid, coenzyme Q10, and oral collagen hydrolysate.

While with age the needs for types and quantities of nutrients change, it has been found that as many as 50% of older adults have a vitamin and mineral intake less than the Recommended Dietary Allowance, and as many as 30% of the elderly population have subnormal levels of vitamins and minerals.

Guidance for Supplementation in High-Risk Subgroups

Sometimes, patients with hair loss present with comorbidities that put them at high risk for nutritional deficiencies. As dermatologists and doctors we must look at the patient from a more generalized perspective, and also take care of deficiencies or at least draw the patient's attention to them, that may not be directly related to the complaint of hair loss.

Gluten Sensitivity: Iron, folic acid, vitamin B12.

Obesity: Iron, vitamin B1 (thiamine), vitamin B12, vitamin D.

Bariatric Surgery: Protein, vitamin B1 (thiamine), vitamin B12, folate, fat-soluble vitamins (A, D, E, and K), vitamin C, iron, zinc, copper, magnesium, calcium.

Anorexia and Bulimia: Calories, calcium, potassium, magnesium, selenium, zinc, vitamin A, folic acid.

Alcoholism: Vitamin B1 (thiamine), vitamin B6, vitamin B12, folic acid, niacin, biotin, vitamin C, vitamin A, vitamin D, vitamin E, vitamin K, selenium, zinc, copper.

Smoking: Vitamin C, biotin, L-cystine, vitamin B6.

Oncologic Patient: Calories, protein, vitamin D, selenium, zinc.

Caveat: The success of treatment and the healing process in cancer patients are significantly influenced by the nutritional status of patients. Yet, from the oncological viewpoint, there have been concerns that dietary supplements may decrease the effectiveness of chemotherapy and radiotherapy. Therefore, there is a need of an open dialogue between oncologists and cancer patients, addressing the needs of the patient while dealing with issues related to the efficacy and safety of nutritional supplements.

Medications: Nutrients relevant to healthy hair that may be affected by medications include iron (antacids, aspirin, and NSAR), zinc (antacids, ACE inhibitors, diuretics), copper (zinc), selenium (statins), biotin (antacids, antibiotics, isotretinoin, valproic acid), vitamin B12 (antacids), niacin (isoniazid), and vitamin D, and possibly the sulfur amino acids (paracetamol), and essential fatty acids (orlistat).

Veganism: Omega 3-fatty acids, vitamin B12, iron, zinc, calcium.

Guidance for Supplementation in Specific Hair Conditions

Androgenetic Alopecia and Aging Hair: Androgenetic alopecia is the most frequent cause of hair loss. It is understood to represent a hereditary, androgen-dependent thinning of scalp hair in a defined pattern, though there exist significant differences in frequency, age of onset, and pattern between men and women. The limited success rate of the hair growth-promoting agent minoxidil and of modifiers of androgen metabolism means that further pathogenic pathways may be taken into account. Premature senescence of androgenetic dermal papilla cells in vitro in association with increased sensitivity to environmental stress identifies alternative pathways. Further in vitro findings suggest that there may be a role for oxidative stress in pathogenesis.

Vitamin D, zinc, folic acid, antioxidants; some may benefit from supplemental fenugreek, saw palmetto, black cohosh, soy, ginseng, green tea, and hydrolyzed collagen.

Telogen Effluvium: Telogen effluvium results from increased shedding of hairs in telogen. While telogen effluvium represents a monomorphic reaction pattern of the hair follicle, the underlying pathologic dynamics are varied. Cyclic hair growth activity occurs in a random mosaic pattern with each follicle possessing its individual control mechanism over the evolution and triggering of the successive phases, though systemic and external factors linked to the environment have influence, such as hormones, cytokines and growth factors, toxins, and deficiencies of nutrients. A sufficient supply of protein, energy, vitamins, and trace metals is essential for the biosynthetic and energetic metabolism of the hair follicle.

L-Cystine, vitamin B1 (thiamine), pantothenic acid (vitamin B5), vitamin B6, vitamin B12 (if associated with scalp dysesthesia), L-methionine, L-lysine, biotin, iron, zinc, copper, millets, nutritional yeast, silica (horsetail).

Alopecia Areata: Alopecia areata is a non-scarring, organ-specific autoimmune disease of the hair follicle on a genetic background. While there is no cause relationship between nutritional deficiencies and alopecia areata, several deficiencies may either be associated with alopecia areata or have a disease-modifying effect.

Vitamin D, vitamin B12, iron, zinc.

Premature Graying: Hair graying is closely related to chronological age, and the age of its onset is largely controlled by genetics. Hair is said to gray prematurely if it occurs before the age of 20 in Caucasians, 25 in Asians, and 30 in Africans. While premature graying most commonly appears without underlying pathology, inherited in an autosomal dominant manner, it has also been linked to a similar cluster of autoimmune disorders observed in association with alopecia areata, i.e., pernicious anemia, and autoimmune thyroid disease. Reports linking cigarette smoking with premature hair graying have drawn on the one hand the attention to gray hair as a marker for the general health status, and on the other to the role of oxidative stress on hair growth and pigmentation.

Vitamin B12, folate, biotin, L-cystine, L-methionine, para-aminobenzoic acid (PABA), essential fatty acids, antioxidants, zinc, copper.

In every art, there are many techniques, but few principles. The only way to achieve success is to have a firm foundation of principles to build upon, and the right attitude about achieving one's goals [15]. In the chapters of this book, a guidance has been provided to the understanding and practice of nutrition for healthy hair. In the first two chapters, it has been reflected upon the history of human nutrition and today's understanding of nutrition basics. In the following two chapters, an overview has been given on the hair growth cycle's relation to nutrition and energy and on the nutritional disorders, both the specific single-nutrient deficiencies and the complex nutritional disorders, and how they may affect the hair. Finally, the last three chapters have attempted at separating the chaff from the grain in the practice of nutrition-based interventions for healthy hair through a review of safety and efficacy issues, and conclude with guidance for supplementation by life stage, health risks, and specific hair conditions.

From experience, the patient complaining of hair loss takes a low position in the scale of popularity in dermatological practice [16]. Few dermatologic problems carry as much emotional overtones as the care of hair loss, and the patient often suspects a nutritional culprit, while the physician tends to downplay this issue from a lack of comprehension and respective education.

As with any medical problem the patient complaining of hair loss requires a careful medical and drug history, physical examination, and appropriate laboratory evaluation to identify the cause. Prerequisite for delivering appropriate patient care is an understanding of the underlying pathologic dynamics of hair loss and a potential multitude of cause relationships, including nutritional factors, such as deficiencies of proteins, calories, vitamins and minerals, and environmental toxins.

The quantity and quality of hair are closely related to the nutritional state of an individual. Normal supply, uptake, and transport of proteins, calories, trace elements, and vitamins are of fundamental importance in tissues with a high biosynthetic activity such as the hair follicle. Because hair shaft is composed almost entirely of protein, protein component of diet is critical for production of normal healthy hair. The rate of mitosis is sensitive to the calorific value of diet, provided mainly by the carbohydrates, and a sufficient supply of vitamins and trace metals is essential for the biosynthetic and energetic metabolism of the follicle.

It would appear that on a typical Western diet, the hair follicle should have no problem in producing an appropriate hair shaft. Nevertheless, vitamin and nutritional deficiencies are not uncommonly observed in adolescents with eating disorders, people on fad diets, alcoholics, and the chronically ill, and are especially common in the elderly population. Moreover, the hair and scalp are exposed to an increasing number of noxious environmental factors.

The examination of the patient complaining of hair loss begins with an all-inclusive patient history:

- Date of onset of the hair loss problem and chronology of events
- Previous investigations and treatments
- Present and past medical history
- Medications
- Dietary habits
- Alcohol abuse
- Smoking
- Occupational and recreational hazards
- Associated symptoms relating to the general health status
- Associated symptoms relating to the condition of the scalp

These lay the foundations for further systematic investigations into the culprits to include a comprehensive clinical examination of the hair, skin, nails, and mucous membranes; a trichogram; a diagnosis-oriented blood nutritional screening program (nutrigram); and toxicologic studies as indicated. Finally, the presence of potential comorbidities must be considered, and the dermatologist may eventually choose to participate with other medical disciplines in the management of hair problems as they may relate to systemic disease [17]. Once the culprits are identified, treatment appropriate for the condition is likely to control the problem and restore healthy hair. *Appetitus rationi pareat.*

References

1. Kantor ED, Rehm DC, Du M, White E, Giovannucci EL. Trends in dietary supplement use among US adults from 1999-2012. JAMA. 2016;316:1464–74.
2. Weldon KJ, Botta MD, Benson JM, Blendon RJ. Users' views of dietary supplements. JAMA Intern Med. 2013;173:74–6.
3. Kelly JP, Kaufman DW, Kelley K, Rosenberg L, Anderson TE, Mitchell AA. Recent trends in use of herbal and other natural products. Arch Intern Med. 2005;165(3):281–6.
4. Dickinson A, Shao A, Boyon N, Franco JC. Use of dietary supplements by cardiologists, dermatologists and orthopedists: report of a survey. Nutr J. 2011;10:20.
5. Kolasa KM, Rickett K. Barriers to providing nutrition counseling cited by physicians: a survey of primary care practitioners. Nutr Clin Pract. 2010;25:502–9.
6. Groopman J. How doctors think. Boston, New York: Houghton Mifflin; 2007.
7. Morris NP. The neglect of nutrition in medical education: a firsthand look. JAMA Intern Med. 2014;174:841–2.
8. Ashar BH, Rice TN, Sisson SD. Physicians' understanding of the regulation of dietary supplements. Arch Intern Med. 2007;167:966–9.
9. Goodwin JS. Tangum MR Battling quackery: attitudes about micronutrient supplements in American academic medicine. Arch Intern Med. 1998;158:2187–91.

10. Morris MC, Tangney CC. A potential design flaw of randomized trials of vitamin supplements. JAMA. 2011;305:1348–9.
11. Kunz M, Seifert B, Trüeb RM. Seasonality of hair shedding in healthy women complaining of hair loss. Dermatology. 2009;219:105–10.
12. Wolf S. The pharmacology of placebos. Pharmacol Rev. 1959;11:689–704.
13. Dupré A, Lassère J, Christol B, et al. Traitement des alopécies diffuses chroniques par le panthénol et la D.biotine injectables. Rev Med Toulouse. 1977;13:675–7.
14. Chartres N, Fabbri A, Bero LA. Association of industry sponsorship with outcomes of nutrition studies: a systematic review and meta-analysis. JAMA Intern Med. 2016;176:1769–77.
15. Dale C. The quick & easy way to effective speaking. Modern techniques for dynamic communication. New York: Pocket Books, a division of Simon & Schuster, Inc; 1977.
16. Trüeb RM. The difficult hair loss patient: a particular challenge. Int J Trichology. 2013;5:110–4.
17. Jakovljević M, Ostojić L. Comorbidity and multimorbidity in medicine today: challenges and opportunities for bringing separated branches of medicine closer to each other. Psychiatr Danub. 2013;25(Suppl 1):18–28.

Index

© Springer Nature Switzerland AG 2020
R. M. Trüeb, *Nutrition for Healthy Hair*,
https://doi.org/10.1007/978-3-030-59920-1

Printed in the United States
by Baker & Taylor Publisher Services